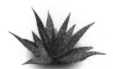

Clinical decision making in
**complementary**
**and alternative medicine**

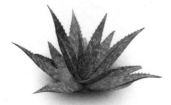

# Clinical decision making in
# complementary
# <sub>AND</sub> alternative medicine

Matthew Leach

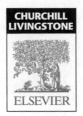

CHURCHILL
LIVINGSTONE

ELSEVIER

Sydney    Edinburgh    London    New York    Philadelphia    St  Louis    Toronto

**ELSEVIER**

Churchill Livingstone
is an imprint of Elsevier

Elsevier Australia. ACN 001 002 357
(a division of Reed International Books Australia Pty Ltd)
Tower 1, 475 Victoria Avenue, Chatswood, NSW 2067

National Library of Australia Cataloguing-in-Publication Data

---

Author: Leach, Matthew.

Title: Clinical decision making in complementary and alternative medicine / Matthew Leach.

ISBN: 9780729539333 (pbk.)

Subjects: Alternative medicine--Decision making.

Dewey Number: 615.5

---

Publisher: Sophie Kaliniecki
Developmental Editor: Sabrina Chew and Neli Bryant
Publishing Services Manager: Helena Klijn
Project Coordinator: Geraldine Minto
Edited by: Sandra Goldbloom-Zurbo and Ruth Matheson
Proofread by: Kerry Brown
Cover and internal design by: Lisa Petroff
Index by: Jon Forsyth
Typeset by: TnQ Books and Journals
Printed by: China Translating & Printing Service Ltd

# Foreword by Professor Nicola Robinson

Delivery of safe, effective, appropriate and timely healthcare is a challenge to both the patient and the practitioner. Patients are increasingly proactive when seeking the healthcare options available and are more and more informed regarding the healthcare choices available. In the search for the best care available, the use of complementary and alternative medicine (CAM) has also continued to increase, and, as a result, patients' expectations of healthcare practitioners have increased.

Those of us who are practitioners and researchers in the field recognise the advantages of providing CAM alongside conventional medicine and the importance of an integrative approach. This comprehensive and practical approach to clinical decision making provides an important and useful clinical tool for the CAM practitioner. It is a valuable practical resource for those using CAM, both within conventional healthcare settings and in private practice.

The author provides a decision-making framework to help CAM and integrative practitioners – the DeFCAM. DeFCAM enables practitioners to deliver care using a consistent, systematic, critical and transparent approach, which adheres to the principles of evidence-based practice. The six stages of the DeFCAM process chart and divide the consultation into rapport, assessment, diagnosis, planning, assessment and review. These stages are designed to address the core principles and philosophy used in CAM, while firmly acknowledging the evidence base and the links to mainstream medicine. The use of this consultative and investigative framework is particularly highlighted in the book's ten case scenarios, which cover various chronic long-term conditions. These scenarios provide the reader with examples, which can guide their use of the DeFCAM approach to practically inform their own clinical decision making.

This book demonstrates the opportunities to integrate knowledge from different sources and will stimulate the reader to incorporate a critical technique and approach to their practice. It also emphasises the importance of collaborative and interprofessional inquiry when making clinical decisions.

The reader is encouraged to explore the relevance of CAM to their clinical practice, the options, challenges and opportunities available, and how these can be integrated into their day-to-day practice.

The book also provides a real and practical insight into the contribution that CAM can make to healthcare decision making; no one system of care has all the answers and all have a part to play. More importantly, it promotes the delivery of professional excellence in CAM and I hope that this can help drive and facilitate CAM professionalisation.

Professor Nicola Robinson
Professor of Complementary Medicine
Centre for Complementary Healthcare and Integrated Medicine
Thames Valley University

# Foreword by Professor Marja Verhoef

*What is CAM? Does it work? Is it safe? Would it work for this particular patient? When? Why?* These are probably the most commonly asked questions about complementary and alternative medicine (CAM). Yet most books on CAM focus only on some of these questions; many describe CAM therapies in general and some address methods and strategies to study CAM. However, very few address the connection between CAM research and practice, and, most importantly, how to make safe treatment decisions that are evidence-based and take into account patient and contextual factors. Therefore, I was delighted to see this book, which focuses on clinical decision making guided by a framework (DeFCAM) and enables practitioners to deliver compassionate care that is individualised and safe, and uses current scientific evidence.

*Clinical Decision Making in Complementary and Alternative Medicine* intimately links research and practice, using a decision-making framework that captures the many components that are relevant to CAM practice. Within this framework, effective and safe treatments that meet patients' needs are based on a comprehensive assessment and carefully formulated diagnosis in the context of a trusting relationship. The author also effectively stresses the necessity of scientific evidence, as well as financial, social and cultural aspects, which are highly relevant in the current healthcare climate. The framework presented in this book goes well beyond CAM practice and will be of great importance to physicians, nurses, physiotherapists and other allied health professionals as well.

The book is well organised, well written and presented in a language that is suitable to various audiences. It introduces concepts and a logic for treatment decision making that may differ from what practitioners were taught in their training program. This may be overwhelming at first; however, the DeFCAM framework provides a solid basis and step-by-step approach upon which to develop an understanding of how a patient-centred approach can be applied in practice. Transforming the way one practises by integrating the various steps of the framework may lead to many benefits, expected as well as unanticipated, related to patient and provider satisfaction, greater wellness and greater involvement in the recovery process. This approach may be time consuming at first, but for many practitioners it may facilitate practising in a more efficient manner that is true to the philosophy underlying many CAM approaches.

Through this book, Dr Leach has made a very important contribution to the CAM literature and the professionalisation of CAM practice. I hope that many will read this book, and will engage in the various useful learning activities. I anticipate that this book will inspire practitioners to practise in a more reflective, comprehensive, holistic and evidence-based/informed manner, resulting in the provision of highly effective and humanistic care to their patients and clients.

Professor Marja Verhoef
Professor and Canada Research Chair in Complementary Medicine
Department of Community Health Sciences
University of Calgary

# Contents

# List of figures

# List of tables

# Preface

Over the past few decades there has been a resurgence of interest in complementary and alternative medicine (CAM), with more than half of the Western population reporting the use of these therapies and at least one in 10 accessing CAM services. During this time, many CAM occupations have transformed from often humble beginnings as cottage industries to what are now recognised as important providers of healthcare and vital members of the integrative healthcare team. Although these changes have been slow in coming, they have been progressive.

The increased demand for CAM products and services in the late 20th century was partly driven by a shift in consumer attitudes and need, specifically, the need for holistic, individualised and participatory care, and the need for greater choice in healthcare. Regulatory bodies have also shaped the CAM industry, through educational reform, increased regulation of CAM products and the reimbursement to the client of the cost of CAM services through private health insurance providers. The changing face of many CAM occupations, particularly the system-based disciplines such as naturopathy, Western herbalism and traditional Chinese medicine, suggests that these specialties are in the midst of transforming from occupations to professions.

While much progress has been made over the past few decades to facilitate the professionalisation of several CAM disciplines, there are still many shortcomings that prevent these occupations from achieving full professional status. There is, for instance, a need for greater unity within and across CAM disciplines, although the fractionated nature of the industry does not yet lend itself to unification. Closer alignment with the scientific or evidence-based paradigm is also essential for the professional advancement of CAM occupations. Yet according to findings from a recent Australian survey,[1] there is still much to be done before system-based CAM practitioners embrace evidence-based practice to its full extent. Another criterion necessary to the professionalisation of CAM occupations is the development and standardisation of knowledge. While most CAM disciplines share similar philosophies and a unique body of knowledge, a systematic and consistent approach to CAM practice within and across disciplines is still missing.

*Clinical Decision Making in Complementary and Alternative Medicine* endeavours to address these shortfalls by introducing a decision-making framework for complementary and alternative medicine (DeFCAM), as well as adding to the unique body of knowledge for CAM. This framework, which consists of six stages, is primarily aimed at guiding CAM practitioner thinking, assessment and care, without detracting from the philosophical underpinnings of CAM. Specifically, DeFCAM enables practitioners to deliver care in a systematic, critical, transparent, efficient and consistent manner, while adhering to the principles of evidence-based practice. In so doing, it is anticipated that DeFCAM will improve cross-disciplinary communication, clinical outcomes and the quality of client care.

In terms of structure, the text is divided into two parts. Part 1, Theoretical foundations, describes the theoretical foundations of DeFCAM. In this part, each stage of the framework is discussed in detail. Chapter 2 discusses rapport, chapter 3 assessment, chapter 4 diagnosis, chapter 5 planning, chapters 6 and 7 application, and chapter 8 review. Part 2, Practical application (chapter 9), is dedicated to the clinical application of DeFCAM. This part, exemplified by a number of clinical scenarios, demonstrates to readers how DeFCAM can be applied in clinical practice.

As well as promoting the delivery of professional excellence in CAM, it is hoped that this text will serve as an impetus for positive change in the CAM industry and, by forging unity among the many CAM disciplines, help to facilitate the professionalisation of these occupations.

Dr Matthew Leach

## Reference

1 Leach MJ. Gillham D. (2009) Attitude and use of evidence-based practice among complementary medicine practitioners: a descriptive survey. 2nd North American Research Conference on Complementary and Integrative Medicine, Minneapolis, 12–15 May.

# About the author

Dr Matthew J Leach RN, DipAppSci (Nat), DipClinNutr, BN (Hons), PhD, Registered Nurse, Naturopath, Research Fellow, University of South Australia, Adelaide, is a research fellow in the health economics and social policy group at the University of South Australia and was previously a registered nurse, naturopath and lecturer in naturopathy and health sciences. Dr Leach completed his Bachelor of Nursing degree in 1994, followed by a Diploma of Applied Science (Naturopathy) in 1998, a Bachelor of Nursing (Honours) degree in 2000 and a Diploma of Clinical Nutrition in 2008. His PhD, which he completed in 2005, examined the clinical feasibility of horsechestnut seed extract in the management of venous leg ulceration. Since then, he has been driven to improving the evidence base of complementary and alternative medicine (CAM), as well as the professionalisation of CAM services. This is evidenced by the type of research conducted by Dr Leach, the papers and book chapters he has published in these areas and the many forums, seminars and international conferences he has presented at.

# Acknowledgements

Many years have passed since the idea for this book was first conceived. But with much planning, research, time, effort and writing, the idea has developed into an informative text for the complementary and alternative medicine (CAM) profession. However, no man is an island unto himself, and this text would not have been possible without the support of some exceptional individuals.

First and foremost I need to acknowledge the tremendous support provided by my family, specifically, my wife Pam, son Haiden and daughter Mikaela. In spite of the many late nights and very early mornings, and the constant requests for one more minute of time, they were always there for me, and for that, I am extremely thankful. Their unconditional love and faith in me was also a constant reminder of the most important thing in my life – my family. And, of course, I cannot dismiss my two study companions, my dogs Arum and Raphael, who were often by my side on those many late nights.

To my friends, students and colleagues, thank you for your encouragement and for believing in me, listening to me and sharing your wisdom, thoughts and insights into CAM, health and healthcare. For this I will be forever grateful.

I am also grateful for the support, understanding and guidance offered by the Elsevier team, especially Sophie Kaliniecki and Sabrina Chew, who have been there right from the start.

Thank you to Rachel Arthur, Liesl Blott, Jenny Wilkinson and Emily Bradley, the reviewers of this book whose valuable feedback helped shape the text.

To the current and future generations of CAM practitioners, it is for you that I dedicate this book, and it is in you that I wish to instil hope and passion for the professional advancement of the greater CAM profession.

Parts of this book have been reproduced from previous works of the author with written permission from Elsevier, the *Journal of the Australian Traditional Medicine Society*, Blackwell Publishing and the Berkeley Electronic Press.

Dr Matthew Leach

# Reviewers

**Rachel Arthur,** BHSc BNat(Hons) (SCU) MACCNEM MNSA MNHAA MANTA, Lecturer, School of Health and Human Sciences, Southern Cross University, NSW, professional and corporate educator, private practitioner, NSW.

**Liesl Blott,** BHSc (WHerbal Med) (ACNM), AdvDipNat (ACNM) BPharm (UWits), PGDip MM (UNISA), Lecturer, Faculty of Health Science, Curtin University, WA.

**Jenny Wilkinson,** BSc (Hons) (Qld), PhD (Macq), GradDipFET (SQld), MHEd (Macq), Associate Professor in Physiology, Charles Sturt University, NSW.

**Emily Bradley,** ND (SSNT), MANTA, Lecturer and Clinical Supervisor, Naturopathy Department, Endeavour College of Natural Health and Southern School of Natural Therapies, practising naturopath, Melbourne.

# PART 1

# Theoretical foundations

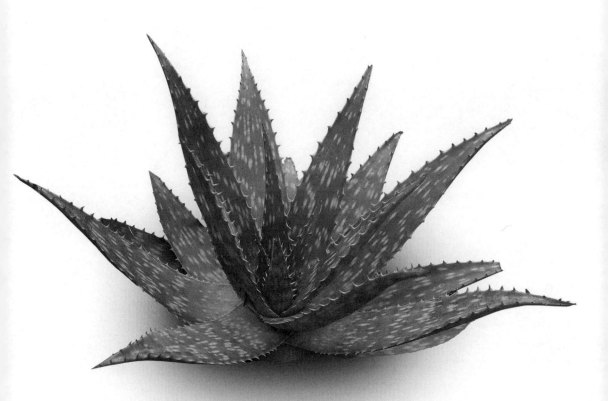

# 1
# A decision-making framework for complementary and alternative medicine

## Chapter overview
The safe, effective and efficient delivery of client care is informed primarily by sound clinical decision making. Strategies that guide practitioners through the process of decision making may not only foster professional excellence in complementary and alternative medicine (CAM) practice, but also help to improve the quality of client care. An example of such a strategy is the decision-making framework for complementary and alternative medicine (DeFCAM). In this first chapter, an overview of DeFCAM is provided, which aims to assist readers in understanding the context of the following chapters and the circumstances in which the framework can be applied to CAM practice.

## Learning objectives
The content of this chapter will assist the reader to:
- identify a range of decision-making frameworks used in clinical practice
- understand the sequence and purpose of each stage of DeFCAM
- recognise the benefits and limitations of DeFCAM
- understand how DeFCAM can facilitate clinical decision making.

## Chapter outline
- Introduction
- CAM philosophy
- Clinical decision-making models
- The decision-making framework for complementary and alternative medicine (DeFCAM)
- Rapport
- Assessment
- Diagnosis
- Planning
- Application
- Review
- Summary

## Introduction

'Complementary and alternative medicine' (CAM) is an overarching term that encapsulates a diverse range of modalities considered to be outside the scope of orthodox medicine. According to the National Center for Complementary and Alternative Medicine in the US[1] and the National Institute of Complementary Medicine in Australia,[2] both of which are leading authorities in CAM research, these therapies can be divided into five distinct categories, including whole medical systems (such as naturopathy, homeopathy, Western herbalism, Ayurveda, indigenous and traditional Chinese medicine (TCM)); energy medicine (including therapeutic touch, flower essences and Reiki); biologically based interventions (such as nutrients, plant and animal products); manipulative therapies (including massage, chiropractic, osteopathy and reflexology), and mind–body interventions (such as tai chi, yoga, meditation and progressive relaxation).

Given the recent trend towards integrative medicine, the line separating CAM from orthodox medicine is becoming less distinct. This is further perpetuated by vague definitions of CAM. NCCAM,[1] for example, defines CAM as 'a group of diverse medical and healthcare systems, practices, and products that are not presently considered to be part of conventional medicine'. Defining CAM by what it is not is no longer appropriate given the changing face of healthcare and the integration of CAM into medical, nursing and allied health curricula. CAM is more fittingly defined as a diverse group of health-related modalities that promote the body's innate healing ability in order to facilitate optimum health and wellbeing, while retaining a core focus on holism, individuality, education and disease prevention.

Consumer interest in these therapies has escalated over the past few decades. In fact, more than fifty per cent of the Western population,[3] including the Australian,[4,5] US[6] and Japanese populations,[7] have used CAM at least once over a 12-month period. Biologically based interventions, such as nutrient supplements and herbal medicines, and manipulative therapies, such as massage and chiropractic, are among those demonstrating the highest level of use. Over the same period, close to ten per cent of UK adults,[8] twelve per cent of US adults,[6] and twenty-three[9] to forty-four per cent of Australians[5] have consulted a CAM practitioner; chiropractic and osteopathy were the most commonly used services. The growing interest in CAM across the globe can be attributed to a number of factors. Although earlier studies signalled consumer dissatisfaction with orthodox medicine as a leading cause of CAM use,[3] more recent reports indicate that an aspiration for active healthcare participation, greater disease chronicity and severity, holistic healthcare beliefs, and an increase in health-awareness behaviour are more likely to predict CAM use.[10–12] These transformations in consumer attitude and health behaviour have parallelled changes in the way many CAM specialties practise.

The shift towards evidence-based practice, along with issues concerning education and regulation, are now shaping the future of many system-based modalities, particularly naturopathy, Western herbalism and TCM. These changes suggest that the aforementioned specialties may be in the process of professionalisation, that is, transforming from occupation to profession. Unification of the CAM profession, controlled entry into the vocation (i.e. occupational closure), closer alignment to the mainstream scientific-evidence-based practice paradigm, and the development and standardisation (or codification) of knowledge are all essential criteria for the professionalisation of CAM occupations.[13,14] Although codification involves claiming a unique body of knowledge, it also requires an understanding of how that knowledge can be applied to practice.[15] Clinical decision-making models play a pivotal part in this translational process. This chapter will therefore introduce the reader to a decision-making framework for complementary and alternative medicine (DeFCAM), and demonstrate how this framework may facilitate the application of CAM knowledge into clinical practice. The uptake of such a model may also help to espouse the ongoing development of CAM and enhance the professionalism of CAM practitioners.

## CAM philosophy

The practice of CAM is guided by the art, science and principles of each profession. Even though the art and science of the CAM therapies are distinctly different from each other, many of these professions share similar philosophies. Some of the core principles underlying these philosophies that are shared by therapies such as naturopathy, Ayurveda, TCM, chiropractic, osteopathy, Western herbalism and homeopathy,[16-24] are as follows:

- CAM is client-centred and individualised
- CAM treats each person holistically
- CAM identifies and manages the underlying cause of the person's condition
- CAM supports the body's innate healing ability and/or vital energy
- CAM helps to restore balance or homeostasis
- CAM should not cause harm
- CAM alleviates suffering
- CAM focuses on the prevention of illness
- CAM optimises health, wellness and wellbeing.

These principles are central to understanding the unique approach of CAM. More importantly, these principles serve to inform clinical decision making, particularly decisions relating to the assessment and treatment of an individual patient (including the identification of the underlying cause of the condition and the provision of holistic care). Even so, these doctrines are neither systematic nor process oriented and, as such, are unable to methodically direct practitioners through the CAM consultation or decision-making process. For graduates of CAM, the absence of a clear framework could make transition from student to clinician difficult. One way to facilitate this transition is by bridging the gap between the philosophical foundations of CAM and the requirements of modern-day clinical practice (i.e. avoiding client harm by adopting the best available evidence, formulating client-centred treatment goals, evaluating care to ensure balance has been restored), through the provision of a CAM-specific clinical decision-making framework.

## Clinical decision-making models

Over the past few decades, a number of decision-making models have emerged within the healthcare sector. The general aim of these frameworks was to guide practitioners through the process of decision making in often complex clinical environments. Examples of some of the more common models used in clinical practice are highlighted in Table 1.1. Many of these frameworks were originally designed to improve documentation in the healthcare sector rather than guide clinical decision making. SOAP, DAP, OHEAP and SNOCAMP, for example, while providing a simple, systematic and consistent approach to documentation in the clinical environment, provide very little direction for practitioners in the management of client problems. Fortunately, several models have since emerged that attempt to address this problem.

One of the earliest participative decision-making frameworks to surface in orthodox medicine was that developed by Ballard-Reisch (1990).[25] Originally designed for physicians, the eight-stage participative decision-making model aimed to provide a more client-centred and structured approach to client care. Although the need for a participative approach was timely and well justified, the stages of the model lacked

| Table 1.1: Clinical decision-making models used in the healthcare sector | |
|---|---|
| DAP | Data, assessment, plan |
| FARM | Findings, assessment, recommendations/resolutions, management |
| HOAP | History, observations, assessment, plan |
| Nagelkerk (2001) model | Problem, assessment, diagnoses, diagnostics, single diagnosis, treatment plan |
| Nursing process | Assessment, diagnosis, planning, implementation, evaluation |
| Nutrition care process | Assessment, diagnosis, implementation, monitoring and evaluation |
| Participative decision-making model (Ballard-Reisch 1990) | Information gathering, information interpretation, exploration of treatment alternatives, criteria establishment for treatment, weighing of alternatives against criteria, alternative treatment selection, decision implementation, evaluation of implemented treatment |
| Prion (2008) model | Situation prime, gather cues, determine relevant/non-relevant cues, cue grouping, problem identification, patient status, cause hypothesis, intervention, gather more information |
| OHEAP | Orientation, history, exam, assessment, plan |
| SNOCAMP | Subjective data, nature of presenting complaint, objective data, counselling, assessment, medical decision making, plan of treatment |
| SOAP | Subjective data, objective data, assessment, plan |

sufficient description. There is also little evidence to indicate that, to date, this process has been accepted or taken up by the wider medical community. This is not to say that other participative models have not been adopted by physicians, only that the use of such frameworks has not been well published.

A well-documented decision-making framework is the nursing process. This model has been widely accepted by the nursing community and is recognised internationally and integrated into most nursing curricula.[26] In essence, the process provides a client-centred framework for nursing practice 'by which nurses use their beliefs, knowledge, and skills to diagnose and treat the client's response to actual and potential health problems'.[26]

The benefits that the nursing process delivers to the nursing profession have been recognised by other disciplines, including the dietetics community, which has led to the subsequent development of the nutrition care process.[27,28] It is not surprising, therefore, that there is considerable overlap between the two processes. In fact, there are many similarities between most decision-making models, including the Prion[29] clinical reasoning model, Nagelkerk[30] diagnostic reasoning process and the aforementioned frameworks. The key themes that arise from all of these models are assessment, diagnosis, planning, implementation and evaluation.

Another concept that is implied in the Ballard-Reisch model[25] but not explicitly stated in any other decision-making process, yet a component that is critical to all client–practitioner interactions, is rapport. Incorporating rapport into a clinical decision-making framework, together with the five themes listed above, would in effect create a more complete, systematic and structured approach to the management of client problems. DeFCAM is therefore one of only a few, if not the only known model to adequately capture all of these themes within one process. Although the development of such a model could be perceived by some as merely following the trends of other professions, there is in fact real merit for the CAM profession in adopting such a framework, which the following section alludes to.

## The decision-making framework for complementary and alternative medicine (DeFCAM)

DeFCAM is a systematic clinical reasoning framework developed by the author specifically for CAM and integrative healthcare practitioners. The six stages of the process include rapport, assessment, diagnosis, planning, application and review (Figure 1.1). The process is primarily aimed at guiding CAM practitioner thinking, assessment and care, and, as such, is likely to generate benefits for the CAM practitioner, the client and members of the integrative healthcare team, including:

- an increase in professional autonomy, status and accountability[31]
- improvements in client outcomes
- greater consistency with clinical documentation
- clearer treatment priorities
- improvements in quality of care[32]
- a reduction in decision-making error [32]
- greater transparency of decision-making process
- greater efficiency and improved focus of consultations
- improvements in intra- and interprofessional communication.

While DeFCAM is displayed in a linear fashion, and maybe applied as such, the process is not unidirectional. In fact, each stage of the process is interlinked because just as in clinical practice, the acquisition of new information requires a CAM practitioner to shift between various stages of assessment, diagnosis and planning until an appropriate treatment plan is developed. Still, the six stages of DeFCAM are

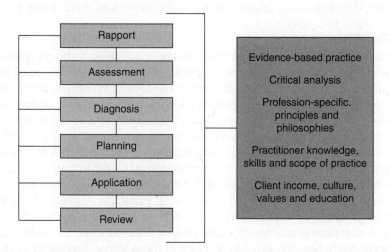

**Figure 1.1:** The decision-making framework for complementary and alternative medicine (DeFCAM)

presented in a logical order because each phase of the process acts as a prerequisite for subsequent stages.

As illustrated in Figure 1.1, there are a number of concepts that overarch DeFCAM. This is because each of these constructs exercises significant influence on a CAM practitioner's decision making. In particular, each factor directs how a clinician should assess a client, how the data should be interpreted and what interventions should be selected. By taking these elements into consideration, a CAM practitioner can make attempts to resolve any limitations in their decision-making style in order to deliver more effective clinical care.

To summarise at this point, DeFCAM enables CAM practitioners to systematically assess, diagnose, plan, treat and review client-centred health problems in accordance with CAM philosophy. An introduction to each of the six-stages of DeFCAM, including how these phases address the core principles of CAM philosophy, will now follow.

## Rapport

Establishing client rapport is the first and most important phase of DeFCAM. By developing rapport with the client, communication between the practitioner and client may improve, as may assessment, treatment compliance and the achievement of expected treatment outcomes.[33,34] Even though a therapeutic relationship may develop throughout the consultation, it is important that time is allocated at the beginning of the visit to build client trust. In order to develop trust and decrease client anxiety, the practitioner should introduce themselves to the client and allow the individual to verbalise what they expect from the consultation.[33] The CAM practitioner may also build trust and strengthen client rapport by being open, empowering, empathetic, objective, honest, non-judgemental, flexible, consistent, committed and interested in the health and welfare of the client.[33-35] These attributes should not only be expressed verbally, but also non-verbally through facial expressions, eye contact and posture.[33-35] Effective communication and optimal client–practitioner interaction may be further facilitated by identifying and respecting differences in client age, gender, developmental stages, cognitive ability, values, beliefs and culture.[35]

## Assessment

The assessment phase of DeFCAM involves the acquisition, validation and organisation of client information, and the identification of factors that may influence client health and wellbeing. Given that assessment informs every succeeding stage of DeFCAM, the accuracy and inclusivity of the process will almost certainly impact on client outcomes. By following a transparent and systematic assessment process, clinicians may be able to enhance the quality of clinical assessment by reducing the potential for data omission. One way CAM practitioners may approach clinical assessment is through the use of theoretical models, such as Maslow's hierarchy of human needs[36] or the Neuman systems model.[37] Even though these models are useful for recognising pertinent physiological, social or psychological needs of a client, they do little to guide the practitioner through the clinical assessment process overall. This is also the case for traditional clinical methods, including the head-to-toe and body systems approaches. The CAM assessment process addresses these limitations by providing a more complete, holistic and systematic approach to clinical assessment, incorporating not only the health history and physical examination, but also pertinent diagnostics, thereby enabling CAM practitioners to effectively identify the underlying cause of the presenting condition. The collection of detailed information also gives rise to a more informed CAM practitioner, who is capable of making prompt and appropriate decisions about the need for referral. This process is described in greater detail in chapter 3.

## Diagnosis

In the third phase of DeFCAM, data acquired from the client assessment are clustered into logical groups, which enables hypotheses or diagnoses to be generated. This process, known as diagnostic reasoning,[35] is critical to the generation of clinical diagnoses. Even though CAM practitioners and other non-medical health professionals are not legally permitted to formulate 'medical' diagnoses, at least not in Australia,[38] some professions, including nursing and dietetics, have overcome this practice limitation by developing a list of diagnoses that they can legally identify and treat. CAM practitioners could follow a similar path to that of these professions and establish their own set of CAM diagnoses in order to avoid litigation around claims of practising medicine.

As with nursing and nutrition diagnoses, a CAM diagnosis also consists of a client-centred problem (actual or potential) and the aetiology of the problem.[33,39] Such an approach benefits practitioners because the problem component indicates what the client outcome should be at the review stage, whereas the aetiology component directs the clinician towards the cause of the condition, and thus points the practitioner towards an appropriate approach to treatment.[26] As a result, CAM diagnoses may provide a framework for the delivery of CAM treatment,[39] and thereby link CAM philosophy to clinical practice (i.e. identifying and treating the cause of the complaint), and improve client prognosis and management.

## Planning

The planning phase of DeFCAM focuses on the development of goals in order to identify and prioritise strategies that may prevent, reduce or resolve client problems, or that facilitate or augment client function. But before these goals can be developed, client problems must first be prioritised. One model that is often used to prioritise client problems is Maslow's hierarchy of needs.[26] However, Maslow's model does not inform practitioners how to prioritise within each of the six needs; for instance, what physiological problems should a practitioner treat first? Determining what CAM diagnosis to initially address should be ascertained by the level of risk that the problem poses to the client, with conditions demonstrating a higher risk of harm demanding a higher priority of care.[35,39]

Once CAM diagnoses have been prioritised, the most important diagnosis can then be used to formulate the goals of treatment. These goals should be client-centred, individualised, observable, measurable, mutually derived and realistic, with each goal addressing only one problem and one outcome.[35,39] Treatment goals must also take into consideration the cost of treatment, available resources, client age, environment, values, beliefs and culture, as well as social status, client self-efficacy, motivation and readiness to change, and the client's cognitive, physical and emotional capacity.[40,41]

## Application

After CAM diagnoses have been formulated and treatment goals and expected outcomes established, appropriate interventions may then be commenced. As with the planning phase, the treatment options need to be negotiated between the CAM practitioner and the client in order to enhance independence, control, dignity and self-esteem.[40] Client involvement in clinical decisions may also improve treatment compliance and thus facilitate progression towards expected outcomes. The treatments should also be aimed at achieving the goals identified in the planning stage.

Due to the eclectic nature of CAM practice, the diversity of CAM education around the globe and personal preference, very few CAM practitioners are likely to employ the same approach, so it would be inappropriate to dictate which therapies CAM practitioners should prescribe for specific conditions, though it is recommended that the choice of interventions be based on the best available evidence so as to maximise improvements in client outcomes and the quality of care, and to minimise harm and suffering.[42] This concept of evidence-based practice and how it applies to CAM practice is discussed in greater detail in chapter 6. Therapies that are supported by clinical evidence, which may be integrated into CAM practice, are outlined in chapter 9.

## Review

The review stage of the decision-making framework utilises assessment techniques to determine whether the treatment approach was effective, if the expected outcomes of client care were achieved,[35] if illness was prevented and whether homeostasis was restored. Clinicians need to appreciate that clients may find it difficult to achieve the expected outcomes of treatment if a practitioner's knowledge base and level of skill are inadequate, and if the client lacks understanding, self-efficacy or is not involved in the treatment process.[35,43] The achievement of treatment goals may be facilitated by involving clients in DeFCAM, and by CAM practitioners engaging in reflective practice. This rational and conscious process of systematically and rigorously reflecting on one's practice enables clinician's to challenge existing approaches and to learn from one's actions.[44]

## Summary

At present, there is a paucity of universally recognised, clearly constructed, systematic decision-making frameworks to guide the practice of system-based CAM. In order for many systems of CAM to develop professionally, a body of knowledge must be developed and codified. The development of DeFCAM endeavours to facilitate the professionalisation of these CAM systems and to improve clinical reasoning in CAM practice by providing a structured process for clinical care. DeFCAM consists of six interrelated stages, including rapport, assessment, diagnosis, planning, application and review. These stages are best remembered by the acronym RADPAR. It is envisaged that this framework will provide the necessary foundations for the development of a codified knowledge base for CAM disciplines in order to improve professional status, quality of care and client outcomes. The close alignment of DeFCAM with CAM philosophy also ensures that the core principles of CAM practice have not been discounted. The assessment phase of DeFCAM, for example, addresses the principle of holism and the need to identify the cause of the presenting condition; CAM diagnosis focuses on treating the primary cause of the complaint, as well as preventing illness; the planning approach maintains client-centredness and individualism; application applies the concept of evidence-based practice to minimise harm, optimise health and wellbeing, and alleviate suffering; and review assesses whether the prevention of illness and the restoration of homeostasis has been attained. A more detailed discussion of each of these stages is presented in the chapters that follow, beginning with rapport.

## Learning activities

1 Compare and contrast the structures of different models of clinical decision making.
2 Identify, and briefly describe, each of the six stages of DeFCAM.
3 Describe some of the benefits of DeFCAM to the practitioner, profession and the client.
4 Outline some of the possible limitations of DeFCAM.
5 In relation to your own specialty, explain how DeFCAM is compatible and/or incompatible with the principles and philosophy of your profession.
6 If you could add another stage to DeFCAM, what would that stage be? Explain how this stage would enable DeFCAM to improve CAM practitioner thinking, assessment and care.

# References

1. National Center for Complementary and Alternative Medicine (NCCAM). (2000) What is CAM? NCCAM, Maryland. Accessed at <http://nccam.nih.gov/health/whatiscam/overview.htm>, 1 March 2009.
2. National Institute of Complementary Medicine (NICM). (2009) About complementary medicine. Sydney: NICM. Accessed at <www.nicm.edu.au/content/view/14/17/>, 1 March 2009.
3. Leach MJ. (2004) Public, nurse and medical practitioner attitude and practice of natural medicine. Complementary Therapies in Nursing and Midwifery, 10(1): 13–21.
4. MacLennan AH. Myers SP. Taylor AW. (2006) The continuing use of complementary and alternative medicine in South Australia: costs and beliefs in 2004. Medical Journal of Australia, 184(1): 27–31.
5. Xue CCL et al (2007) Complementary and alternative medicine use in Australia: a national population-based survey. Journal of Alternative and Complementary Medicine, 13(6): 643–50.
6. Barnes PM et al (2004) Complementary and alternative medicine use among adults: United States, 2002. Seminars in Integrative Medicine, 2(2): 54–71.
7. Hori S et al (2008) Patterns of complementary and alternative medicine use amongst outpatients in Tokyo, Japan. BMC Complementary and Alternative Medicine, 8: 14–23.
8. Thomas K. Coleman P. (2004) Use of complementary or alternative medicine in a general population in Great Britain. Results from the National Omnibus survey. Journal of Public Health, 26(2): 152–7.
9. Lin V et al (2006) The Practice and Regulatory Requirements of Naturopathy and Western Herbal Medicine. Melbourne: Government of Victoria, Department of Human Services.
10. Busato A et al (2006) Health status and healthcare utilisation of patients in complementary and conventional primary care in Switzerland: an observational study. Family Practice, 23(1): 116–24.
11. Robinson A. Chesters J. Cooper S. (2007) People's choice: complementary and alternative medicine modalities. Complementary Health Practice Review, 12(2): 99–119.
12. Sirois FM. Purc-Stephenson RJ. (2008) Consumer decision factors for initial and long-term use of complementary and alternative medicine. Complementary Health Practice Review, 13(1): 3–20.
13. Cant S. Sharma U. (1996) Professionalization of complementary medicine in the United Kingdom. Complementary Therapies in Medicine, 4: 157–62.
14. Hirschkorn KA. (2006) Exclusive versus everyday forms of professional knowledge: legitimacy claims in conventional and alternative medicine. Sociology of Health and Illness, 28(5): 533–57.
15. Sharma U. (1995) Professions, power and the patient: some more useful concepts. In: Complementary medicine today: practitioners and patients. Sharma U, editor. London: Routledge.
16. Cassidy CM. (2001) Social and cultural context of complementary and alternative medical systems. In: Fundamentals of complementary and alternative medicine. Micozzi MS, editor. Philadelphia: Churchill Livingstone.

17. Ebrall PS. (2003) Chiropractic. In: An introduction to complementary medicine. Robson T, editor. Sydney: Allen & Unwin.
18. Howden I. (2003) Homeopathy. In: An introduction to complementary medicine. Robson T, editor. Sydney: Allen & Unwin.
19. Lucas N. Moran R. (2003) Osteopathy. In: An introduction to complementary medicine. Robson T, editor. Sydney: Allen & Unwin.
20. Matthews S. (2003) Ayurveda. In: An introduction to complementary medicine. Robson T, editor. Sydney: Allen & Unwin.
21. Myers S et al (2003) Naturopathic medicine. In: An introduction to complementary medicine. Robson T, editor. Sydney: Allen & Unwin.
22. Pizzorno JE. Murray MT. (2006) Textbook of natural medicine. 3rd ed. Philadelphia: Elsevier.
23. Patching van der Sluijs CG. Bensoussan A. (2003) Traditional Chinese medicine. In: An introduction to complementary medicine. Robson T, editor. Sydney: Allen & Unwin.
24. Wohlmuth H. (2003) Herbal medicine. In: An introduction to complementary medicine. Robson T, editor. Sydney: Allen & Unwin.
25. Ballard-Reisch DS. (1990) A model of participative decision making for physician–patient interaction. Health Communication, 2(2): 91–104.
26. Iyer PW. Taptich BJ. Bernocchi-Losey D. (1995) Nursing process and nursing diagnosis. 3rd ed. Philadelphia: WB Saunders.
27. Bueche J et al (2008) Nutrition care process and model Part I: the 2008 update. Journal of the American Dietetic Association, 108(7): 1113–17.
28. Lacey K. Pritchett E. (2003) Nutrition care process and model: ADA adopts road map to quality care and outcomes management. Journal of the American Dietetic Association, 103(8): 1061–72.
29. Prion S. (2008) The case study as an instructional method to teach clinical reasoning. In: Clinical reasoning in the health professions. 3rd ed. Higgs J, editor. Amsterdam: Elsevier/Butterworth Heinemann.
30. Nagelkerk J. (2001) Clinical decision-making in primary care. In: Diagnostic reasoning: case analysis in primary care practice. Nagelkerk J, editor. Philadelphia: WB Saunders.
31. Higgs J. (2008) Clinical reasoning in the health professions. In: Clinical reasoning in the health professions. 3rd ed. Higgs J, editor. Amsterdam: Elsevier/Butterworth Heinemann.
32. Dowding D. Thompson C. (2002) Decision analysis. In: Clinical decision making and judgement in nursing. Thompson C, Dowding D, editors. Edinburgh: Churchill Livingstone: 131–45.
33. DeLaune SC. Ladner PK. (2006) Fundamentals of nursing: standards and practice. 3rd ed. Albany: Thomson Delmar Learning.
34. Leach MJ. (2005) Rapport: a key to treatment success. Complementary Therapies in Clinical Practice, 11(4): 262–5.
35. Harkreader H. Hogan MA. Thobaben M. (2007) Fundamentals of nursing: caring and clinical judgement. 3rd ed. Philadelphia: Elsevier Saunders.
36. Taylor C et al (2008) Fundamentals of nursing: the art and science of nursing care. 6th ed. Philadelphia: Wolters Kluwer/Lippincott Williams & Wilkins.
37. Ume-Nwagbo PN. DeWan SA. Lowry LW. (2006) Using the Neuman systems model for best practices. Nursing Science Quarterly, 19(1): 31–5.
38. Weir M. (2007) Complementary medicine: ethics and law. 3rd ed. Ashgrove: Prometheus Publications.
39. Crisp J. Taylor C. (2008) Potter and Perry's fundamentals of nursing. 3rd ed. Sydney: Elsevier.
40. Kozier B et al (2004) Fundamentals of nursing: concepts, process, and practice. 7th ed. Upper Saddle River: Pearson Education.
41. Treasure J. Maissi E. (2007) Motivational interviewing. In: Cambridge handbook of psychology, health and medicine. 2nd ed. Ayers S et al, editors. Cambridge: Cambridge University Press.
42. Leach MJ. (2006) Evidence-based practice: a framework for clinical practice and research design. International Journal of Nursing Practice, 12: 248–51.
43. Leach MJ. (2007) Revisiting the evaluation of clinical practice. International Journal of Nursing Practice, 13(2): 70–4.
44. Rolfe G. Freshwater G. Jasper D. (2001) Critical reflection for nursing and the helping professions: a user's guide. Basingstoke: Palgrave.

# 2
# Rapport

## Chapter overview

Rapport is a concept often ignored in the current literature. As a result, the importance of this relationship may be overlooked. To address this concern, this chapter will highlight the probable effects that rapport has on client satisfaction, treatment compliance and client outcomes, which serves to underline the importance of rapport at the beginning and throughout DeFCAM. Strategies that practitioners can employ to facilitate the development of this relationship are also discussed.

## Learning objectives

The content of this chapter will assist the reader to:
- define rapport
- state the reasons for establishing client–practitioner rapport
- identify the factors that foster the development of client–practitioner rapport
- outline the factors that may constrain client–practitioner rapport.

## Chapter outline
- Introduction
- Definitions
- Importance of rapport
- Factors that facilitate and constrain client rapport
- Summary

## Introduction

The first and most important objective of any client–practitioner interaction is the establishment of client rapport. Aside from facilitating communication between the practitioner and client, good rapport can also improve client assessment and the achievement of expected treatment outcomes.[1] Development of this relationship requires time and skill.[2] As the therapist's contribution to rapport is often overlooked in the literature,[3] the purpose of this chapter will be to inform readers of the importance of establishing a strong therapeutic relationship with their clients and to provide CAM practitioners with useful strategies to improve client rapport in clinical practice. These skills may also enable practitioners to develop more effective working relationships with other healthcare providers.[4] First though, an exploration of the terms used to describe rapport will enable readers to understand the context in which this chapter is situated.

## Definitions

Many terms exist that describe the bond between a client and practitioner. The terms most frequently used are 'therapeutic alliance', 'therapeutic relationship' and 'client rapport'. By definition, a therapeutic alliance is ' a conscious and active collaboration between the patient and therapist'.[3] Similarly, a therapeutic relationship is 'a trusting connection and rapport established between therapist and client through collaboration, communication, therapist empathy and mutual understanding and respect'.[4] Rapport is defined as a 'harmonious relationship'.[5] As each of these terms incorporate similar underlying themes, including collaboration, reciprocity, parity and growth, they are considered interchangeable.

The therapeutic alliance and other similar terms are frequently cited in the psychology literature. This may be because the concept of 'alliance' is an integral component of many counselling models, such as the 'here and now' focused counselling model,[6] the lifestyle-oriented nutrition counselling model[7] and the four stages of therapy process.[8] The latter model suggests that therapist techniques, client involvement in care and the therapeutic alliance are inextricably linked. According to Hill,[8] this means that a practitioner is unable to use techniques effectively if a client is not involved in the care and there is no alliance, that a client is not likely to be involved in the care if a therapist does not skilfully use techniques and there is no therapeutic alliance, and that alliance cannot exist without a competent clinician and a participating client. In essence, what this theory suggests is that a competent practitioner who adopts a client-centred, participative and empowering practice style is likely to develop a strong therapeutic alliance. This is a somewhat simplistic interpretation of this relationship, because like other aforementioned models, it does not take into consideration the myriad factors that affect the development of this alliance, as will be elucidated throughout this chapter.

## Importance of rapport

There are many reasons why CAM practitioners should be encouraged to develop rapport with their clients. On the whole, building and maintaining rapport leads to positive client outcomes.[9–14] A survey exploring the views of 129 Connecticut occupational therapists on therapeutic relationships supports this claim.[4] While descriptive surveys are not the most appropriate design for evaluating causal relationships, clinical evidence is beginning to mount that validates the association between good rapport and positive client outcomes.

A cohort study involving 354 patients in a community-based non-profit drug treatment program and 223 patients from a private for-profit program found lower levels of client rapport during counselling treatment resulted in poorer treatment outcomes, including greater cocaine use and criminality.[15] Likewise, studies of patients with non-chronic schizophrenia,[16] depression,[14,17] post-traumatic stress disorder[18] and alcoholism[19] show that good client rapport improves treatment outcomes.

Although these studies suggest that the development of rapport may benefit clients receiving psychotherapy, data on the effect of good client rapport on the outcomes of interventions in other healthcare fields are lacking. In particular, further research is required to ascertain whether changes in CAM practitioner behaviour can improve treatment success and reduce unnecessary demand on existing health services.

A reason why well-established rapport may contribute to improved client outcomes may be explained by increased treatment compliance.[20] In support of this statement, mothers attending a Los Angeles children's hospital reported greater treatment compliance when highly satisfied with a physician's attitude.[21] Similarly, perioperative patients who reported a higher level of satisfaction with their care were more likely to take responsibility for their decisions.[22]

The positive relationship between client satisfaction and treatment compliance has also been reported among patients with chronic pain,[23] dermatological disorders[24] and diabetes.[25] Thus, client satisfaction appears to be a strong motivator of treatment compliance and, as such, maybe fundamental to treatment success. In other words, good rapport may be responsible for improving client satisfaction and treatment compliance,[26] and ameliorating client outcomes.

Even though the needs of clients are a priority in any consultation, there are also professional implications associated with building client–practitioner rapport. First, strong therapeutic relationships between clients and clinicians may improve the public's perception of a practitioner group.[4] Second, by increasing client rapport and satisfaction, the risk of litigation might be reduced. Although this claim is speculative, Eastaugh [27] and Panting[28] agree that improving client trust and communication, such as that developed through good rapport, results in fewer malpractice claims. Indeed, effective communication could reduce the risk of litigation by increasing rapport and treatment compliance.[10,21,29] Alternatively, since good client rapport is critical to formulating adequate diagnoses,[21,30] practitioners may misdiagnose less frequently.

Because the practitioner is predominantly responsible for developing and maintaining client rapport,[31] the following section will highlight some useful strategies that clinicians can use to strengthen therapeutic relations and improve client outcomes.

## Factors that facilitate and constrain client rapport

The clinician's behaviour and communication style can have significant impact on the practitioner–client relationship. Therapists who are warm, friendly (p = 0.01), affirming and understanding (p = 0.05) demonstrate greater rapport with their clients than those who do not manifest these qualities.[32] These attributes may also increase client compliance[21] and improve treatment outcomes.[33] Another essential ingredient in the development of rapport is time.

### Consultation time

Developing client rapport within the first few minutes of a consultation builds client trust[34] and minimises defensive attitudes by blurring the transition from small talk to formal assessment.[21,35] Constraints on practitioner time, such as escalating workloads, costs, and organisational and political pressures diminish the opportunity for practitioners to build a strong rapport with their clients.[4,36]

Evidence from a recent survey of 186 outpatients attending a Japanese psychiatric clinic lends support to the postulated relationship between consultation time and rapport. The study found session concentration (or session duration divided by session frequency) to be positively correlated with patient satisfaction of physician communication style (p<0.05). Higher levels of patient satisfaction also predicted lower levels of depression and anxiety. The authors concluded that communication satisfaction, which was predicted by consultation duration and frequency, was indicative of a good therapeutic relationship.[37] The correlation between increased consultation duration and improved physician communication is consistent with findings from an earlier study of general practitioners.[38]

Because time constraints are likely to have a negative impact on client outcomes,[4] adequate consultation time is as important as effective communication skills. Thus, practitioners of professions that necessitate longer consultations, such as CAM, may have the capacity to establish greater rapport with their clients than practitioners constrained by time. For clinicians whose time is scarce, strategies such as providing a quiet environment, actively listening, avoiding interruptions and displaying non-hurried actions[31] may portray to the client that the practitioner has time to listen, which may in turn facilitate greater disclosure of client concerns. Even though these strategies may assist in developing rapport between practitioner and adult clients, children may require a more distinctive approach.

In a study of 64 3.5-year-old children, the effects of practitioner–child interaction on the establishment of rapport were investigated.[39] Children left alone in a playroom remained with a stranger longer when the stranger greeted the child quickly but interacted with the child for a greater period of time. Conversely, children who were approached gradually but only interacted with the individual for a brief period of time were also less likely to leave the playroom. Unlike adults, too much time spent trying to establish rapport with a child may inversely affect the establishment of this relationship.

## Consultation style

A collaborative consultation style is also essential to building rapport.[3,20] Such an approach may empower the individual to participate in their own care and enable the client to grow.[5,40] Clinicians adopting a technical or parental role as opposed to a collaborative role may compromise client rapport, respect, compliance and treatment outcomes by invoking negative client attitudes.[36] Hence, a relationship in which the practitioner takes control and in which the client follows orders is neither conducive to client growth nor the development of good rapport.

The delivery of a collaborative consultation style requires CAM practitioners to adopt a client-centred approach, develop mutually agreed upon goals with the client[41] and involve the client's family and/or significant others in the consultation.[4] A critical first step to achieving these outcomes is understanding how a clinician's interview style can impede or foster collaborative consultation, particularly a practitioner's phrasing of questions and statements. This is exemplified in Table 2.1.

By adopting a collaborative approach, practitioners also ensure that a client's right to make decisions about the choice of treatment is retained and respected. This, together with informed consent, is not only crucial to the delivery of ethical care, but is also conducive to establishing good client–practitioner rapport. Equally important is the need for effective communication.

**Table 2.1:** Questions or phrases that hinder or facilitate client–practitioner collaboration

| Hindering (paternal) phrases | Facilitating (collaborative) phrases |
|---|---|
| What can **I** do for you? | What are **your** concerns? |
| How can **I** help you? | What brought **you** here today? |
| What **you should** concentrate on is … | What condition concerns/affects **you** the most? |
| What **you need to** do is … | What **we** could do is … |
| I am going to prescribe for you … **you will** need to… | These are the different treatment approaches **we** could take … do you have any thoughts or preferences about these? |
| **I do not want** you to … **I want you** to … | If we could work together on reducing or increasing … this may help us to … |

## Communication skills

CAM practitioners choosing to develop good rapport with their clients will need to possess skills that facilitate effective communication. Skills such as listening and responding are fundamental to the exchange of information, as are open questioning, reflecting, paraphrasing and summarising.[41] Effective communication and optimal client–practitioner interaction also require the clinician to identify and respect individual differences in gender, developmental stages, cognitive ability, values, beliefs, priorities, culture, social circumstance and health literacy.[4,34] The latter is particularly pertinent, as physician explanations of conditions and processes of care are often in language that is too technical or in other ways not tailored to the individual with poor health literacy,[42] which can result in a lack of understanding and, consequently, poor treatment compliance. Thus, it is important that CAM practitioners adapt their language to the needs of the client, and to ensure that they do not speak in language that is too technical for people with poor health literacy. Likewise, practitioners should avoid oversimplifying information for people with good health literacy, such as health professionals and people well versed in their disease, as this could be perceived as condescending and may act as a potential barrier to the establishment of rapport. Other strategies that foster communication between clinician and client are listed in Table 2.2.

| Table 2.2: Practitioner strategies and behaviours that improve client trust, communication and rapport ||
| --- | --- |
| Maintain | an open posture<br>attentiveness<br>a collaborative relationship<br>client comfort<br>confidentiality and trust<br>enthusiasm<br>eye contact<br>interest in client concerns<br>objectivity. |
| Avoid | an authoritarian demeanour<br>interruptions<br>jargon and technical language<br>passing judgement. |
| Be | altruistic<br>confident<br>dependable<br>empathetic<br>empowering<br>engaging and interactive<br>flexible<br>friendly<br>genuine<br>honest<br>open minded<br>reassuring and supportive<br>respectful of client wishes and needs<br>sensitive<br>sincere<br>warm. |
| Use | open-ended questions<br>rationales for procedures, treatments and decisions. |

Effective communication is particularly reliant on the establishment of client trust. It is through trust and respect that a practitioner can enhance communication and facilitate the development of rapport.[40,43] However, client trust is not a skill that can be acquired, but an attribute that must be developed. Practitioners who are clinically competent, consistent, honest and committed to the client[44] may accelerate the development of this trust and, in turn, improve client communication, rapport and clinical outcomes.

Awareness of the signs of increasing or worsening rapport may enable practitioners to better evaluate the strength of this relationship. Signs of growing rapport may be manifested in an increased flow of conversation, the disclosure of sensitive information, relaxed body language, increased eye contact, and improvements in listening and responding. Poor client rapport may present as long periods of silence, sudden withdrawal of conversation,[45] lack of eye contact, brief responses and defensive body language.

## Clinical environment

Another modifiable factor that may influence the development of client–practitioner rapport is the clinical environment. This milieu, which incorporates the consultation room as well as the waiting area, encompasses elements such as lighting, temperature, odour, décor, colours, audiovisual media and sounds. Each of these factors almost certainly affect client comfort, experience, mood and satisfaction, as well as practitioner health, wellbeing and performance.

Music therapy, for instance, has been shown, albeit modestly, to reduce pain intensity levels,[46] elevate mood[47] and reduce anxiety.[48] Exposure to music therapy has also been reported by most patients receiving postanaesthesia care to be a pleasant to very pleasant experience, with a favourable attitude towards music therapy being positively correlated with the degree of relaxation and satisfaction ($p<0.05$). Despite insufficient data on the effect of music therapy on patients within non-hospital environments being available, it is likely that exposure to music within the clinical setting will improve client comfort, mood and satisfaction to some degree, and thus hasten the development of client rapport. The provision of ambient music in clinic waiting areas, in conjunction with other noise control measures such as soundproofing of walls and doors, may also help to preserve client confidentiality and privacy. Therefore, whether it is for ethical, legal or clinical reasons, there appears to be some merit in adopting this approach.

Other measures that may improve client satisfaction and mood and thus help to foster rapport include shortened waiting times ($p = 0.005$), increased exposure to educational interventions ($p<0.001$),[49] and aromatherapy, particularly the presence of diffused orange essential oil in the waiting room.[50] Ambient room temperature is another important consideration; undesirable room temperature may adversely affect client comfort, exacerbate specific symptoms and/or affect the accuracy of clinical assessments, such as capillary perfusion.[51] An example of a clinical environment that fosters client–practitioner rapport is illustrated in Figure 2.1.

In cases where rapport fails to develop, practitioners may need to critically reflect on their techniques, the environment and the client to isolate the factors that impede the growth of client rapport. The CAM practitioner may also choose to utilise the strategies listed in Table 2.2 to facilitate the development of this relationship.[1–5,10,20,26,30,34,41,43,52]

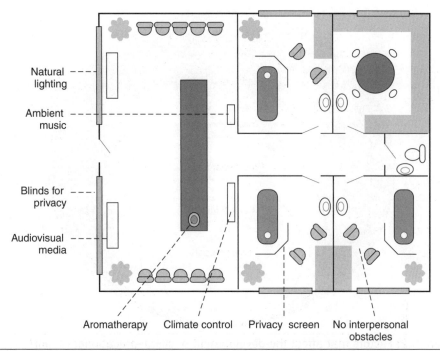

Natural lighting

Ambient music

Blinds for privacy

Audiovisual media

Aromatherapy   Climate control   Privacy screen   No interpersonal obstacles

**Figure 2.1:** A CAM practice floorplan that fosters client–practitioner rapport

## Summary

The development of client–practitioner rapport and the subsequent production of positive client outcomes are dependent on trust, effective communication skills, the clinical environment, practitioner behaviour, consultation style and time. As illustrated in Figure 2.2, these elements can be conceptualised as layers, ranging from intrinsic client-related factors, to more extrinsic environmental factors. By adopting the techniques identified in this chapter, practitioners may significantly improve client health and wellbeing, as well as the efficiency of CAM services. Rapport has widespread implications for the client, the practitioner, the community and the healthcare system, although further research is still needed to evaluate the effect rapport has on the outcomes of CAM interventions. While the initial stages of the clinical consultation are critical to building client rapport, the development of this relationship continues throughout the entire consultation process, particularly during the second stage of DeFCAM – the clinical assessment.

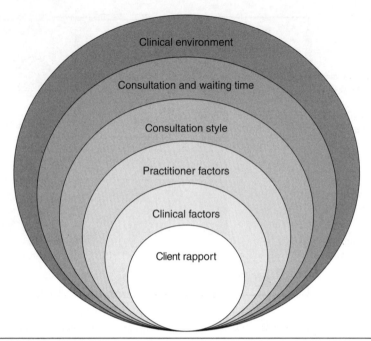

**Figure 2.2:** Factors that affect the development of client–practitioner rapport

## Learning activities

1 Describe in your own words the meaning of rapport.
2 Compare the benefits of rapport for the client, the CAM practitioner and the wider community.
3 What features of CAM practice are conducive to the development of client–practitioner rapport? How do these elements compare with allied health, nursing and medical practice?
4 What features of CAM practice are likely to constrain the development of rapport? How do these elements compare with allied health, nursing and medical practice?
5 Discuss how poorly established client–practitioner rapport may affect the other stages of DeFCAM, including assessment, diagnosis, planning, application and review.

# References

1. DeLaune SC. Ladner PK. (2006) Fundamentals of nursing: standards and practice. 3rd ed. Albany: Delmar Cengage Learning.
2. Kennedy M. (2000) In doc we trust: building rapport with young patients takes time and skill. Wisconsin Medical Journal, 99(2): 33–6.
3. Ackerman SJ. Hilsenroth MJ. (2003) A review of therapist characteristics and techniques positively impacting the therapeutic alliance. Clinical Psychology Review, 23(1): 1–33.
4. Cole MB. McLean V. (2003) Therapeutic relationships re-defined. Occupational Therapy in Mental Health, 19(2): 33–56.
5. Spink LM. (1987) Six steps to patient rapport. AD Nurse, 2(2): 21–3.
6. Weaver J. (2002) 'Here and now' focussed counselling: a model for nurses. Contemporary Nurse, 13(2–3): 239–48.

7. Horacek TM. Salomon JE. Nelsen EK. (2007) Evaluation of dietetic students' and interns' application of a lifestyle-oriented nutrition-counseling model. Patient Education and Counseling, 68: 113–20.

8. Hill C. (2005) Therapist techniques, client involvement, and the therapeutic relationship: inextricably intertwined in the therapy process. Psychotherapy: Theory, Research, Practice, Training, 42(4): 431–42.

9. Martin DJ. Garske JP. Davis MK. (2000) Relation of the therapeutic alliance with outcome and other variables: a meta-analytic review. Journal of Consulting and Clinical Psychology, 68(3): 438–50.

10. Mejo SL. (1989) Communication as it affects the therapeutic alliance. Journal of the American Academy of Nurse Practitioners, 1(1): 20–2.

11. Karver MS et al (2006) Meta-analysis of therapeutic relationship variables in youth and family therapy: The evidence for different relationship variables in the child and adolescent treatment outcome literature. Clinical Psychology Review, 26: 50–65.

12. Paley G. Lawton D. (2001) Evidence-based practice: accounting for the importance of the therapeutic relationship in the UK National Health Service therapy provision. Counselling and Psychotherapy Research, 1(1): 12–17.

13. Shirk SR. Karver M. (2003) Prediction of treatment outcome from relationship variables in child and adolescent therapy: a meta-analytic review. Journal of Consulting and Clinical Psychology, 71(3): 452–64.

14. Zuroff DC. Blatt SJ. (2006) The therapeutic relationship in the brief treatment of depression: contributions to clinical improvement and enhanced adaptive capacities. Journal of Consulting and Clinical Psychology, 74(1): 130–40.

15. Joe GW et al (2001) Relationships between counselling rapport and drug abuse treatment outcomes. Psychiatric Services, 52(9): 1223–9.

16. Frank AF. Gunderson JG. (1990) The role of the therapeutic alliance in the treatment of schizophrenia. Relationship to course and outcome. Archives of General Psychiatry, 47(3): 228–36.

17. Krupnick JL et al (1996) The role of the therapeutic alliance in psychotherapy and pharmacotherapy: findings in the national institute of mental health treatment of depression collaborative research program. Journal of Consulting and Clinical Psychology, 64(3): 532–9.

18. Cloitre M. Stovall-McClough KC. Chemtob CM. (2004) Therapeutic alliance, negative mood regulation, and treatment outcome in child abuse-related posttraumatic stress disorder. Journal of Consulting and Clinical Psychology, 72(3): 411–16.

19. Connors GJ et al (1997) The therapeutic alliance and its relationship to alcoholism treatment participation and outcome. Journal of Consulting and Clinical Psychology, 65(4): 588–98.

20. Crellin K. (1999) Communication briefs. Nursing Management, 30(1): 49.

21. Jarratt L. Nord W. (1985) Establishing patient rapport and communication. South Dakota Journal of Medicine, 38(1): 19–23.

22. Larsson US et al (1992) Patient involvement in decision-making in surgical and orthopaedic practice: effects of outcome of operation and care process on patients' perception of their involvement in the decision-making process. Scandinavian Journal of Caring Sciences, 6(2): 87–96.

23. Hirsch AT et al (2005) Patient satisfaction with treatment for chronic pain: predictors and relationship to compliance. Clinical Journal of Pain, 21(4): 302–10.

24. Renzi C et al (2002) Association of dissatisfaction with care and psychiatric morbidity with poor treatment compliance. Archives of Dermatology, 138(3): 337–42.

25. Alazri MH. Neal RD. (2003) The association between satisfaction with services provided in primary care and outcomes in Type 2 diabetes mellitus. Diabetic Medicine, 20(6): 486–90.

26. O'Connor GT. Gaylor MS. Nelson EC. (1985) Health counselling: building patient rapport. Physician Assistant, 9(3): 154–5.

27. Eastaugh SR. (2004) Reducing litigation costs through better patient communication. The Physician Executive, 30(3): 36–8.

28. Panting G. (2004) How to avoid being sued in clinical practice. Postgraduate Medical Journal, 80(941): 165–8.

29. Davis CM. (2006) Patient practitioner interaction: An experiential manual for developing the art of health care. 4th ed. Thorofare: SLACK Incorporated.

30. Franke J. (1996) Communication tune-up: forty tips to improve rapport with your patients. Texas Medicine, 92(3): 36–42.

31. Purtilo R. Haddad A. (2002) Health professional and patient interaction. 6th ed. Philadelphia: WB Saunders.

32. Najavits LM. Strupp HH. (1994) Differences in the effectiveness of psychodynamic therapists: a process-outcome study. Psychotherapy, 31(1): 114–23.

33. Williams DDR. Garner J. (2002) The case against 'the evidence': a different perspective on evidence-based medicine. British Journal of Psychiatry, 180: 8–12.

34. Harkreader H. Hogan MA. Thobaben M. (2007) Fundamentals of nursing: caring and clinical judgement. 3rd ed. Philadelphia: Elsevier Saunders.

35. Gumenick NR. (2003) Classical five-element acupuncture. Acupuncture Today, 4(2).

36. Crepeau EB. Cohn ES. Schell BAB. (2008) Willard and Spackman's occupational therapy. 11th ed. Philadelphia: Lippincott Williams & Wilkins.

37. Igarashi H et al (2008) Consultation frequency and perceived consultation time in a Japanese psychiatric clinic: their relationship with patient consultation satisfaction and depression and anxiety. Psychiatry and Clinical Neurosciences, 62(2): 129–34.

38. Roland MO et al (1986) The 'five minute' consultation: effect of time constraint on verbal communication. British Medical Journal, 292(6524): 874–6.

39. Donate-Bartfield E. Passman RH. (2000) Establishing rapport with preschool-age children: implications for practitioners. Children's Health Care, 29(3): 179–88.

40. Fox V. (2002) Therapeutic alliance. Psychiatric Rehabilitation Journal, 26(2): 203–4.

41. MacDonald P. (2003) Developing a therapeutic relationship. Practice Nurse, 26(6): 56–9.

42. Schillinger D et al (2004) Functional health literacy and the quality of physician–patient communication among diabetes patients. Patient Education and Counseling, 52: 315–23.

43. Myers DG. (2006) Psychology. 8th ed. New York: Worth Publishers.

44. Usherwood T. (1999) Understanding the consultation: evidence, theory and practice. Buckingham: Open University Press.

45. Latey P. (2000) Placebo: a study of persuasion and rapport. Journal of Bodywork and Movement Therapies, 4(2): 123–36.

46. Cepeda MS et al (2006) Music for pain relief. Cochrane Database of Systematic Reviews, issue 2.

47. Maratos AS et al (2008) Music therapy for depression. Cochrane Database of Systematic Reviews, issue 1.

48. Evans D. (2001) Music as an intervention for hospital patients: a systematic review. Joanna Briggs Institute for Evidence Based Nursing and Midwifery: 1–58.
49. Oermann MH. (2003) Effects of educational intervention in waiting room on patient satisfaction. Journal of Ambulatory Care Management, 26(2): 150–8.
50. Lehrner J et al (2000) Ambient odor of orange in a dental office reduces anxiety and improves mood in female patients. Physiology and Behaviour, 71(1–2): 83–6.
51. Gorelick MH. Shaw KN. Baker MD. (1993) Effect of ambient temperature on capillary refill in healthy children. Pediatrics, 92(5): 699–702.
52. Ramjan LM. (2004) Nurses and the 'therapeutic relationship': caring for adolescents with anorexia nervosa. Journal of Advanced Nursing, 45(5): 495–503.

# 3
# Assessment

## Chapter overview
Clinical assessment is an important component of DeFCAM. As discussed in the preceding chapter, the quality of this assessment is heavily influenced by the quality of the client–practitioner relationship. It is also argued that without an appropriate clinical assessment, every step of the decision-making framework that follows will be compromised, including the accuracy and relevance of differential diagnoses, treatment goals, expected outcomes and selected interventions. Therefore, a systematic and holistic clinical assessment that is inclusive of a comprehensive health history, physical examination and relevant diagnostics may help to minimise clinical error, as well as subsequent delays in client progress. An example of such an approach is described throughout this chapter.

## Learning objectives
The content of this chapter will assist the reader to:
- describe the types of data that may be obtained during a clinical assessment
- identify the principles of rigorous clinical assessment
- describe the CAM assessment process
- recognise key assessment techniques pertinent to each major body system

## Chapter outline
- Introduction
- Types of assessment data
- CAM assessment process
- Cardiovascular system assessment
- Respiratory system assessment
- Gastrointestinal system assessment
- Urinary system assessment
- Reproductive system assessment
- Integumentary system assessment
- Endocrine system assessment
- Nervous system assessment
- Musculoskeletal system assessment
- Summary

## Introduction

Competency in clinical assessment (in varying degrees) is an essential requirement of any practising healthcare professional, including practitioners of CAM. This is because assessment data directly inform clinical decision making, determining for instance when a clinician should initiate, continue or cease treatment, or when to refer or involve others in the multidisciplinary team. Even though the acquisition of pertinent knowledge and skills in clinical assessment is a vital first step to developing competence in this area, it is important to note that assessment is not just a step-by-step data collection exercise, but a process that requires a high level of critical thinking. Put simply, assessment should not be about ticking all the boxes, but about analysing and evaluating the data to determine what additional techniques and tests would support or refute suspected or possible diagnoses. This ongoing evaluation of the data is known as critical analysis, which is vital given that many client health problems can be complex and fraught with uncertainty. Integrating critical analysis into a comprehensive and systematic clinical assessment framework also promotes the efficient use of practitioner and client time, and healthcare resources. Before discussing such a framework, it is important to understand the types of data that can contribute to the clinical assessment.

## Types of assessment data

There are several types of data that can be acquired during a clinical assessment. Each form can be distinguished by the means in which it is collected, interpreted and utilised. Recognising the merits and limitations of these different types of data is critical to understanding the assessment process. The first of these types is subjective data. This category of data is defined as that which is informed by personal opinion, feelings and perceptions. Subjective data are typically obtained during client and family interviews, and are the predominant form of data collected during a health history. While subjective data provide valuable information about a client's lived experience, such as the duration and severity of a symptom, this form of data is easily confounded by personal bias, which raises concern about the accuracy and consistency of such information.[1,2]

The other major form of data that can be collected during the assessment process is objective data, which is defined as that which is observable, verifiable, measurable and not distorted by subjective impressions. Objective data are often acquired using recognised measures such as pathology tests, radiological imaging and physical examination techniques; as a result it is less likely to be tainted by personal bias. As such, the validity and reliability of objective data are greater than that obtained by subjective data. What this means is that clinicians should give higher priority to the collection of objective data over subjective information during the clinical assessment.[3,4]

The differences in these types of data is analogous to the levels of evidence in evidence-based practice (EBP), with objective data being comparable to relatively higher levels of evidence (such as level II or III) and subjective data similar to level V (expert opinion) evidence. As with EBP, the strength of the data is also relevant, with consistent findings from multiple objective data sources likened to level A or B evidence, and consistent subjective information equivalent to level D evidence. Of course, measures that quantify or objectify subjective data could help to reduce risk of bias and improve the validity and reliability of this information.

## CAM assessment process

Clinical assessment is a pivotal component of DeFCAM in that it directly informs every succeeding stage of the process. For this reason it is necessary that client assessments are comprehensive and complete, and that they follow the principles of rigorous clinical assessment (see Table 3.1). One way practitioners can minimise the risk of omitting important data is to adopt a systematic approach to clinical assessment. The head to toe and body systems approaches are two such processes used in clinical practice. The problem with these methods is that neither presents a comprehensive approach to clinical assessment. The CAM assessment process is a more complete assessment process, not only because it integrates additional elements of the health history (such as socioeconomic background) and physical examination (such as olfaction), but also because it encompasses an essential diagnostics phase. These interrelated stages of the process and the non-linear nature of the approach are illustrated in Figure 3.1.

| **Table 3.1:** Principles of rigorous clinical assessment | |
| --- | --- |
| **Data should be** | accurate |
| | complete |
| | comprehensive |
| | interpreted appropriately |
| | corroborated by supporting evidence |
| | objective |
| | systematic |
| **Methods should be** | ethically sound |
| | reliable |
| | safe |
| | sensitive |
| | specific |
| | valid |

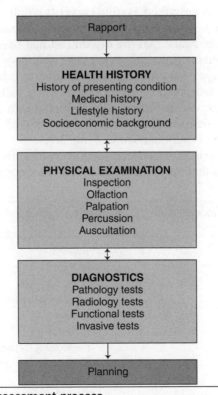

**Figure 3.1:** The CAM assessment process

## Health history

Implementing measures that build client rapport before and during the clinical consultation are critical to developing client trust, improving communication and enhancing the accuracy of acquired information.[5] This is particularly important when completing a health history because subjective data often dominate this stage of assessment. It is probable that the quality of clinical assessments will be improved if clinicians become more consciously aware of the many factors that improve client rapport (see Table 2.1) and, more importantly, attempt to address these elements throughout the consultation.

Once measures have been put in place to build rapport, the clinician can begin to explore the client's health history. During the initial stages of the interview, the practitioner will need to obtain sufficient information about the history of the presenting condition, which includes establishing what the client's primary problem is and, from that, developing a more comprehensive understanding of the complaint. To fulfil these requirements, the clinician will need to acquire information about the location, quality, severity, onset, radiation, duration and frequency of the symptoms, otherwise known as the where, what and when of the complaint. The identification of concomitant symptoms, as well as factors that aggravate and ameliorate the symptom, including previous and existing treatments, foods, body position, activity, environmental conditions, temperature and emotions, will further improve the description of the presenting complaint and enable the practitioner to narrow down the causes of the condition. The following example illustrates this point.

Asking a clinician to speculate on the aetiology of a disease when the history of a presenting complaint is described as mild (severity), dull ache (quality) to the left lower abdominal quadrant (location) would be difficult and inappropriate. On the other hand, if the history added that the discomfort had been present for the past 3 months (onset), occurred intermittently every day (frequency) for approximately 1–2 hours at a time (duration), was non-radiating (radiation), improved by defecation (ameliorating factors), worsened by stress (aggravating factors) and was accompanied by bloating and flatus (concomitant symptoms), then a clinician may be able to consider possible hypotheses, such as irritable bowel syndrome. This description of the presenting complaint is summarised in Table 3.2.

Once the presenting condition has been adequately described the clinician can start to explore other factors that may contribute to the chief complaint, the client's state

| **Table 3.2:** Core components of the presenting complaint description (ReLOAD FACQS) | |
|---|---|
| **Re** | Radiation |
| **L** | Location |
| **O** | Onset |
| **A** | Aggravating factors |
| **D** | Duration |
| **F** | Frequency |
| **A** | Ameliorating factors |
| **C** | Concomitant symptoms |
| **Q** | Quality |
| **S** | Severity |

of health and wellbeing, and the overall plan of care. These determinants can be separated into medical, lifestyle and socioeconomic factors. With reference to the medical determinants, these include family history of illness, allergies and sensitivities to foods, medications and environmental agents, over-the-counter and prescribed medications, complementary medicines and supplements, current and previous medical conditions or illnesses, and history of surgical or investigational procedures (see Table 3.3). For paediatric clients, it is important to also consider immunisation, birth, breastfeeding, growth and development history.

Another important component of the health history is the client's lifestyle history. A lifestyle history includes details about diet and fluid intake (including quality and quantity of consumed goods), illicit drug use (including type, route and frequency of use), smoking status (including strength and quantity), frequency and duration of exercise, alcohol use (including type, quantity and frequency), quality and duration of sleep, and entertainment and recreation choices (see Table 3.4).

The final part of the health history, socioeconomic background, is a particularly important component as many of the factors within this category are likely to affect a client's capacity to understand and/or comply with treatment. This category includes information about the client's family environment (including living arrangements, proximity of family, family dynamics), occupation and employment status, religion and cultural background, level of social support from family, friends and/or external agencies, level of educational attainment (including primary, secondary and tertiary level education), and residential and/or work environment (see Table 3.5). For paediatric clients, information also should be obtained about childcare arrangements and school performance.

In an attempt to quantify the severity and/or impact of the presenting condition, some practitioners choose to use one of a number of clinical assessment tools, such as pain, depression, anxiety, stress and irritable bowel syndrome scales. Although such tools may be useful in providing clear, concise and measurable data about the presenting problem, which may help in the evaluation of client care, the validity

**Table 3.3:** Medical components of the health history (FAMMS)

| | |
|---|---|
| F | Family history |
| A | Allergies and sensitivities |
| M | Medications |
| M | Medical conditions |
| S | Surgical and investigational procedures |

**Table 3.4:** Lifestyle components of the health history (DISEASE)

| | |
|---|---|
| D | Diet and fluid intake |
| I | Illicit drug use |
| S | Smoking status |
| E | Exercise frequency and duration |
| A | Alcohol use |
| S | Sleep quality and duration |
| E | Entertainment or recreation choices |

| Table 3.5: Socioeconomic components of the health history (FORSEE) | |
| --- | --- |
| F | Family environment |
| O | Occupation and employment status |
| R | Religion and cultural background |
| S | Social support |
| E | Education |
| E | Environment (work and residential) |

and reliability of many evaluation tools are not well established. If the accuracy of a tool can be determined and the data are found to be reasonably consistent, then that assessment instrument may have a place in the CAM assessment process. Examples of tools that can be used in the assessment of conditions pertinent to each body system are outlined in the second half of this chapter.

## Physical examination

A complete and comprehensive health history should provide the clinician with a detailed description of the client's presenting condition and enable the practitioner to formulate a number of assumptions about the aetiology of the complaint. To determine which, if any, of these hypotheses are likely to become probable diagnoses, the clinician will need to test the assumptions by acquiring additional data. The source of such data can be derived from the physical examination (for a more detailed discussion of assumption or hypothesis processing, see chapter 4).

The physical examination is pivotal in corroborating findings from the more subjective health history, partly by adding much-needed objective data to the clinical assessment. For the examination to be accurate and reliable it needs to be systematic and all-inclusive. Using a system-based approach in conjunction with the inspection, olfaction, palpation, percussion and auscultation (IOPPA) strategy, enables a practitioner to fulfil these requirements.

The physical examination generally involves some degree of physical contact between the practitioner and client, so it is critical that the clinician establishes some level of rapport and trust with the client (see chapter 2) and has at least obtained verbal consent from the client prior to commencing the examination. Appropriate hand washing, infection control measures, privacy, client conversation, instrument use, draping, level of client contact and exposure are also important measures for reducing a client's risk of physical or psychological harm. Because inappropriate physical contact and professional misconduct are major causes of complaint against CAM practitioners,[6–8] these strategies may also serve to protect clinicians from unnecessary professional and legal action. To further protect the client and practitioner from immediate and enduring harm, it is important that clinicians also recognise their professional boundaries and the limits to their scope of practice, and, where appropriate, refer clients to relevant health professionals for further assessment. For paediatric clients, it is important that a parent or guardian is present whenever possible.

Once these factors have been taken into consideration, a practitioner can commence the physical examination. The first part of this assessment, which begins from the time the practitioner makes visual contact with the client, is inspection. This visual assessment of the client incorporates a general and a specific component. The general inspection examines the client's broad state of health by observing features such as posture, gait, affect, body language, physical guarding and functional capacity, which can alert the clinician to possible causes of the presenting condition as well as related comorbidities. Specific inspection focuses on the presenting complaint and associated body systems, and requires the clinician to make observations about pertinent structural and functional manifestations (including normal and atypical signs), such as a flat or distended abdomen and pink or pale skin colour.

An important element of the physical examination often dismissed in the literature is olfaction, in particular, the detection of pathognomonic odours. Apart from enabling clinicians to develop a better understanding of the presenting complaint, smell helps to identify health concerns that are neither reported nor detectable by sight, sound or touch. The presence of urine odour, for example, may indicate a client is suffering from a urinary tract infection or is having difficulty self-managing care, whereas halitosis may be a sign of dental, neurological, respiratory or gastro-oesophageal disease.

The tactile component of the physical examination, known as palpation, uses deep and light touch, where relevant, to acquire information about the size, depth, texture, temperature, mobility, firmness and tenderness of the presenting condition.[9] Apart from corroborating observed data, palpation adds necessary detail about the condition of the underlying structures, including muscles, bones, organs and blood vessels. The tactile examination of pulses, masses, lesions and areas of localised pain are some examples of where this technique maybe applied. Palpation also provides supporting evidence for pathological processes, such as inflammation, infection and carcinogenesis. A good case in point is erythema. The presence of localised erythema to the lower limb, for instance, says very little about the aetiology of the condition, but when combined with palpable heat and tenderness, suspicions of inflammation and/or infection may be confirmed.

Complementing palpation is percussion, an examination technique that uses touch (i.e. tapping the area of interest) and sound, specifically, vibration, to define the density of the underlying structure, in particular, whether the structure is gas, fluid or solid.[10] This information can help a clinician distinguish between certain pathologies without relying on invasive or costly diagnostic tests in the early stages of assessment. A particularly important place for percussion is in the early detection of pneumonia, pneumothorax, internal bleeding and organomegaly. With reference to respiratory disease, percussion can be especially helpful in differentiating between generally less fatal conditions such as lobar pneumonia (manifested by percussive dullness), and life-threatening emergencies such as pneumothorax (manifested by hyper-resonance).

The final component of the physical examination is auscultation. Auscultation uses sound to detect changes in physiological function, such as blood flow (i.e. bruits, blood pressure, cardiac murmurs), bowel motility and respiratory function (i.e. breath sounds). While auscultation is most frequently assessed using a stethoscope, the value of ultrasound and the naked ear should not be dismissed. The naked ear is useful for detecting a number of minor and potentially serious complaints, such as crepitus, audible wheeze and borborygmi, whereas ultrasound can be used to identify changes not detectable by the human ear, including fetal heart sounds and peripheral blood flow.

The data collected from a comprehensive health history and physical examination can be particularly helpful in informing the CAM practitioner about possible diagnoses, as well as the need for referral. The following example illustrates this point further. A brief clinical assessment that identifies the presence of cough and chest discomfort may mislead a practitioner into believing that a client has asthma or respiratory tract infection. A more detailed assessment that identifies the additional presence of haemoptysis, hoarseness, weight loss, dyspnoea, digital clubbing and supraclavicular lymphadenopathy, may direct a practitioner to a more probable diagnosis of lung cancer, resulting in prompt referral to an allopathic medical practitioner and the avoidance of unnecessary delays in treatment. Other clinical manifestations that should alert a clinician to the possibility of more serious pathology, and the need for prompt referral to an appropriate practitioner, are bleeding (such as haemoptysis, melaena and haematuria), escalating pain (including central chest pain, cephalgia and abdominal pain), altered levels of consciousness, seizures, unresolving masses, rapid weight loss and petechiae.

## Diagnostics

The final aspect of the clinical assessment is the diagnostics phase. Depending on the practitioner's level of expertise, this stage of assessment may require clinicians to request, perform and/or interpret findings from a range of pathology, radiology, functional, invasive and miscellaneous tests. Even though the use of such tests can be justified where there are inadequate data from the health history or physical examination to support or refute possible hypotheses, or when the outcomes of treatment need to be monitored, issues relating to access, cost, comfort, competency and convenience may be significant obstacles to ordering these investigations. Effective interdisciplinary communication, as well as appropriate referrals to pertinent health professionals, may be necessary to execute this stage of assessment.

Each type of diagnostic test is capable of addressing important gaps in the clinical assessment and of adding valuable objective data to the pool of clinical information. Laboratory investigations of blood, urine, semen, hair, wound and sputum specimens, for instance, can provide critical information about the functional status of the client (and in some cases the possible cause of the clinical picture), including data about hepatic, renal, endocrine and haematopoietic function. The thyroid function test (TFT) is a good case in point. The clinical manifestation of low libido, weight gain and depression, for instance, may be indicative of hypothyroidism. Without performing a TFT, however, it would be difficult to determine whether the client has abnormal levels of circulating thyroid hormone (and therefore hypothyroidism), and whether the condition is attributable to thyroid disease or pituitary gland dysfunction.

Functional tests also serve to explore the functionality of specific tissues, organs or systems, including the musculoskeletal, digestive, endocrine and immunological systems. These investigations generally fall into two broad categories:

1 comprehensive pathology profiles (e.g. cardiovascular profile), and
2 detailed physiological assessments (e.g. functional skin integrity testing).

Radiological tests enable a practitioner to visualise structural and functional aspects of the presenting complaint, such as bone and tissue integrity, tissue content and fluid dynamics. Medical images are created using different sources of energy, including electromagnetic radiation (i.e. computed tomography), ultrasound, and magnetic and radiofrequency energy (i.e. magnetic resonance imaging), and are enhanced with the use of contrast media (i.e. barium enema) and radionuclide (i.e. scintigraphy).

Investigations not typically performed by CAM practitioners, but for which clinicians may need to interpret findings or refer clients on, are invasive procedures. These investigations, often used in conjunction with pathology tests, provide important information about the structure, function and/or pathology of the presenting complaint, although when compared with other diagnostic methods, most invasive tests pose a greater risk of harm to the client, including an increased risk of pain, infection and haemorrhage.

The other category of diagnostic investigation, which is commonly used by CAM practitioners, is the miscellaneous tests. Despite the long history of use of these tests within CAM, particularly methods such as iridology, kinesiology, Vega testing and pulse diagnosis, there is insufficient clinical evidence to support their use. This is not to say that these methods are ineffective or should be dismissed in clinical practice, only that further research is needed to evaluate the validity and reliability of these procedures. Miscellaneous tests are not confined to CAM diagnostics: this category also captures investigations that do not nest within the other four diagnostic categories, including electrodiagnostics and sleep studies. Examples of tests that fall into the five diagnostic categories are listed in Table 3.6.

**Table 3.6:** Examples of diagnostic tests that may be requested, performed or interpreted in CAM practice

| | |
|---|---|
| **Pathology tests** | Carbohydrate breath test<br>Complete blood examination (CBE)<br>Culture and sensitivity testing (C&S)<br>Glycated haemoglobin (HbA1c)<br>Lipid studies<br>Liver function test (LFT)<br>Nutrient levels (iron studies, hair mineral analysis)<br>Oral glucose tolerance test (OGTT)<br>Semen analysis<br>Thyroid function test (TFT)<br>Urinalysis (UA) |
| **Functional tests** | Adrenal hormone profile<br>Bone metabolism assessment<br>Comprehensive detoxification profile (CDP)<br>Comprehensive digestive stool analysis (CDSA)<br>Intestinal permeability (IP) test<br>Pulmonary function test (PFT)<br>Urodynamic studies |
| **Radiological tests** | Computed tomography scan (CT)<br>Contrast studies<br>Magnetic resonance imaging (MRI)<br>Mammography<br>Positron emission tomography (PET)<br>Radiograph/X-ray<br>Ultrasound (US) |
| **Invasive tests** | Allergy skin testing (prick-puncture test)<br>Arthroscopy<br>Biopsy<br>Colonoscopy<br>Endoscopy<br>Laparoscopy<br>Lumbar puncture (LP) |
| **Miscellaneous tests** | Electrodiagnostics (electrocardiograph)<br>Iridology<br>Plethysmography<br>Pulse diagnosis<br>Quantitative sensory testing (QST)<br>Sleep studies |

To this point, the structure, approach and rationale for the CAM assessment process have been presented, albeit from a general perspective, but as well as understanding the theoretical foundation of the process, a practitioner also needs to consider its application. In the section that follows, the CAM assessment process is applied to each major body system. It is important to note that this section will outline only pertinent assessment methods and investigations for each system. For a comprehensive discussion of examination techniques, particularly for special populations such as pregnant and paediatric clients, refer to a specialist text on physical assessment.

Several of the techniques and diagnostic tests listed in this section may be considered outside the scope of CAM practice, at least for some practitioners. Readers therefore need to be aware of the limitations of their practice when interpreting this information, as well as the skills or tests that are pertinent to their field of practice, the assessment techniques that may best be completed by another health professional and how these methods may or may not fit within the philosophy or context of their discipline. CAM practitioners should also ensure that they keep abreast of the emerging literature on evidence-based diagnostics to make certain that all aspects of their care are evidence-based and not just the interventions they prescribe.

## Cardiovascular system assessment

The cardiovascular system consists of the heart and blood vessels, including arteries, veins and capillaries. The key role of this system is to transport blood (including nutrients, heat, oxygen, hormones and cellular components) throughout the body. Any abnormalities in cardiovascular structure or function are likely to compromise the system's ability to deliver or eliminate vital components to and from cells, which will lead to the manifestation of adverse symptoms.

These points should be taken into account when conducting a comprehensive assessment of the cardiovascular system. An outline of the regions pertinent to cardiovascular system assessment is illustrated in Figure 3.2.

### Health history
#### History of presenting condition
Identify the client's primary problem and establish the location, onset, duration, frequency, quality and severity of the sign or symptom, the presence of radiating symptoms (e.g. chest pain radiating down the left arm or up the neck may

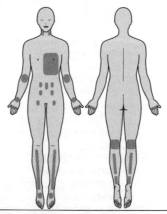

**Figure 3.2:** Cardiovascular assessment cue card

indicate myocardial ischaemia), any aggravating or ameliorating factors (such as walking, stress, rest or leg elevation) and any concomitant symptoms (including shortness of breath, fatigue, chest pain, palpitations, claudication, paresthesias and syncope).

## Medical history
### Family history
Determine if the client has a genetic predisposition to cardiovascular disease (CVD) by assessing the client for any family history of CVD, such as hypertension, dyslipidaemia and coronary artery disease.

### Allergies
Establish whether the client has any allergies or sensitivities to foods (such as caffeine), medications (such as antibiotics or anticonvulsants) and environmental agents (such as latex) that could contribute to the presenting condition or impact on clinical management.

### Medications
Determine whether the client is currently administering or has recently completed any prescribed or over-the-counter medications, supplements, herbs or therapies for CVD, including antihypertensives, hypolipidaemics, diuretics, anticoagulants, antiarrhythmics, antiangina agents and cardiac inotropics. It is also important to establish if the client is receiving any other treatments that may generate cardiovascular symptoms (e.g. antipsychotic drug-induced postural hypotension, or non-steroidal anti-inflammatory drug-induced thromboembolic disease).

### Medical conditions
Ascertain whether the client has any current or previous medical conditions that affect the heart, blood vessels and/or blood, such as hypertension, deep vein thromboses, dyslipidaemia, erectile dysfunction, stroke, coronary artery disease or peripheral vascular disease. It is also important to identify conditions that mimic cardiovascular complaints (such as anxiety, gastro-oesophageal reflux disease, pulmonary and musculoskeletal associated chest pain) or comorbidities that can contribute to the development of CVD (including renal disease, diabetes mellitus and obesity).

### Surgical and investigational procedures
Identify additional or overlooked complaints by asking the client if they have undergone any relevant surgical or investigational procedures, such as vascular surgery, Doppler tests, angiography or an exercise stress test.

## Lifestyle history
Identify any factors that may increase the client's risk of CVD, such as obesity, tobacco use (including number and strength of cigarettes inhaled in a day), alcohol consumption (including number of standard drinks and type of alcoholic beverage consumed in a day), illicit drug use (including type, route and quantity of drug used per day), diet and fluid intake (such as sodium, omega 3 fatty acids, saturated fat,

fibre, fruit and vegetable consumption), quality and duration of sleep (e.g. broken sleep, sleep apnoea) and frequency and duration of exercise.[11]

### Socioeconomic background
Determine whether there are any socioeconomic determinants that may increase the client's risk of CVD, affect their understanding of CVD or affect the management of the disease, such as family environment (i.e. marital status, number and ages of children), occupation and employment status (i.e. day or nightshift, full or part time, number of jobs), religion, ethnicity, race or cultural background (i.e. whether the client follows strict dietary practices or is placed at increased risk of developing CVD as a result of their culture, race or ethnic background), level of social support (i.e. whether the client lives alone and whether the client receives assistance from community services), level of educational attainment (i.e. primary, secondary and/or tertiary education) and residential and/or work environment (i.e. whether the client resides near an industry or arterial road).

## Physical examination
### Inspection
Observe for any signs of impaired cardiovascular function, such as xanthomata (hard, yellow masses that are pathognomonic of familial hypercholesterolaemia),[10] digital clubbing (an abnormal enlargement of the terminal phalanges that may be a sign of chronic hypoxia), splinter haemorrhages of the nail bed (present in infective endocarditis[12]), dyspnoea, pallor or cyanosis (may be observed in hypoxia, anaemia, vasoconstriction or vascular occlusion), Lichstein's sign (oblique, bilateral earlobe crease observed in people over 50 years of age with significant coronary heart disease),[12] dependent oedema (may be indicative of chronic venous insufficiency or right-sided heart failure), leg ulceration (may be indicative of peripheral vascular disease) and lower leg varicose veins and ochre pigmentation (both signs suggest the presence of chronic venous insufficiency). The presence of chest scars (from sternotomy or pacemaker insertion) and/or deformities (such as pectus excavatum or pectus carinatum) may also draw attention to the possibility of cardiovascular defects.

### Olfaction
There are no pertinent olfactory signs known to be indicative of CVD.

### Palpation
Examine major pulses of the neck (carotid), chest (cardiac apex), upper limbs (brachial, radial, ulnar) and lower extremities (femoral, popliteal, posterior tibial, dorsalis pedis) and note the rate, rhythm and amplitude of each pulse, as well as the presence of any thrills or palpable vibratory sensations (thrills are indicative of turbulent blood flow). Assess the peripheries for temperature (cool hands and feet may be indicative of cardiac failure or peripheral vascular disease) and pitting oedema (may indicate the presence of chronic venous insufficiency or right-sided heart failure). In terms of cardiac function, identify the position and diameter of the point of maximum impulse (PMI) (a laterally displaced or enlarged PMI is suggestive of cardiomegaly)[10] and the presence of thrills or increased pulse intensity over the aortic area (may suggest the presence of aortic dilatation), pulmonic area (may be indicative of pulmonary artery dilatation), mitral area (may be indicative of mitral

stenosis or regurgitation) and tricuspid area (may be a sign of tricuspid stenosis or regurgitation).

## Percussion
Use percussion to estimate cardiac size in order to detect the presence of cardiomegaly or to assess left ventricular mass.

## Auscultation
Using a stethoscope, assess the intensity, duration, timing and pitch of heart sounds, the presence of murmurs (abnormal sounds in the cardiac cycle that are indicative of turbulent blood flow through a defective heart valve), bruits (an abnormally harsh sound suggestive of turbulent blood flow through an artery) and pericardial friction rubs (a sign of pericarditis). Auscultation is also used to measure blood pressure by noting the onset and disappearance of Korotkoff sounds.

## Additional signs
Clinical data not derived from the abovementioned physical examination that can provide important information about the aetiology of a presenting condition, as well as the general health and nutritional status of the client, can be derived from assessing core body temperature, weight, height, body mass index (BMI), waist circumference and skinfold thickness.

## Clinical assessment tools
Examples of instruments that may be used to evaluate the severity or effect of cardiovascular complaints, or the effect of treatment on these disorders, are outlined as follows.

### Aberdeen varicose vein questionnaire (AVVQ)
Measures health-related quality of life in clients with varicose veins.

### Canadian cardiovascular scale
Classifies angina according to its level of effect on physical activity. Classifications range from no angina with ordinary physical activity (class I), to angina with any physical activity and/or rest (class IV).

### Claudication scale (CLAU-S)
Evaluates quality of life in clients with peripheral arterial occlusive disease and intermittent claudication.

### Framingham coronary heart disease (CHD) prediction score
Assigns weights to major cardiovascular risk factors, including age, gender, blood pressure, total cholesterol (TC), high-density lipoprotein-cholesterol (HDL-C) and smoking status to predict an individual's risk of developing atherosclerosis and coronary heart disease over a 10-year period.

### MacNew heart disease health-related quality of life questionnaire
Assesses the effect of coronary heart disease and its treatment on physical, emotional and social functioning, and on activities of daily living.

### New York Heart Association (NYHA) grading of heart failure

Assesses the severity of chronic heart failure (CHF) according to the level of physical activity needed to manifest symptoms, ranging from class I (ordinary physical activity does not cause symptoms) to class IV (symptoms of CHF manifest at rest).

### Newcastle stroke-specific quality of life measure (NEWSQOL)

Assesses quality of life in people who have suffered from stroke.

### Venous clinical severity score (VCSS)

Measures the severity of nine hallmark signs of venous disease and the need for compression therapy.

## Diagnostics
### Pathology tests
#### Apolipoprotein-B:Apolipoprotein-A$_1$ ratio

Apolipoproteins are the major protein component of lipoproteins, with apolipoprotein-B a major component of LDL and apolipoprotein-A1 a key component of HDL. Apo-B:Apo-A$_1$ is an independent and significant predictor of CVD, in particular, fatal and non-fatal myocardial infarction.[13]

#### Asymmetric dimethylarginine (ADMA)

ADMA is a by-product of protein methylation. Elevated levels of ADMA are associated with smooth muscle cell proliferation and platelet aggregation. ADMA is also an endogenous inhibitor of nitrous oxide; elevated levels are linked to endothelial dysfunction and small vessel disease.[14]

#### C-reactive protein (CRP)

CRP is a marker of inflammatory activity, which is implicated in the development and complications of atherosclerosis.[15] CRP is independently related to future cardiovascular events.[15]

#### Cardiac enzymes/proteins

These are released from the myocardium during injury, such as in myocardial infarction. Because many of these enzymes or proteins are also present in skeletal tissue, it is recommended that cardiac-specific enzymes or proteins be ordered, including cardiac-specific troponin T and I, and the isoenzyme creatine phosphokinase-MB.[16]

#### Complete blood examination (CBE)

A CBE provides important information about the cellular elements of the blood, including haemoglobin, haematocrit, the number, volume, haemoglobin concentration and width of erythrocytes, white blood cell count, and the number and volume of platelets. As a cardiovascular screening tool the CBE may assist in the diagnosis of vascular or haematological pathologies, such as anaemia, infection, dehydration and blood loss.

#### Hair, urine, serum and blood nutrient levels

These tests may be indicated when presenting clinical manifestations are suggestive of nutrient deficiency or toxicity, when the presenting condition is likely to be caused by nutrient deficiency or toxicity or when the condition is likely to contribute to the development of nutrient deficiency or toxicity. Nutrient tests that are particularly relevant to cardiovascular assessment are hair mineral analysis, serum vitamin $B_{12}$, serum magnesium, serum coenzyme Q10, serum zinc, red blood cell folate and iron studies.

### Homocysteine (Hcy)
Hcy is an amino acid derived from methionine. Even though Hcy plays an important role in protein synthesis, elevated levels are associated with smooth muscle cell proliferation, platelet aggregation and impaired endothelial derived nitric oxide induced vasodilatation, all of which promote atherosclerosis.[17,18]

## Lipid studies
### High-density lipoprotein-cholesterol (HDL-C)
HDL-C is a class of lipoprotein that transports cholesterol from the tissues and circulation to the liver. Increased levels of serum HDL-C are inversely related to the development of atherosclerosis and coronary artery disease.[15]

### Low-density lipoprotein-cholesterol (LDL-C)
LDL-C is a class of lipoprotein that transports cholesterol from the liver to the peripheral tissues. Elevated levels of serum LDL-C are positively correlated with the incidence of cardiovascular disease.[15]

### Total cholesterol (TC)
TC is a structural component of cell membranes and plasma lipoproteins. Elevated serum TC is a predictor of CVD.[19]

### Triglycerides (TG)
TG are the main storage form of lipids within the human body. Elevated serum TG is predictive of future cardiovascular events.[15]

## Radiology tests
### Angiography/venography
This is an invasive radiological procedure in which a blood vessel is injected with contrast media and a series of X-ray images taken. By assessing blood flow dynamics and blood vessel defects, this procedure can support suspicions of aneurysm, vessel stenosis or occlusion, and vascular malformation.[16]

### Computed tomography (CT)
CT uses multiple X-ray beams to produce cross-sectional images of the head, chest, abdomen and pelvis to provide information about cardiovascular structure. CT imaging is particularly useful for identifying aneurysms, vessel occlusion or stenosis (with angiography), arteriovenous malformations, haematomas and haemorrhage.[20]

### Doppler/ultrasound
This test uses sound waves to assess blood flow velocity and direction, and blood flow disturbances of major blood vessels, including the carotid arteries and the arteries and veins of the extremities. It is a procedure that is useful for detecting aneurysms, vessel occlusion or stenosis, deep vein thrombosis, Raynaud's disease, chronic venous insufficiency and varicose veins.[18]

### Echocardiography

Echocardiography uses ultrasonic waves to evaluate cardiac structure and function, including information about heart size, position, walls, valves and chambers, the pericardium and masses. This procedure can help in the diagnosis of valvular regurgitation or stenosis, thrombus formation, endocarditis, myxoma, septal or congenital heart defects, cardiomyopathy and ventricular hypertrophy.[18]

### Magnetic resonance imaging (MRI)

MRI uses magnetic and radiofrequency energy to produce images of the heart and vasculature, including information on structure and function. MRI is particularly useful for detecting aneurysms, congenital heart defects, myocardial infarction/ischaemia, pericardial changes, vascular malformations and arterial occlusive disease, and for determining cardiac chamber and ventricular function.[18]

### Positron emission tomography (PET)

PET provides anatomical and functional information about the heart. Following the administration of an inhaled or intravenous radionuclide, areas of radionuclide accumulation, which reflect the level of cellular metabolic activity, are tracked by CT imaging and positron detectors. A reduction in positron emission, and thus cardiac metabolism, can occur in conditions such as myocardial infarction or scarring.[16] Increased cellular metabolism may be a sign of carcinoma. Other abnormal states that may be detected by PET include heart chamber disorders and ventricular enlargement.[18]

### X-rays or radiographs

X-rays use electromagnetic radiation to produce images of the heart (providing information about size, shape and location), pericardium (particularly the presence of inflammation or effusion), large blood vessels (such as the aorta) and, in conjunction with angiography, smaller blood vessels. Without contrast media, X-rays are limited to detecting cardiac enlargement, pericarditis, pericardial effusion and large vessel dilatation or stenosis.[20]

## Functional tests
### Comprehensive cardiovascular profile

This profile identifies a number of lipid-independent risk factors that are related to cardiovascular disease, such as Hcy, CRP and fibrinogen.

## Invasive tests
### Transoesophageal echocardiography (TOE)

TOE assesses the size, position, chambers, valves and movements of the heart, as well as the condition of proximal blood vessels. This procedure is useful for detecting coronary artery disease, congenital heart defects, aneurysms, valve and septal defects, thrombi and congestive cardiac failure.[18]

## Miscellaneous tests
### Arterial/venous plethysmography

This procedure measures volume changes in the blood vessels of the upper and lower extremities to determine the presence of occlusive disease such as venous thrombosis, arterial embolisation and Raynaud's disease.[18]

### Electrocardiograph (ECG)

An ECG measures the electrical activity of the heart. The reading can be used to detect cardiac arrhythmias, myocardial ischaemia, electrolyte imbalances, conduction defects, pericarditis, cor pulmonale and ventricular hypertrophy.[16]

### Exercise stress test

An exercise stress test assesses the response of the heart and the vessels of the lower limb to physical stress. The results can be used to identify the presence of intermittent claudication, occlusive coronary artery disease, exercise-induced hypertension and cardiac dysrhythmias.[16]

### Iridology

Iridology can be used to detect the presence of arcus senilis (a whitish ring at the perimeter of the cornea), which is highly suspicious of hypercholesterolaemia in clients under 40 years of age.[10] The sign is also predictive of CVD and coronary artery disease in older people, yet, given that arcus senilis is strongly associated with increasing age, the sign may be misleading in this population.[21]

## Respiratory system assessment

The respiratory system is divided into two sections – the upper and lower respiratory tracts. The upper tract consists of the nose, paranasal sinuses, nasal cavity and pharynx, while the lower tract includes the larynx, trachea, bronchi, bronchioles, alveoli and lungs. The respiratory system is primarily responsible for gas exchange, in particular, the uptake of oxygen from the atmosphere and the elimination of carbon dioxide into the external environment. When the functional capacity of this system is comprised, hypoxia, hypercapnia and waste accumulation can occur.

A practitioner should consider these points when conducting a comprehensive assessment of the respiratory system. An outline of the regions pertinent to respiratory system assessment is illustrated in Figure 3.3.

## Health history

### History of presenting condition

The practitioner should ascertain the client's primary problem and determine the location, onset, duration, frequency, quality and severity of the sign or symptom,

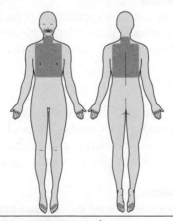

**Figure 3.3:** Respiratory assessment cue card

the presence of radiating symptoms, any aggravating or ameliorating factors (such as exercise, cold air, cigarette smoke, dietary factors or medication) and any concomitant symptoms (including fatigue, dyspnoea, dyspepsia, pain, cough, nasal discharge, haemoptysis, fever and hoarseness).

## Medical history
### Family history
Ascertain whether the client is at risk of respiratory illness or if the presenting condition can be explained by genetic predisposition by assessing if there is a family history of respiratory complaints such as asthma, chronic obstructive pulmonary disease (COPD) and atopic disease.

### Allergies
Establish whether the client has any sensitivities or is allergic to medications (such as antibiotics), foods (such as peanuts) and environmental substances (such as pollen, animal dander or dust mite) that could contribute to the presenting complaint or affect on clinical management.

### Medications
Establish whether the client is currently taking or has recently completed any over-the-counter or prescribed medications, herbs, supplements or therapies for respiratory illness, including bronchodilators, antibiotics, inhaled corticosteroids, expectorants, decongestants, antitussives and oxygen. It is also essential to determine if there are any treatments that may generate respiratory-type symptoms (i.e. angiotensin conventing enzyme (ACE) inhibitor-induced cough, fluoxetine-induced pneumonia, amiodarone-induced pneumonitis).

### Medical conditions
Identify any current or previous medical conditions that involve the upper and lower respiratory tracts, such as asthma, bronchitis, bronchiectasis, pneumonia, emphysema, rhinosinusitis, tonsillitis, pharyngitis, laryngitis or neoplastic disease. In addition, determine if there are any conditions that could yield respiratory-type symptoms or mimic respiratory disease (including anaemia, anxiety, gastro-oesophageal reflux disease, musculoskeletal complaints or cardiac failure).

### Surgical and investigational procedures
Determine whether the client has undergone any surgical or investigational procedure in the past (such as rhinoplasty, thoracotomy, bronchoscopy or tracheotomy) to ascertain if there are any other respiratory conditions that may have been overlooked in the health history.

## Lifestyle history
Identify any lifestyle determinants that may exacerbate, prolong or increase a client's risk of upper or lower respiratory tract illness, particularly tobacco use (including number and strength of cigarettes inhaled in a day) and level of physical activity,[22] and diet and fluid intake (i.e. sodium, tea, fruit and vegetable consumption).[23]

## Socioeconomic background
Ascertain if there are any socioeconomic factors that may increase the client's risk of respiratory disease, affect their understanding of the condition or the management

of the disease, such as residential and/or work environment (i.e. whether the client resides near an industry or arterial road, whether they are exposed to dust, asbestos, silica, chemicals or other respiratory irritants or whether any people in the household smoke), family environment (i.e. marital status, number and ages of children), occupation and employment status (i.e. day or nightshift, full or part time, number of jobs), religion, ethnicity, race or cultural background (i.e. whether the client follows strict dietary practices, whether the client's culture, race or ethnic background place the client at increased risk of developing respiratory disease), level of social support (i.e. whether the client lives alone or receives community services) and level of educational attainment (i.e. primary, secondary and/or tertiary education).

## Physical examination
### Inspection
Assess the quality of respirations, taking particular note of the rate (an accelerated respiratory rate may be a sign of anxiety, fever, metabolic acidosis or airway obstruction; bradypnoea may signify liver failure, diabetic ketoacidosis or increased intracranial pressure), rhythm (an irregular breathing pattern, such as Cheyne-Stokes or Biot's breathing, may suggest brain damage or drug-induced respiratory depression),[10] depth (hyperpnoea, or deep breathing, may occur in metabolic acidosis; shallow breathing can be a sign of pneumonia, pulmonary oedema, COPD or pleurisy) and effort of respirations (laboured breathing may occur in chronic obstructive pulmonary disease). The clinician should also observe for signs of clubbing (an abnormal enlargement of the terminal phalanges that may be indicative of chronic hypoxia), central cyanosis (a bluish tinge to the lips and tongue that may signify reduced arterial oxygenation, which can occur in severe airflow limitation or pulmonary fibrosis),[12] finger or fingernail staining (brown-yellow staining of the fingers can indicate a history of cigarette smoking), nasal flaring, accessory muscle use and intercostal retraction (these signs are indicative of airway obstruction and/or respiratory distress), tracheal asymmetry (tracheal deviation may occur in upper lobe lung disease, such as tension pneumothorax),[24] chest wall asymmetry (asymmetrical movement of the chest may signify impaired air entry from localised pulmonary consolidation, collapse, fibrosis or effusion)[24] and chest wall deformities (pectus carinatum may develop following severe respiratory illness in childhood; barrel chest may occur in chronic obstructive pulmonary disease).[12] Other noteworthy observations that may allude to previous respiratory dysfunction include body position (whether the client finds it difficult to breathe when lying down on the examination table), flow of conversation (whether the client can maintain a normal conversation without becoming short of breath), pharyngeal mucosa (whether there is pharyngeal erythema or tonsillar enlargement), scarring (whether there is evidence of previous thoracic surgery (i.e. thoracoplasty) and trauma (whether there are chest drain scars from previous pneumothorax or haemothorax). For paediatric clients, the practitioner should also observe for the presence of foreign bodies in the ear, nose and throat.

### Olfaction
During the clinical examination, the clinician should note the presence of halitosis, or foul-smelling breath. This symptom may allude to the existence of dental, gingival, sinus, oral, oesophageal or respiratory pathology. In terms of the latter, this can include respiratory tract infection, lung abscesses and bronchiectasis.

## Palpation

Palpate the paranasal sinuses (localised tenderness may indicate sinusitis), the position of the trachea (tracheal deviation may suggest a mediastinal shift), the presence of chest wall masses, sinus tracts and discomfort (chest/intercostal tenderness may be associated with pleurisy and/or underlying musculoskeletal disease; sinus tracts may indicate tuberculosis or actinomycosis),[9] and the size, shape, mobility and tenderness of lymph nodes (tender and mobile lymph nodes are suggestive of infection and/or inflammation).[9] The degree of symmetry of respiratory expansion is another important technique that can aid the detection of localised pulmonary disease, such as pneumonia or bronchial obstruction. The density of underlying tissue can be determined by palpating the chest wall for tactile fremitus (vibrations transmitted from voice sounds to the chest wall may be reduced in the presence of liquid, gas and excess adipose tissue, and increased in solid or consolidated areas).[10]

## Percussion

Much like tactile fremitus, percussion is also used to assess the density of underlying tissues up to a depth of 5–7 centimetres. Percussion can help to confirm or refute any abnormal findings identified during palpation. Percussive tones that may be detected include flatness (short, high pitch tone over a fluid-filled region, such as pleural effusion), dullness (medium duration and medium pitch tone over a solid area, such as pneumonia), resonance (long, low pitch tone over normal lung) and hyperresonance (long, low pitch tone over an air-filled structure, such as pneumothorax).[24]

## Auscultation

The auscultation of breath sounds is an important component of the respiratory assessment as it provides valuable information about airflow. Using the diaphragm of a stethoscope, examine the quality, location, intensity and duration of breath sounds, including the presence of vesicular breath sounds (soft, low pitch breath sounds normally heard over most parts of the lungs) and bronchial breath sounds (the presence of these loud, high-pitch sounds over areas other than the manubrium may indicate lung consolidation).[24] Additional cues about underlying pathology can be determined from adventitious sounds such as stridor (due to narrowing or obstruction of the larynx or trachea), crackles (from excess airway secretions, as in respiratory tract infection and pulmonary oedema), wheezes (resulting from narrowed or obstructed airways), rhonchi (from transient airway plugging, as in bronchitis) and pleural rub (due to pleural inflammation).[10] Auscultation also can be used to assess the density of underlying tissue by examining the quality of transmitted voice sounds. The existence of bronchophony (when the spoken words 'ninety-nine' become loud and clear), aegophony (when the spoken sound 'ee' sounds like 'ay') and/or whispered pectoriloquy (when the whispered words 'ninety-nine' become loud and clear) over any part of the chest is suggestive of lung consolidation.[9]

## Additional signs

Clinical data not derived from the abovementioned physical examination, which can support suspicions of infectious disease, can be derived from assessing core body temperature.

## Clinical assessment tools
Examples of instruments that may be used to evaluate the severity or effect of respiratory complaints, or the effect of treatment on these conditions, are as follows.

### Asthma control scoring system (ACSS)
Quantitatively evaluates the level of asthma control by providing percentage scores for clinical, physiologic and inflammatory parameters.

### Clinical chronic obstructive pulmonary disease questionnaire (CCQ)
Measures the severity, degree of functional limitation and level of clinical control in clients with COPD.

### Cystic fibrosis questionnaire (CFQ)
Measures the effect of cystic fibrosis on overall health, activities of daily living and wellbeing.

### Influenza symptom severity (ISS) scale
Assesses the intensity of influenza symptoms.

### Rhinosinusitis disability index (RDI)
Evaluates the physical, functional and emotional effects of nasal and sinus disorders on health-related quality of life.

### Wisconsin upper respiratory symptom survey (WURSS)
Assesses the severity and functional effect of the common cold, as well as changes in symptoms over time.

## Diagnostics
### Pathology tests
#### Arterial blood gases (ABG)
An ABG test is useful in assessing ventilatory function and acid–base balance. The test measures the pH, oxygen saturation, bicarbonate level and partial pressures of oxygen ($pO_2$) and carbon dioxide ($pCO_2$) in the blood. ABG findings pertinent to the respiratory system are as follows:
- elevated pH (may occur in respiratory alkalosis, cystic fibrosis, pulmonary emboli, acute pulmonary disease)
- decreased pH (suggestive of respiratory acidosis and respiratory failure)
- increased $pCO_2$ (indicative of COPD)
- reduced $pCO_2$ (may occur in pulmonary emboli).[16]

#### Hair, urine, serum and blood nutrient levels
These nutrient tests may be indicated when presenting clinical manifestations are suggestive of nutrient deficiency or toxicity, when the presenting condition is likely to be caused by nutrient deficiency or toxicity or when the condition is likely to contribute to the development of nutrient deficiency or toxicity. Nutrient tests that are particularly relevant to respiratory assessment are hair mineral analysis, serum vitamin A, serum pyridoxine and serum calcium.

### Sputum culture and sensitivity testing

Testing of a fresh sputum specimen enables sufficient numbers of the organism to be isolated, identified and quantified, and the antibiotics to which the microbial strains are sensitive or resistant to be determined. This test may be ordered for the purpose of aiding the diagnosis and treatment of bacterial, viral or fungal infection of the respiratory tract.[16]

## Radiology tests
### Chest X-ray (CXR)

CXR uses electromagnetic radiation to produce images of the chest wall, lung fields, bones and diaphragm; it can also be used to detect abscesses, atelectasis, bronchitis, COPD, lymphadenopathy, tumours, pleural effusion, pleuritis, pneumonia, pulmonary oedema, haemo/pneumothorax, pulmonary fibrosis and tuberculosis.[20]

### Computed tomography (CT)

CT uses multiple X-ray beams to produce cross-sectional images of the lungs, mediastinum, bronchi, pleural space and bones; it is also a useful radiological test for identifying tumours, lesions, cysts, pleural effusion, pneumonitis, lymphadenopathy, inflammatory nodules and bronchial stenosis or dilatation.

### Magnetic resonance imaging (MRI)

MRI uses magnetic and radiofrequency energy to generate images of the lungs, pleural space, soft tissues and bones, and together with appropriate agents, can also assess lung perfusion and ventilation. While MRI can be used to detect pleural effusion, tumours, lung malformations, pneumonia, asbestosis and lung fibrosis, motion artefacts are a current concern with chest MRI.[25]

### Ventilation–perfusion (VQ) scan

A VQ scan uses intravenous radioactive material to assess pulmonary blood flow and perfusion, and an aerosolised agent (such as Krypton gas) to measure the patency of pulmonary airways. A VQ mismatch (i.e. normal ventilation and abnormal perfusion) is indicative of pulmonary embolus, whereas abnormal ventilation and perfusion findings are suggestive of pneumonia, emphysema and/or pleural effusion.[16]

## Functional tests
### Pulmonary function tests (PFTs)

PFTs are often performed to evaluate the presence and severity of respiratory disease. The PFT can incorporate any number of different measures of lung volume and capacity, including total lung capacity, tidal volume, forced vital capacity (FVC), forced expiratory volume in 1 second ($FEV_1$), maximal mid-expiratory flow (MMEF), maximal volume ventilation (MVV), peak inspiratory flow rate (PIFR) and peak expiratory flow rate (PEFR). Reductions in many of these measures are often evident in asthma, emphysema, chronic bronchitis, bronchiectasis and other obstructive pulmonary diseases.[16]

## Invasive tests
### Bronchoscopy

This is an endoscopic procedure that enables direct visualisation of the trachea, larynx, bronchi, bronchioles and alveoli. As a diagnostic tool, bronchoscopy is useful in detecting tumours, inflammatory disease, foreign bodies, structural anomalies, abscesses, interstitial pulmonary disease, strictures, tuberculosis and opportunistic lung infections. Bronchoscopy also plays an important role in the collection of tissue biopsies.[20]

### Thoracentesis, or pleural tap
In this procedure, a needle is inserted into the pleural cavity for the purpose of removing fluid or gas. As a diagnostic tool, thoracentesis is used to determine the aetiology of a pleural effusion such as empyema, pneumonia, tuberculosis, pulmonary infarction, malignancy and haemothorax.[16]

## Gastrointestinal system assessment
The gastrointestinal system consists of a number of structures that can be categorised into two parts. The first of these is the gastrointestinal (GI) tract, which incorporates the mouth, oesophagus, stomach, duodenum, jejunum, ileum, caecum, colon, rectum and anus. The remaining parts are collectively known as the accessory structures, which include the tongue, teeth, salivary glands, pancreas, gallbladder and liver. The principle roles of the GI system are ingestion, digestion, absorption, secretion and elimination.

Any deviation from normal GI integrity or physiology may manifest as abnormal changes in these functions. These points should be taken into consideration when conducting a comprehensive assessment of the gastrointestinal system. An outline of the regions pertinent to gastrointestinal system assessment is illustrated in Figure 3.4.

### Health history
#### History of presenting condition
After establishing the client's primary problem, ascertain the location, duration, frequency, onset, quality and severity of the sign or symptom, the presence of radiating symptoms (i.e. right upper quadrant pain radiating to the right inferior scapula is suggestive of cholelithiasis),[26] any aggravating or ameliorating factors (such as emotional stress, alcohol, dietary components, exercise, defecation, meal consumption, cigarette smoking, distinct odours, medications or movement) and any concomitant symptoms (including fatigue, fever, diarrhoea, constipation, nausea, vomiting, odynophagia, halitosis, weight change, pain, flatulence, bloating, dysphagia, tenesmus, dyspepsia, anorexia, abdominal distension and cramping).

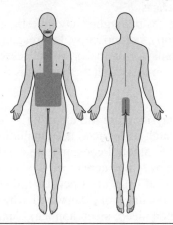

**Figure 3.4:** Gastrointestinal assessment cue card

## Medical history

### Family history

Determine whether the client is at risk of GI disease or if the presenting condition can be explained by genetic predisposition by asking if there is any family history of GI illness, such as inflammatory bowel disease (IBD), colon cancer, irritable bowel syndrome (IBS), gastroenteritis or coeliac disease.

### Allergies

Ascertain whether the client has any allergies or sensitivities to foods (such as lactose, gluten, soy, nuts, corn, dairy or eggs), medications (such as antibiotics) and environmental substances (such as molds or pollens) that could contribute to the presenting complaint or affect on clinical management.

### Medications

Determine whether the client is currently administering, or has recently completed, any over-the-counter or prescribed medications, supplements, herbs or therapies for a GI complaint (i.e. aperients, antibiotics, antispasmodics, antidiarrhoeals, antacids, digestive enzymes, probiotics, anorectal agents, gastric acid suppressants). The clinician should also note if there are any treatments that may generate GI symptoms (i.e. antibiotic-associated diarrhoea, aperient-associated diarrhoea, non-steroidal anti-inflammatory drug-induced gastritis).

### Medical conditions

Ascertain if there are any previous or current medical conditions that involve the GI tract and accessory structures, including appendicitis, carcinoma, coeliac disease, cirrhosis, cholelithiasis, constipation, cystic fibrosis, dental caries, diverticulosis, dyspepsia, gastritis, gastroenteritis, gastro-oesophageal reflux disease, gingivitis, haemorrhoids, hepatitis, IBD, IBS, liver failure, pancreatitis, peptic ulceration and peritonitis. Also establish if there are any complaints that could yield GI-type symptoms or mimic GI illness (such as anxiety, aperient abuse, depression, diabetes mellitus, eating disorders, electrolyte disturbance, neuromuscular disease, nutrient deficiency or thyroid disorder).

### Surgical and investigational procedures

Establish whether the client has undergone any investigational or surgical procedure in the past (such as endoscopy, colonoscopy, laparoscopy, laparotomy, appendicectomy, cholecystectomy, stoma formation or bowel resection) to discover other GI conditions that may have been missed in the health history.

## Lifestyle history

Identify any factors that may increase the client's risk of GI illness or exacerbate the presenting complaint, such as tobacco use (including number and strength of cigarettes inhaled in a day),[27] alcohol consumption (including number of standard drinks and type of alcoholic beverage consumed in a day),[28] illicit drug use (including type, route and quantity of drug used per day), diet and fluid intake (such as fibre, fruit and vegetable consumption, dairy and wheat intake),[26,29] quality and duration of sleep (e.g. broken sleep, sleep apnoea),[30] and frequency, duration and type of exercise.[31]

## Socioeconomic background

Determine whether there are any socioeconomic factors that may increase the client's risk of GI illness, affect their understanding of the condition or the management of the complaint, such as occupation and employment status (i.e. day or nightshift; full or part time, number of jobs, hours worked each week), residential and/or work environment (i.e. do these environments create significant emotional stress?), family environment (i.e. marital status, number and ages of children), religion, ethnicity, race or cultural background (i.e. whether the client follows stringent dietary practices, whether the client's culture, race or ethnic background place the client at increased risk of developing GI disease), level of social support (i.e. whether the individual lives alone or receives community services) and level of educational attainment (i.e. primary, secondary and/or tertiary education).

# Physical examination

## Inspection

Observe for any signs of previous or existing impairment to GI structure and/or function, beginning with examination of the oral cavity, including the lips (i.e. angular stomatitis), tongue (i.e. candidiasis, carcinoma, glossitis), palate (i.e. torus palatinus), gingivae (i.e. gingivitis, ulceration, bleeding), teeth (i.e. caries) and oropharynx (i.e. tonsillitis, pharyngitis). This examination is particularly important as these structures play an essential role in chemical and mechanical digestion, and furthermore, can manifest early signs of nutritional imbalance and/or deficiency. Inspection of the skin and sclera may also detect the presence of jaundice that may be secondary to haemolysis or liver disease.[24] For paediatric clients, the buccal mucosa should be assessed for the presence of Koplik's spots (small white spots indicative of measles), the soft palate should be inspected for Forschheimer's spots (small dusky red spots that may arise at the onset of rubella), and the number and condition of the teeth recorded.[10]

The abdomen should then be observed for scars (from previous surgery or trauma), striae (such as the pink purple striae of Cushing's syndrome), dilated veins and/or spider naevi (due to liver disease), everted umbilicus (due to late pregnancy, ascites or large mass), ecchymosis (bluish discolouration of the flanks and/or periumbilicus secondary to haemoperitoneum), rashes, peristalsis (visible peristalsis may indicate intestinal obstruction), lesions, asymmetry (due to organomegaly or masses), contour and herniation.[9] Where appropriate, the anus and perianal region should be inspected for signs of underlying pathology, such as haemorrhoids (may be indicative of constipation), lichenification (suggestive of pinworm infection), excoriation (a manifestation of chronic diarrhoea) and fistula formation (a sign of IBD). Because of the potential risk of litigation with this technique, this aspect of the examination should be restricted to clinicians who are qualified to perform this assessment.

## Olfaction

The presence of abnormal odours from the GI tract may highlight signs of underlying pathology. Fetid smelling stools, for instance, may suggest the presence of malabsorption syndrome, steatorrhoea, cystic fibrosis, coeliac disease, intestinal dysbiosis or GI infection. Halitosis may be indicative of tobacco use, poor oral hygiene, dental disease, mouth ulceration, liver disease, dry mouth, carcinoma, GORD, bowel obstruction or infection.[24]

## Palpation

Light and deep palpation is used to assess the position, shape, mobility, consistency, tenderness and size of the liver, spleen and abdominal contents, as well as any masses.[9] Particularly useful signs of underlying pathology are Murphy's sign (the existence of right upper quadrant pain subsequent to right subchondral pressure and deep inspiration, which is suggestive of cholecystitis), Rovsing's sign (the occurrence of right lower quadrant pain following the application of left lower quadrant pressure, which is a sign of appendicitis) and rebound tenderness (the presence of abdominal pain following the rapid withdrawal of deep pressure, which may be indicative of peritoneal irritation). The presence of voluntary guarding and/or involuntary muscle spasm or rigidity is also suggestive of an irritated peritoneum.[10] Qualified clinicians may choose to perform a rectal examination to detect the presence of haemorrhoids, rectal prolapse, fissures, fistulas and carcinoma of the anus.[24]

## Percussion

This technique can be applied to assess the size and location of masses and organs (which produce a dull percussive tone), and fluid or air-filled regions (which produce a tympanic percussive tone).[9]

## Auscultation

The pitch and frequency of bowel sounds can allude to changes in GI function. Hyperactive bowel sounds, for instance, may be suggestive of diarrhoea or early intestinal obstruction, whereas hypoactive or absent bowel sounds may indicate peritonitis and paralytic ileus.[24]

## Additional signs

Clinical data not derived from the physical examination, which can provide important information about the aetiology of a presenting condition, as well as the general health and nutritional status of the client, can be derived from the assessment of core body temperature, weight, height, BMI, waist circumference and skinfold thickness.

## Clinical assessment tools

Examples of instruments that can be used to evaluate the severity or impact of GI complaints, or the effect of treatment on these conditions, are summarised below.

### Bristol stool scale (BSS)

BSS classifies faecal form and consistency into one of seven categories, ranging from type 1 (separate hard lumps) to type 7 (entirely liquid).

### Chronic liver disease questionnaire (CLDQ)

CLDQ assesses the symptomatic, physical and emotional effect of chronic liver disease on health-related quality of life.

### Cystic fibrosis questionnaire (CFQ)

CFQ measures the effect of cystic fibrosis on overall health, activities of daily living and wellbeing.

### Gastro-oesophageal reflux disease symptom frequency questionnaire (GSFQ)
GSFQ measures symptom frequency and the effect of these symptoms on eating, sleeping and other activities of daily living in clients with GORD.

### Inflammatory bowel disease questionnaire (IBDQ)
IBDQ evaluates health-related quality of life in clients with IBD.

### Irritable bowel syndrome – quality of life questionnaire (IBS-QOL)
IBS-QOL assesses the effect of IBS and its treatment on health-related quality of life.

## Diagnostics
## Pathology tests
### Amylase
Amylase is an enzyme located within the pancreatic acinar cells. Trauma, pancreatitis, pancreatic carcinoma and/or pancreatic cysts can cause damage to these cells, resulting in excess amounts of this enzyme entering the circulation.[32]

### Carbohydrate breath test
Assesses carbohydrate malabsorption, orocecal transit time and small intestinal bacterial overgrowth (SIBO). The test requires the client to consume a specified dose of carbohydrate (lactulose, lactose, fructose, glucose), which the intestinal bacteria metabolise into hydrogen and/or methane. After ingestion, a series of breath samples is taken over a 2–4 hour period. The increased presence of exhaled hydrogen and/or methane (typically over 20 parts per million) is suggestive of carbohydrate malabsorption and possibly SIBO. The sensitivity and specificity of this test for SIBO is currently inadequate for routine clinical use.[33]

### *Helicobacter pylori* breath test or urea breath test
A highly specific and sensitive test for detecting *H. pylori* infection as a cause of peptic ulceration, gastric carcinoma and gastritis that requires the oral administration of radiolabelled carbon and urea, which, in the presence of *H. pylori*, is converted into $CO_2$. The radiolabelled $CO_2$ is exhaled after 30 minutes, collected and tested.[26]

### Culture and sensitivity testing
This type of testing of a fresh stool specimen enables sufficient numbers of an organism to be isolated, identified and quantified, and the antibiotics that the microbial strains are sensitive or resistant to, to be determined. This test may be ordered to aid the diagnosis and treatment of bacterial, viral, fungal, protozoan or parasitic enterocolitis.[16]

### Faecal analysis
This test examines a number of stool characteristics, including appearance, colour, occult blood (present in carcinoma, inflammatory bowel disease, upper GI disease and diverticular disease), epithelial cells (elevated in IBD), leucocytes (increased in intestinal infections), carbohydrates (present in malabsorption syndromes), fat (a sign of fat malabsorption), meat fibres (present in altered protein digestion)

and trypsin (reduced in malabsorption syndromes, cystic fibrosis and pancreatic deficiency).[18]

### Hair, urine, serum and blood nutrient levels

These tests may be indicated when presenting clinical manifestations are suggestive of nutrient deficiency or toxicity, when the presenting condition is likely to be caused by nutrient deficiency or toxicity or when the condition is likely to contribute to the development of nutrient deficiency or toxicity. Nutrient tests that are particularly relevant to GI assessment are hair mineral analysis, iron studies, red blood cell folate, serum α-tocopherol, serum vitamin A, serum vitamin $B_{12}$, serum vitamin C, serum calcium, serum cholecalciferol, serum magnesium, serum phylloquinone, serum pyridoxine and serum zinc.

### Liver function test (LFT)

A LFT provides information about liver function (i.e. total protein, albumin, bilirubin, ammonia) and hepatocyte integrity (i.e. alkaline phosphatase (ALP), gamma glutamyl transpeptidase (GGT), alanine amino transferase (ALT), aspartate amino transferase (AST)). Results of the LFT can assist in the diagnosis of alcohol abuse, cirrhosis, hepatitis, liver disease, biliary disease, malnutrition and malabsorption.[34]

## Radiology tests

### Abdominal X-ray

Uses electromagnetic radiation to generate images of the abdominal cavity and organs, which can detect conditions such as hepatomegaly, bowel obstruction, abscesses, perforation, paralytic ileus and tumours.[20]

### Computed tomography (CT)

CT uses multiple X-ray beams to generate cross-sectional images of the abdomen and pelvis, thus enabling the detection of tumours, cysts, bowel obstruction, bleeding, pancreatitis, cirrhosis, fatty liver, diverticulitis, colonic polyps, cholelithiasis and ductal obstruction or dilatation.[18]

### Lower GI series, or barium enema

Provides serial X-ray images of the colon and distal ileum using rectally administered barium contrast media to enhance visualisation. A lower GI series can be ordered to facilitate a diagnosis of carcinoma, IBD, polyps, diverticula, structural defects, perforation, fistula formation, appendicitis and herniation.[16]

### Magnetic resonance imaging (MRI)

MRI uses magnetic and radiofrequency energy to produce images of the organs and soft tissues of the abdomen and pelvis that can be useful in detecting tumours, pancreatitis, cholangitis, peritonitis, abscesses, cirrhosis, fatty liver, diverticulitis, cholelithiasis and ductal obstructions or dilatation.[18]

### Ultrasound

Ultrasound uses sound waves to assess the size, position, contour and texture of the organs of the abdomen and pelvis in order to detect conditions such as pancreatitis, ductal obstructions or dilatation, cysts, tumours, cirrhosis, cholecystitis, cholelithiasis, hepatitis and peritonitis.[18]

### Upper GI series, or barium swallow
Provides serial X-rays of the lower abdomen, stomach and duodenum using orally administered barium contrast media to enhance visualisation. This test is particularly useful for detecting tumours, oesophageal varices, hiatus hernia, perforation, strictures, congenital defects, peptic ulceration, motility disorders and diverticula.[20]

## Functional tests
### Comprehensive detoxification profile, or functional liver detoxification profile
Measures the rate of phase I and phase II liver detoxification following caffeine, aspirin and paracetamol challenge. Findings from this test, such as a reduction in the rate of substance clearance, can provide important insight into a client's liver function, specifically, whether a client is able to effectively clear toxic metabolites from the blood.[35]

### Comprehensive digestive stool analysis (CDSA)
CDSA obtains data on enzymatic digestion, fatty acid absorption, microbiological balance and metabolic markers of disease, and may help to determine the presence of intestinal dysbiosis, intestinal candidiasis, nutrient malabsorption and indigestion.[36]

### Intestinal permeability test
This test assesses small intestine absorption and permeability by measuring urinary elimination of lactulose and mannitol 6 hours after oral administration. Increased elimination of these non-metabolised sugars in the urine may be indicative of leaky gut syndrome and impaired intestinal permeability, whereas reduced urinary elimination may suggest malabsorption.[37]

## Invasive tests
### Abdominal paracentesis, or peritoneal tap
Requires the insertion of a sterile needle into the peritoneal cavity for the purpose of removing fluid. As a diagnostic tool, the procedure is used to determine the aetiology of peritoneal effusion, such as carcinoma, peritonitis, pancreatitis, tuberculosis, lymphoma and perforation.[16]

### Biopsy
A biopsy involves the excision of a small sample of tissue and the subsequent microscopic examination of the sample in order to identify cell morphology and tissue abnormalities. A biopsy of GI tissue may assist in the diagnosis of cancer, infection, inflammation, cirrhosis, coeliac disease and lactose deficiency.[18]

### Colonoscopy
Permits direct visualisation of the colon, ileocecal valve and terminal ileum through the use of a flexible fiberoptic colonoscope. Colonoscopy can be used to determine the presence of tumours, polyps, inflammation, diverticula, haemorrhoids, ulceration and bleeding.[20]

### Endoscopic retrograde cholangiopancreatography (ERCP)
ERCP enables direct and radiographic visualisation of the biliary and pancreatic ducts through the use of a fiberoptic endoscope, X-ray imaging and contrast media. As a diagnostic procedure, ERCP can identify the presence of obstructive jaundice, duodenal papilla carcinoma, pancreatitis and pancreatic or biliary duct abnormalities, calculi, stenosis or cysts.[16]

### Gastric acid stimulation test
Measures the volume and pH of gastric acid before and after administration of a gastric acid stimulant, such as pentagastrin. Nasogastric aspirates of stomach acid are analysed to determine the cause of peptic ulceration, pernicious anaemia or gastrinoma, the efficacy of ulcer treatment and the presence of hyper- or hypochlorhydria.[18]

### Laparoscopy
Through the use of a rigid fibreoptic laparoscope, enables direct visualisation of the peritoneal cavity and abdominal organs, including the stomach, liver, gallbladder, pancreas and intestines. The procedure is helpful in detecting tumours, adhesions, cirrhosis, lymphomas, perforation, inflammation and infection.[20]

### Oesophagogastroduodenoscopy (OGD)
OGD uses a fibreoptic endoscope to examine the upper GI tract, including the oesophagus, stomach and duodenum. Capsule endoscopy, which uses an orally administered capsule camera, is also capable of visualising the jejunum and ileum. Both endoscopic procedures are useful in detecting oesophageal varices, diverticula, duodenitis, oesophagitis, gastritis, hiatus hernia, peptic ulceration, tumours, bleeding, stenosis and polyps.[18]

### Sigmoidoscopy
Uses a flexible or rigid sigmoidoscope to directly visualise the anus, rectum and sigmoid colon, which can be helpful in detecting tumours, polyps, haemorrhoids, ulceration and bleeding.[16]

## Urinary system assessment
The urinary system comprises the kidneys, ureters, urinary bladder and urethra. While the urinary system is primarily responsible for the elimination of waste products, it is also essential for maintaining homeostasis. Hence, adverse changes to the structure or function of this system will almost certainly lead to an inability to fulfil these roles and the subsequent manifestation of adverse signs and symptoms.

These considerations should be borne in mind when conducting a comprehensive assessment of the urinary system. An outline of the regions pertinent to urinary system assessment is illustrated in Figure 3.5.

## Health history
### History of presenting condition
Identify the client's primary problem and establish the quality, severity, onset, location, duration and frequency of the sign or symptom, the presence of radiating symptoms (i.e. pain radiating from the flank, across the abdomen and down the inner thigh is suggestive of urinary calculi),[26] any aggravating or ameliorating factors (such as

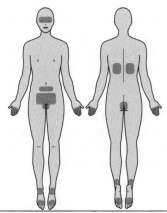

**Figure 3.5:** Urinary assessment cue card

fluid consumption, constipation, body position, cigarette smoking, spices, alcohol or caffeine) and any concomitant symptoms (including urinary frequency, urgency, tenesmus, dysuria, nocturia, enuresis, haematuria, hesitancy, dribbling, incontinence, loin pain, pneumaturia, polyuria, pyrexia, oliguria, oedema, and any changes in urine colour, odour, turbidity, force and calibre of stream).

## Medical history
### Family history
Establish whether the individual has a genetic predisposition to urinary tract disease by assessing whether the client has any family history of urological illness, including polycystic kidney disease, carcinoma of the urinary tract, interstitial cystitis, nephrotic syndrome or pyelonephritis.

### Allergies
Discover whether the client has any sensitivities or allergies to medications (such as antibiotics), foods (such as gluten) and environmental substances (such as insect stings) that could contribute to the presenting condition or affect clinical management.

### Medications
Ascertain whether the client is presently administering, or has recently finished, any over-the-counter or prescribed medications, supplements, herbs or therapies for a urological complaint, including urine alkalinisers or acidifiers, diuretics, antibiotics, antispasmodics, urinary antiseptics and 5-alpha reductase inhibitors. The practitioner should also note the use of treatments that may contribute to urinary tract symptoms, such as anticholinergic drug-induced urinary retention, diuretic-induced polyuria, and prazosin-associated urinary incontinence.

### Medical conditions
Establish if there are any current or previous medical conditions that involve the kidney, bladder or urinary tract, such as cancer, cystitis, benign prostatic hypertrophy, hydronephrosis, glomerulonephritis, nephritic/nephrotic syndrome, nephropathy, polycystic kidney disease, pyelonephritis, renal failure, urinary tract infection, urinary calculi or urinary incontinence. The presence of conditions that could yield

urinary-type symptoms or mimic urological disease (including bowel–urinary tract fistula, dehydration, diabetes insipidus, epididymitis, neuromuscular disease, pregnancy and vaginitis) should also be ascertained. A history of urethral/suprapubic catheterisation or renal dialysis may also allude to the presence of other urological defects.

### Surgical and investigational procedures
Determine whether the client has undergone any pertinent surgical or investigational procedures in the past (such as biopsy, cystoscopy, pyelogram, laparoscopy, removal of urinary calculi or transurethral resection of the prostate) to identify other urological conditions that may have been overlooked in the health history.

## Lifestyle history
Establish if there are any factors that may increase the individual's risk of urological disease or worsen the presenting complaint, such as obesity,[38] tobacco use (including number and strength of cigarettes inhaled in a day),[39] alcohol consumption (including number of standard drinks and type of alcoholic beverage consumed in a day),[40] illicit drug use (including type, route and quantity of drug used per day), diet and fluid intake (such as fruit and vegetable consumption, simple sugar intake, omega 3 fatty acid consumption),[39,40] quality and duration of sleep (e.g. broken sleep, sleep apnoea)[41] and frequency, duration and type of exercise.[42]

## Socioeconomic background
Explore whether there are any socioeconomic factors that might increase the client's risk of urological disease, affect their understanding of the condition or the management of the condition, such as family environment (i.e. marital status, number and ages of children), religion, ethnicity, race or cultural background (i.e. whether the client abides by strict dietary practices, whether the client's culture, race or ethnic background place the client at increased risk of developing urological disease), level of social support (i.e. whether the client lives alone or receives community services), occupation and employment status (i.e. day or nightshift, full or part time, number of jobs, hours worked each week), residential and/or work environment (i.e. whether these environments create significant emotional stress), and level of educational attainment (i.e. primary, secondary and/or tertiary education).

## Physical examination
### Inspection
Signs that may be indicative of underlying urinary dysfunction include abnormal skin colour (individuals with chronic renal failure may develop dirt-brown skin pigmentation due to impaired urinary pigment excretion and/or anaemia secondary to reduced erythropoietin secretion),[24] gouty tophi (the manifestation of white chalky masses of urate crystals on the hands, feet and joints may occur in hyperuricaemia),[26] nail markings (leuconychia, the presence of white transverse opaque lines on the nails, may be a sign of hypoalbuminaemia stemming from glomerular disease),[24] scars (such as a nephrectomy scar) and long-term urinary drainage devices (such as a urostomy, suprapubic catheter or indwelling urethral catheter). Observation of the client's urine, including the colour (i.e. red urine related to haematuria, colourless urine due to diabetes insipidus, dark orange-amber urine related

to dehydration), odour (as discussed below) and transparency (i.e. cloudy urine from bacteria, urate deposits or leucocytes) can also capture valuable information about an individual's urological function. Observe also for signs of fluid retention, such as a distended abdomen, puffy eyelids and pedal oedema, as these may be indicative of glomerular disease or renal failure.[26] In pertinent cases, inspection may also detect congenital defects of the male urethra, such as hypospadias or epispadias.[10]

## Olfaction
Certain body odours can be indicative of urological or systemic disease. Malodorous urine, for instance, can be a sign of urinary tract infection (faecal or fishy odour), dehydration (strong ammonia odour), diabetes mellitus (sweet odour), phenylketonuria (musty odour) or maple syrup urine disease (sweet maple syrup odour). The consumption of particular foods and medications, including asparagus, vitamin B supplements and antibiotics, can also be responsible for abnormal urine odour.[24] An ammonia or fishy breath odour (uraemic fetor) may allude to the presence of uraemia from chronic renal failure.[43]

## Palpation
Palpation over the costovertebral angle (kidney region) and suprapubic area (bladder region) can help to identify the size, contour and tenderness of underlying structures. Signs of tenderness, for instance, may allude to the presence of infection or inflammation, while masses may be indicative of cysts or tumours and unequal kidney size suggestive of hydronephrosis.[44] A suitably qualified clinician may also conduct a digital rectal examination in order to assess the size, texture and firmness of the prostate. A tender prostate gland may, for instance, be suggestive of prostatitis, while an indurated and/or nodular prostate may be indicative of prostatic carcinoma.[10]

## Percussion
The application of conventional percussion over the suprapubic region enables the clinician to visualise the border of the bladder, thus aiding the detection of urinary retention. The application of Murphy's kidney punch can be useful in detecting renal tenderness from conditions such as glomerulonephritis and glomerulonephrosis.[44]

## Auscultation
Auscultation, which plays a minor part in urological assessment, is used primarily to assess the presence of renal bruits. These abnormally harsh sounds, together with hypertension, are suggestive of renal artery stenosis.[44]

## Additional signs
Clinical data not derived from any of the abovementioned physical examinations that can provide important information about the aetiology of a presenting condition, as well as the general health and nutritional status of the client, can be derived from assessing core body temperature, blood pressure, weight, height, BMI, waist circumference and skinfold thickness.

## Clinical assessment tools
Examples of instruments that may be used to evaluate the severity or effect of urinary complaints or the effect of treatment on these conditions are listed below.

### Kidney disease quality of life (KDQOL)

Measures the effect of kidney disease on physical, mental and emotional health, disease burden and daily activities.

### International prostate symptom score (IPSS)

Assesses urinary frequency, urgency, stream, hesitancy, intermittence, nocturia and bladder emptying in clients with benign prostatic hyperplasia (BPH).

### Interstitial cystitis symptom index and problem index

Measures the severity and effect of urinary symptoms in clients with interstitial cystitis.

### Male urinary symptom impact questionnaire (MUSIQ)

Evaluates social health, psychological health and perceptions of function and well-being in men with urinary incontinence.

### Urinary incontinence – specific quality of life instrument (I-QOL)

Measures the effect of avoidance and limiting behaviour, psychosocial factors and social embarrassment on health-related quality of life in women with urinary incontinence.

## Diagnostics

## Pathology tests

### Culture and sensitivity testing of urine

This test allows sufficient numbers of a pathogenic organism to be isolated, identified and quantified, and the antibiotics the microbial strains are sensitive or resistant to, to be determined. This test may be ordered to aid the diagnosis and treatment of urinary tract infection.[16]

### Blood urea nitrogen (BUN)

A BUN test measures the level of urea nitrogen, an end product of protein catabolism, in the blood. Elevated levels of urea may be indicative of impaired renal excretory function. Urological causes of azotemia can be classified as prerenal (e.g. burns, dehydration, excessive protein ingestion or catabolism), renal (e.g. acute tubular necrosis, glomerulonephritis, pyelonephritis, renal failure) and postrenal (e.g. ureteric or bladder outlet obstruction).[16]

### Creatinine

Creatinine is a product of creatine metabolism, an amino acid stored predominantly in skeletal muscle. If skeletal and dietary factors can be eliminated, serum and urine creatinine levels can be a useful measure of glomerular and renal function. Above normal levels of creatinine may, for instance, be a sign of acute tubular necrosis, dehydration, glomerulonephritis, nephritis, nephropathy, nephrosclerosis, obstructive uropathy, polycystic kidney disease, pyelonephritis, renal calculi and renal failure.[18]

### Hair, urine, serum and blood nutrient levels

May be indicated when presenting clinical manifestations are suggestive of nutrient deficiency or toxicity, when the presenting condition is likely to be caused by nutrient deficiency or toxicity, or when the condition is likely to contribute to the development of nutrient deficiency or toxicity. Nutrient tests that are particularly relevant to urological assessment are hair mineral analysis, iron studies, serum vitamin $B_{12}$, serum vitamin C, serum calcium, serum cholecalciferol, serum magnesium, serum pyridoxine and serum zinc.

### Specific gravity (SG)
SG is a measure of urine concentration, which is determined by the number of solutes (i.e. electrolytes, waste products) in the urine. Reduced concentration capacity of the kidneys may result in more dilute urine or a lower SG, which can manifest in glomerulonephritis or severe renal damage. A high SG may be associated with impaired renal dilution capacity, as in nephrotic syndrome. It is important to note that in the presence of glycosuria and proteinuria SG results may be falsely elevated.[20]

### Uric acid
Uric acid is an end product of purine catabolism. Because uric acid levels are maintained by the kidneys, any changes in renal function may adversely affect serum and urine levels. Reduced urine uric acid levels in the presence of hyperuricaemia may be associated with severe renal disease, such as glomerulosclerosis and glomerulonephritis. Elevated urine uric acid levels in the presence of hypouricaemia may be indicative of impaired renal tubular absorption.[18]

### Urinary haemoglobin (Hb)
Hb should not be present in urine, while red blood cells (RBC) should be present only in very small numbers. Any elevation in urinary Hb or RBC may be indicative of urinary tract disease or injury, including calculi, glomerulonephritis, hydronephrosis, renal infarction, malignancy, prostatitis, pyelonephritis, trauma or urinary tract infection.[34]

### Urinary leucocytes or white blood cells
These are normally present in the urine in very small numbers, but when their level is above normal, it may be a sign of urinary tract infection or inflammation, such as cancer, cystitis, glomerulonephritis, nephritis, pyelonephritis and renal calculi.[20]

### Urinary nitrites
These are formed from urinary nitrates in the presence of nitrate reductase – an enzyme secreted by nitrite-forming bacteria, such as *Escherichia coli*, *Klebsiella* spp., *Proteus* spp. and *Pseudomonas* spp. The presence of urinary nitrites may be indicative of bacteriuria.[16]

### Urinary protein
As these large molecules do not normally pass the glomerular membrane, their presence is an indicator of renal dysfunction. If pre-eclampsia and physical stress can be eliminated as causes, elevated urinary protein levels may be a sign of diabetic nephropathy, glomerulonephritis or nephrotic syndrome.[34]

## Radiology tests
### Computed tomography (CT)
CT uses multiple X-ray beams to create cross-sectional images of the kidneys, ureters and bladder. CT imaging is particularly valuable in detecting calculi, congenital anomalies, cysts, haematomas, obstruction, trauma and tumours.[45]

### Intravenous pyelogram (IVP)

IVP uses intravenous contrast media to provide radiographic visualisation of the kidney, ureter and bladder. It can assess structure and function, and may help in the detection of calculi, congenital defects, cysts, glomerulonephritis, haematomas, hydronephrosis, pyelonephritis and tumours.[18]

### Magnetic resonance urography

Uses magnetic and radiofrequency energy to produce images of the kidney, ureters and bladder following fluid and diuretic challenge. The procedure is useful in the evaluation of suspected congenital anomalies, dilated collecting systems, hydrone-phrosis and obstructive uropathy.[46]

### Plain abdominal X-ray (AXR)

AXR uses electromagnetic radiation to generate images of the kidney, ureter and bladder. This test can be ordered to identify the size, shape and position of these structures, as well as the presence of suspected bladder distension, calculi, congeni-tal defects, haematoma, hydronephrosis, tumours and trauma.[20]

### Renal angiograph

This is an invasive radiological procedure in which the renal artery or vein is injected with contrast media and a series of X-ray images taken of the renal vasculature. The procedure is able to evaluate blood flow dynamics and blood vessel defects, and thus can assist in the detection of arterial stenosis or occlusion, renal artery aneurysm, trauma, tumours and vascular malformation.[16]

### Retrograde pyelography

This procedure provides radiographic visualisation of the renal pelvis, calyces and ureters following cystoscopic-guided ureteric administration of contrast media. The procedure is indicated when abscesses, calculi, congenital anomalies, hydronephro-sis, obstruction, strictures and tumours are suspected.[16]

### Ultrasound

Ultrasound uses high-frequency sound waves to assess the position, size, texture and contour of the kidneys, ureters and bladder. The procedure can be useful in detecting calculi, cysts, bladder diverticulum, congenital anomalies, cystitis, glo-merulonephritis, hydronephrosis, obstruction, organomegaly, pyelonephritis and tumours. Ultrasound can also be used to measure bladder volume and residual urine volume.[18]

## Functional tests
### Urodynamic studies

These studies evaluate bladder and urethral pressure, sensation, volume, capacity and filling pattern (cystometry), as well as the rate of urination (uroflowmetry). Although the procedure is primarily used to classify the type of urinary inconti-nence or the cause of bladder dysfunction, urodynamic studies may also allude to the cause of urinary obstruction or retention, such as carcinoma, congenital defects, prostatic hypertrophy and urethral stricture.[16]

### Invasive tests
#### Biopsy
A biopsy involves the excision of a small sample of tissue and the subsequent microscopic examination of the sample in order to identify cell morphology and tissue abnormalities. A biopsy of urinary tract tissue may assist in the diagnosis of cancer, disseminated lupus erythromatosus, glomerulonephritis, Goodpasture's syndrome, nephrotic syndrome and pyelonephritis.[18]

#### Cystoscopy
This test enables direct visualisation of the urethra, bladder and ureteric orifices through the use of a flexible fibreoptic cystoscope. Cystoscopy can be used as a diagnostic tool to assess the presence of bladder neck contracture, calculi, congenital anomalies, cystitis, diverticulum, foreign bodies, polyps, prostatic hypertrophy, prostatitis, tumours, urethral stricture and urethritis.[20]

## Reproductive system assessment
The male and female reproductive systems are anatomically and physiologically vastly different. As such, each system needs to be summarised separately.

The male reproductive system consists of the scrotum, testes, epididymis, ductus deferens, seminal vesicle, prostate gland, ejaculatory duct, bulbourethral gland, urethra and penis. This system is responsible for synthesising male sex hormones for growth and development, and for producing and storing sperm in preparation for procreation.

The female reproductive system comprises the ovaries, uterine tubes, uterus, cervix, vagina, vestibular glands, clitoris, labia and mammary glands. The role of this system is to synthesise female sex hormones for growth and development, to create an environment that supports fetal development and to provide nourishment for the fetus and newborn. Structural or functional impairments to the male or female reproductive systems are likely to manifest as changes in fertility, sexual health and/or self-image. These points should be taken into account when conducting a comprehensive assessment of the client's reproductive system. An outline of the regions pertinent to reproductive system assessment is illustrated in Figure 3.6.

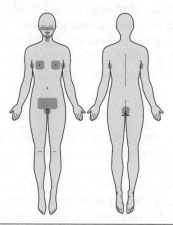

**Figure 3.6:** Reproductive assessment cue card

## Health history
### History of presenting condition
Once the individual's primary problem has been identified, ascertain the location, severity, quality, onset, duration and frequency of the sign or symptom, the presence of radiating symptoms (e.g. back pain radiating down one or both legs may be a sign of pelvic inflammatory disease),[47] any aggravating or ameliorating factors (such as sexual intercourse, menstruation, urination, heat, cold, pressure, constipation, bearing down, anxiety, emotional stress, prolonged sitting or standing, medication or physical activity) and any concomitant symptoms (including abdominal bloating, altered libido, dyspareunia, dysuria, erectile dysfunction, fatigue, haematuria, hesitancy, irritability, incontinence, mood changes, nausea, nocturia, oedema, pain, pyrexia, urethral or vaginal or breast discharge, change in the frequency or volume or duration of menstruation, urinary dribbling and any changes in the force or calibre of the urinary stream).

### Medical history
#### Family history
Explore whether the client has a genetic predisposition to reproductive disease by asking if they have any family history of women's or men's health issues, such as carcinoma, endometriosis, Peyronie's disease or polycystic ovarian syndrome.

#### Allergies
Establish whether the client has any allergies or sensitivities to foods (such as gluten or soy), environmental substances (such as latex, soaps or lubricants) or medications (such as beta-blockers, thiazide diuretics, temazepam, captopril, tetracyclines or antimalarials)[48] that could contribute to the presenting complaint or affect clinical management.

#### Medications
Determine whether the client is currently administering or has recently finished any prescribed or over-the-counter supplements, medications, herbs or therapies for a reproductive system complaint, including analgesics, antibiotics, antifungals, chemotherapy, contraceptive medication or devices, erectile dysfunction agents, fertility treatment, 5-alpha reductase antagonists and hormone replacement therapy. It is also worthy to note the use of treatments that may contribute to reproductive symptoms, such as anticholinergic drug-induced urinary retention, antidepressant-associated loss of libido, antihypertensive-associated impotence and antipsychotic-associated ejaculatory disturbance.

#### Medical conditions
Establish if there are any current or previous medical conditions that involve the male or female reproductive organs or tracts, such as benign prostatic hypertrophy, cancer, endometriosis, epididymitis, erectile dysfunction, infertility, menopause, menstrual disorders, ovarian cysts, pelvic inflammatory disease, number of pregnancies (including complications and birthing outcomes), prostatitis, premenstrual syndrome, salpingitis, sexually transmitted infections, uterine fibroids, vaginitis or varicocoele. Also assess for conditions that can cause reproductive-type symptoms or

mimic reproductive disease, such as eating disorders, endocrine disease, herniation, nutrient deficiency, rectovaginal fistula, substance abuse, urinary tract infection or vesicovaginal fistula.

### Surgical and investigational procedures
Find out whether the individual has received any relevant surgical or investigational procedures (including biopsy, circumcision, colposcopy, cystoscopy, dilatation and curettage, hysterectomy, laparoscopy, mastectomy, orchidectomy, oophorectomy, transurethral resection of the prostate or vasectomy) in the past in order to identify other reproductive disorders that may have been missed in the health history.

### Lifestyle history
Examine the presence of factors that may elevate the client's risk of reproductive disease or exacerbate the presenting condition, such as tobacco use (including number and strength of cigarettes inhaled in a day),[49,50] alcohol consumption (including number of standard drinks and type of alcoholic beverage consumed in a day),[50,51] illicit drug use (including type, route and quantity of drug used per day), diet and fluid intake (such as caffeine, fruit and vegetable consumption, fish and red meat intake, fat consumption),[52] quality and duration of sleep (e.g. interrupted sleep, obstructive sleep apnoea)[53] and frequency, duration and type of exercise.[50]

### Socioeconomic background
Determine whether there are any socioeconomic factors that may increase the client's risk of reproductive disease, affect their understanding of the condition or the management of the condition, such as occupation and employment status (i.e. day or nightshift, full or part time, number of jobs, hours worked each week), residential and/or work environment (i.e. whether these environments create significant emotional stress), family environment (i.e. marital status, number and ages of children), level of social support (i.e. whether the client lives alone or receives community services), religion, ethnicity, race or cultural background (i.e. whether the individual follows firm dietary practices, whether the client's culture, race or ethnic background place the client at increased risk of developing reproductive illness) and level of educational attainment (i.e. primary, secondary and/or tertiary education).

## Physical examination
There are potential legal and ethical implications associated with physical examination of the reproductive system. It is therefore recommended that only suitably qualified practitioners who are not constrained by conditions stipulated within their relevant professional association's code of conduct carry out this physical assessment and, preferably, in the presence of a witness or colleague.

### Inspection
When applicable, look for asymmetry, oedema, inflammation, discharge (including colour, volume, odour and consistency), masses, parasites (such as pubic lice), excoriation, lesions (such as herpes, warts, scars, chancres, psoriasis, ulceration, scabies

and excoriation) and/or congenital defects to the labia (e.g. folliculitis, vulval papillomatosus), vaginal orifice (e.g. vulvovaginitis, leucoplakia), urethral meatus (e.g. epispadias, hypospadias, urethritis), penis (e.g. balanitis, balanoposthitis, phimosis), scrotum (e.g. cryptorchidism, hydrocele, varicocele), abdomen (e.g. ovarian carcinoma, pregnancy), breasts (e.g. carcinoma, gynecomastia, mastitis), anus (e.g. sexually transmitted infections) and perineum (e.g. contact dermatitis, lichen sclerosis).

Also assess signs of normal and atypical endocrine activity, particularly the presence of secondary sex characteristics (such as pubic and other body hair distribution, breast size and penis size relevant to chronological age), hirsutism (androgenic hair distribution in the female may be indicative of adrenal or ovarian pathology, such as polycystic ovarian syndrome and ovarian carcinoma),[10] and virilisation (the manifestation of male secondary sex characteristics in a female, including deepening of the voice, acne and increased muscularity may alert to the presence of adrenal hyperplasia or adenoma).[26]

### Olfaction
Clinicians can use their sense of smell to detect the presence of infection. Vaginal and/or urethral odours, for instance, may be characterised as fishy in urinary tract infection, non-specific vaginitis and trichomoniasis, or yeast-like in candidiasis.[26] Poor personal hygiene may also be identified with olfaction. While poor hygiene practices may simply reflect a client's personal preference, it may also be a telltale sign of underlying socioeconomic, psychological or functional issues.

### Palpation
Palpation is particularly useful in detecting masses, induration, structural defects, tenderness and oedema of the testes (e.g. cryptorchidism, carcinoma, orchitis), scrotal contents (e.g. hydrocele, inguinal hernia, varicocele), penis (e.g. paraphimosis, Peyronie's disease) and breasts (e.g. cysts, carcinoma, fibroadenoma). An internal physical examination by suitably qualified practitioners may also identify pertinent signs of disease in the prostate (such as symmetrical enlargement in benign prostatic hypertrophy; tenderness of prostatitis; induration and nodulation in prostatic carcinoma),[10] vagina (including internal bulging from cystocele or rectocele),[9] cervix (such as tenderness of cervicitis), uterus (such as a large nodular uterus in uterine fibroid disease)[24] and ovaries (including ovarian cysts or tumours).

### Percussion
There is no particular role for percussion in reproductive system assessment.

### Auscultation
There is no role for auscultation in reproductive system assessment, except in the pregnant woman, where fetal heart sounds may be assessed in order to monitor fetal wellbeing.

### Additional signs
Clinical data not derived from the abovementioned physical examination that can provide important information about the aetiology of a presenting condition, as well as the general health and nutritional status of the client, can be derived from assessing core body temperature, blood pressure, weight, height, BMI, waist circumference and skinfold thickness.

## Clinical assessment tools
Examples of instruments that may be used to evaluate the severity or effect of reproductive disorders, or the effect of treatment on these conditions, are described below.

### Endometriosis health profile-30 (EHP-30)
EHP-30 measures the effect of pain, emotional wellbeing, control, self-image and social support on health-related quality of life in women with endometriosis.

### Female sexual function index (FSFI)
FSFI evaluates the level of sexual functioning in women, including sexual satisfaction, orgasm, sexual arousal and pain.

### International index of erectile dysfunction (IIED)
IIED evaluates the severity of erectile dysfunction.

### International prostate symptom score (IPSS)
IPSS assesses urinary frequency, urgency, stream, hesitancy, intermittence, nocturia and bladder emptying in clients with benign prostatic hyperplasia (BPH).

### Menopause rating scale (MRS)
MRS evaluates the impact of psychological, somatovegetative and urogenital symptoms of menopause on health-related quality of life in women.

### Menstrual symptom questionnaire (MSQ)
MSQ measures the concomitant symptoms, aggravating and ameliorating factors, and onset and timing of menstrual symptoms.

### National Institute of Health chronic prostatitis symptom index (NIH-CPSI)
NIH-CPSI measures urinary function, location, severity and frequency of pain, and quality of life in clients with chronic abacterial prostatitis.

## Diagnostics
### Pathology tests
#### Culture and sensitivity testing
The testing of a cervical, urethral or blood specimen enables sufficient numbers of an organism to be isolated, identified and quantified, and the antibiotics the microbial strains are sensitive or resistant to, to be determined. This test may be ordered to aid the diagnosis and treatment of candidiasis, *Chlamydia*, genital warts, gonorrhoea, herpes genitalis, human immunodeficiency virus infection, syphilis and trichomoniasis.[16]

#### Follicle-stimulating hormone (FSH)
FSH is a glycoprotein secreted by the anterior pituitary gland. This hormone is primarily responsible for follicle development and oestrogen production in females and sperm maturation in males.[54] Increased blood levels of FSH can be associated with alcohol abuse, anorchia, hypogonadism, Klinefelter's syndrome, menopause, orchitis, pituitary tumours and Turner's syndrome. Reduced levels of FSH can occur in anorexia nervosa, haemochromatosis, hyperprolactinaemia, pituitary or hypothalamus dysfunction, polycystic ovarian syndrome and pregnancy.[18]

### Hair, urine, serum and blood nutrient levels

These nutrient tests may be indicated when presenting clinical manifestations are suggestive of nutrient deficiency or toxicity, when the presenting condition is likely to be caused by nutrient deficiency or toxicity, or when the condition is likely to contribute to the development of nutrient deficiency or toxicity. Nutrient tests that are particularly relevant to reproductive assessment are hair mineral analysis, iron studies, red blood cell folate, serum vitamin A, serum vitamin C, serum selenium and serum zinc.

### Luteinising hormone (LH)

LH is a glycoprotein secreted by the anterior pituitary gland. In females, LH is responsible for ovulation, corpus luteum development and progesterone production. In males, LH stimulates the release of testosterone.[54] A reduction in circulating LH levels can occur in anorexia nervosa, hypothalamus dysfunction, malnutrition, pituitary dysfunction and stress. Elevated levels of LH can arise from anorchia, hypogonadism, menopause, Klinefelter's syndrome, pituitary adenoma, polycystic ovarian syndrome and Turner's syndrome.[34]

### Oestrogens, including oestrone (E1) and oestradiol (E2)

Oestrogens are steroid hormones secreted primarily by the ovaries. These hormones play a key role in maintaining female sex characteristics, reproductive organ function, and endometrial growth and repair.[54] A reduction in urine or blood oestrogen may be a sign of anorexia nervosa, failing pregnancy, hypogonadism, hypopituitarism, menopause or Turner's syndrome. By contrast, elevated oestrogen levels may be indicative of hyperthyroidism, liver disease, normal pregnancy or an ovarian, testicular or adrenal tumour.[32]

### Progesterone

Progesterone is a steroid hormone produced by the ovaries. Its primary functions are to prepare the endometrium for implantation and the breasts for lactation.[54] Elevated levels of progesterone in the blood or the metabolite pregnanediol in the urine may suggest the presence of hyperadrenalcorticalism, hydatidiform mole, luteal ovarian cysts, ovulation, pregnancy or ovarian carcinoma. Decreased progesterone levels may indicate hypogonadism, ovarian or breast cancer, pre-eclampsia or threatened miscarriage.[16]

### Prostate-specific antigen (PSA)

PSA is a glycoprotein located within prostatic epithelial cells. Even though PSA levels may be used as a screening tool for prostate cancer, PSA has low specificity for this condition and may also be elevated in prostatitis and prostatic hypertrophy.[16]

### Semen analysis

This test is an important measure of male fertility. The test investigates the volume, colour, appearance, liquefaction time and pH of semen, as well as the count, motility and morphology of sperm. Abnormal findings of the analysis may occur in ejaculatory tract obstruction, hyperpyrexia, Klinefelter's syndrome, mumps, orchidectomy, orchitis, testicular atrophy, testicular failure, varicocoele and vasectomy.[18]

## Testosterone

Testosterone is a steroid hormone manufactured primarily by the Leydig cells of the testes; smaller amounts are produced by the ovaries and adrenal glands. The maintenance of male secondary sex characteristics and spermatogenesis are key functions of this hormone. A fall in blood testosterone levels may occur in alcohol abuse, cryptorchidism, Down syndrome, hypogonadism, hypopituitarism, Klinefelter's syndrome, liver disease or orchidectomy. Increased testosterone levels may be a sign of adrenocorticol or ovarian or testicular tumours, androgen resistance syndrome, hyperthyroidism or polycystic ovarian syndrome.[18]

## Radiology tests
### Computed tomography (CT)

CT uses multiple X-ray beams to produce cross-sectional images of reproductive structures contained within the pelvis, including the ductus deferens, ovaries, prostate, seminal vesicle, uterine tubes and uterus. CT can be used to detect abscesses, cysts, ectopic pregnancy, hydrosalpinx, lymphadenopathy, obstruction, prostatic hypertrophy, stricture, tumours and uterine fibroids.[20]

### Magnetic resonance imaging (MRI)

MRI uses magnetic and radiofrequency energy to generate images of the organs and soft tissues of the pelvis. The procedure is useful in detecting abscesses, cysts, infection, inflammation, obstruction, prostatic hypertrophy, stricture, tumours and uterine fibroids.[18]

### Mammogram

This procedure uses electromagnetic radiation to generate images of the breasts. While the procedure is primarily used to examine suspected breast cancer, mammograms are also useful in detecting breast abscesses, cysts, lymphadenopathy and suppurative mastitis.[16]

### Ultrasound

Ultrasound uses high-frequency sound waves to assess the size, texture, position and contour of organs and tissues, including the breasts, ovaries, prostate, scrotum, testes, uterine tubes, uterus and vagina. Conditions pertinent to the reproductive system that may be detected by ultrasound include abscesses, cryptorchidism, cysts, ectopic pregnancy, epididymitis, fibrosis, pelvic inflammatory disease, orchitis, prostatic hypertrophy, prostatitis, tumours, uterine fibroids and varicocoele.[18]

### Uterosalpingography, or hysterogram

This test, which provides radiographic visualisation of the uterine cavity and uterine tubes, is assisted by cervically administered contrast material. The hysterogram is useful for evaluating suspected adhesions, congenital anomalies, ectopic pregnancy, foreign bodies, obstruction, tumours and uterine fistulas.[16]

## Functional tests
### Female hormone profile
This profile measures salivary levels of oestradiol, progesterone, testosterone and dehydroepiandrosterone (DHEA) over a single 28-day menstrual cycle. Abnormal levels of these hormones at different points in the menstrual cycle, and possible correlation with pertinent symptoms, may allude to the cause of altered libido, breast cancer, affective disorders, endometriosis, infertility, menstrual irregularities, polycystic ovary disease and premenstrual syndrome.[55]

### Male hormone profile
From a single serum sample, this test measures the level of DHEA, dihydrotestosterone (DHT), free testosterone, oestradiol, PSA and sex-hormone binding globulin (SHBG). An abnormal profile may be useful in identifying the cause of affective disorders, alopecia, altered libido, cardiovascular disease, myasthenia and prostatic hypertrophy or cancer.[56]

## Invasive tests
### Biopsy
A biopsy involves the excision of a small sample of tissue and the subsequent microscopic examination of the sample in order to identify cell morphology and tissue abnormalities. Biopsy of a reproductive organ or tract may assist in the diagnosis of atrophy, cancer, dysplasia, cysts, erosion, infection, inflammation, leucoplakia and polyps.[18]

### Colposcopy
In this test a colposcope is used to macroscopically examine the vagina and cervix, a procedure that may assist in the detection of atrophy, dysplasia, carcinoma, erosion, infection, inflammation and leucoplakia.[16]

### Cystoscopy
A cystocopy can be used in the male reproductive assessment, as it enables direct visualisation of the male urethra through the use of a flexible fibreoptic cystoscope. As a diagnostic tool, cystoscopy can be used to assess the presence of congenital anomalies, foreign bodies, prostatic hypertrophy, prostatitis, tumours, urethral stricture and urethritis.[20]

### Hysteroscopy
With the assistance of a fibreoptic hysteroscope, a hysteroscopy enables direct visualisation of the cervix and uterine cavity. In conjunction with curettage or biopsy, this procedure can successfully detect endometrial cancer, fibroids, polyps and uterine adhesions.[16]

### Laparoscopy
Laparoscopy uses a rigid fibreoptic laparoscope to directly visualise relevant organs and structures of the pelvis, including the ductus deferens, ovaries, uterine tubes and uterus. The procedure is helpful in detecting adhesions, congenital malformations, cysts, ectopic pregnancy, endometriosis, fibroids, hydrosalpinx, infection, pelvic inflammatory disease, salpingitis and tumours.[20]

**Papanicolaou test, or Pap smear**
This is the collection of a cervical secretion specimen aided by the insertion of a vaginal speculum. Though the procedure is used predominantly for the screening of cervical carcinoma, it may also be used to ascertain the presence of candidiasis, condyloma, endometriosis, sexually transmitted infections and vaginal adenosis.[16]

## Miscellaneous tests
### Basal body temperature, or the temperature of the body upon rising
This is a non-invasive family planning method. By assessing basal temperature at the same time every day, couples can determine when to engage or sustain from sexual intercourse in order to increase or decrease their chances of pregnancy. The rationale behind this method is that a rise in basal body temperature can occur after ovulation due to a rise in serum progesterone.[57]

### Cervical mucus viscosity
Also known as the Billing's method, this is another family planning technique used to determine the point of ovulation in the menstrual cycle. The point of ovulation or fertility is manifested by the presence of transparent slippery cervical mucus, also referred to as fertile oestrogenic mucus.[57]

# Integumentary system assessment
The integumentary system incorporates the hair, nails, mucous membranes and skin, including the epidermis, dermis and subcutaneous layers. The fundamental roles of this system are protection, nutrition, homeostasis and elimination. In the event that the integrity of the integumentary system is compromised, then the ability to maintain these functions will be adversely affected, for which associated signs and symptoms would manifest.

These considerations should be kept in mind when conducting a comprehensive assessment of the integumentary system. An outline of the regions pertinent to integumentary system assessment is illustrated in Figure 3.7.

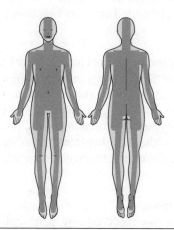

**Figure 3.7:** Integumentary assessment cue card

## Health history
### History of presenting condition
Ascertain the client's primary problem and the location, quality, onset, severity, frequency and duration of the sign or symptom, the existence of radiating symptoms, any aggravating or ameliorating factors (such as alcohol, chemical agents, cold, cosmetics, emotional stress, exercise, fabrics, foods, heat, medications, creams, ointments or lotions, occlusive materials, perspiration, skin friction or trauma or sunlight) and any concomitant symptoms (including arthralgia, exudation, exfoliation, irritability, lymphadenopathy, malaise, oedema, pain, paresthesias, pruritus, pyrexia or sleep disturbance).

## Medical history
### Family history
Establish whether the client has a genetic predisposition to integumentary system disease by assessing whether there is a family history of integumentary illness, including acne, alopecia, eczema, hirsutism, pilonidal sinus and psoriasis.

### Allergies
Ascertain whether the client has any sensitivities or allergies to medications (such as antibiotics), foods (such as dairy, nuts, preservatives or wheat) and environmental substances (such as cosmetics, creams, ointments or lotions, dyes, fabrics, household or occupational chemicals, metal compounds or plants) that could contribute to the presenting condition or affect clinical management.

### Medications
Ask the client if they are presently administering or have recently finished any over-the-counter or prescribed supplements, medications, herbs or therapies for an integumentary condition, including antibiotics, antifungals, antihistamines, anti-inflammatories, antiparasitics, antipruritics, antipsoriatics, barrier creams, cleansers, corticosteroids, emollients, immunomodulators, keratolytic agents and wound dressings. It is also worthy to note the use of treatments that may contribute to integumentary symptoms (e.g. sulfonamide-induced toxic epidermal necrolysis, tetracycline-associated photosensitivity eruption, corticosteroid-induced acneiform lesions, oral contraceptive-associated erythema nodosum).

### Medical conditions
Establish if there are any current or previous medical conditions that involve the skin, nails or hair, such as acne, alopecia, bullous pemphigoid, carcinoma, eczema, fungal or bacterial or viral or parasitic skin infection, ichthyosis, pityriasis rosea, psoriasis, rosacea or skin ulceration. Also ascertain the existence of conditions that might yield integumentary-type symptoms or mimic integumentary illness, such as diabetes mellitus, endocrine disease, hepatobiliary disease, lupus erythromatosus and other connective tissue disorders, nutrient deficiency, renal disease or systemic infectious disease.

### Surgical and investigational procedures
Find out whether the client has received any pertinent surgical or investigational procedures in the past (such as biopsy, cosmetic surgery, curettage, cryotherapy,

dermabrasion, excision of skin lesions or skin grafting) to identify other integumentary disorders that may have been missed in the health history.

## Lifestyle history
Establish whether there are any factors that may increase the client's risk of integumentary disease or worsen the presenting condition, such as tobacco use (including number and strength of cigarettes inhaled in a day),[58] alcohol consumption (including number of standard drinks and type of alcoholic beverage consumed in a day),[59,60] illicit drug use (including type, route and quantity of drug used per day), diet and fluid intake, quality and duration of sleep (e.g. pruritus interrupted sleep),[61] sun exposure, and frequency, duration and type of exercise.[62]

## Socioeconomic background
Identify any socioeconomic factors that may increase the client's risk of integumentary disease, affect their understanding of the complaint or the management of the condition, such as occupation and employment status (i.e. day or nightshift, full or part time, number of jobs, hours worked each week), residential and/or work environment (i.e. whether these environments create significant emotional stress or require prolonged sun exposure, family environment (i.e. marital status, number and ages of children), religion, ethnicity, race or cultural background (i.e. whether the client abides by stringent dietary practices, whether the client's culture, race or ethnic background place the client at increased risk of developing integumentary disease), level of social support (i.e. whether the client lives alone or receives community services) and level of educational attainment (i.e. primary, secondary and/or tertiary education).

## Physical examination
### Inspection
The most valuable technique in integumentary assessment is inspection. This is because many skin conditions can be diagnosed on clinical presentation alone. The condition of the skin is also a good indicator of many nutrient imbalances or deficiencies. Careful observation of the system is therefore essential, including the assessment of skin colour (i.e. erythema, pallor, cyanosis, jaundice and level of skin pigmentation), hair quantity and distribution (including the presence of hirsutism or alopecia), nail quality (including strength, integrity and shape), nail markings (including Beau's lines, Mees' bands, pitting, clubbing, koilonychia and splinter haemorrhages) and skin lesions (including location, distribution, arrangement and colour). The type of lesion should also be identified, which, according to content, size and elevation, may be defined as a macule (small, flat, non-palpable lesion), patch (large, flat, non-palpable lesion), papule (small, solid, elevated mass), plaque (large, flat, elevated lesion), nodule (medium-sized, palpable solid mass), wheal (transient, superficial cutaneous oedema), vesicle (small, elevated, serous-filled lesion), bulla (large, elevated, serous-filled lesion) or pustule (elevated, pus-filled lesion).[10,26] For paediatric clients, also observe for signs of unusual bruising, wounds and scarring as these could be indicative of child abuse.

### Olfaction
The clinician should note the presence of abnormal odours during the physical assessment in order to identify the complaint, or the possible aetiology of the condition.

Specifically, the clinician should take note of the sweet musty odour of tinea pedis,[63] the yeast-like odour of candidiasis, the faecal odour of *Escherichia coli* wound infection, the grape-like sweet odour of *Pseudomonas aeruginosa* wound infection,[64] and bromhidrosis secondary to poor personal hygiene.

## Palpation

Palpation supplements the examination with important information about skin function and underlying disease, particularly the assessment of skin moisture (e.g. skin dryness in hypothyroidism), oiliness (e.g. oily skin in acne vulgaris), texture (e.g. rough skin in hypothyroidism), temperature (e.g. increased skin temperature in pyrexia, local inflammation and hyperthyroidism; reduced skin temperature from cold exposure or hypothyroidism), mobility (e.g. reduced skin mobility in oedema and scleroderma), turgor (e.g. reduced skin turgor in dehydration and advanced age) and hair texture (e.g. dry, coarse hair from hypothyroidism).[9,26]

## Percussion

There is no particular role for percussion in integumentary system assessment.

## Auscultation

There is little role for auscultation in the assessment of the integumentary system other than detecting the presence of crepitus. This dry crackling sound may manifest in subcutaneous emphysema as a result of soft tissue infection or trauma.[65]

## Additional signs

Clinical data not derived from the physical examination, which can provide important information about the aetiology of a presenting condition as well as the general health of the client, can be derived from the assessment of core body temperature.

## Clinical assessment tools

Examples of instruments that may be used to evaluate the severity or effect of integumentary conditions, or the effect of treatment on these disorders, are outlined below.

### Bikowski acne severity index (BASI)

BASI is a standardised grading system for evaluating the type, number and location of acne lesions.

### Diabetic foot ulcer scale (DFS)

DFS assesses the impact of diabetic foot ulceration, and its treatment, on quality of life, in particular, leisure, physical health, emotions, attitude, activities of daily living, family, friends and finances.

### Onychomycosis quality of life questionnaire (ONYCHO)

ONYCHO measures the effect of onychomycosis on health-related quality of life, with specific versions available for fingernails and toenails.

### Patient-oriented eczema measure (POEM)

POEM monitors the level of activity and severity of atopic eczema in children and adults.

### Simplified psoriasis area and severity index (SPASI)

SPASI measures the severity of psoriatic erythema, thickness and scaling, and the area involved.

## Diagnostics
### Pathology tests
### Culture and sensitivity testing

Such testing of skin lesion specimens enables sufficient numbers of the pathogenic organism to be isolated, identified and quantified, and the antibiotics the microbial strains are sensitive or resistant to, to be determined. This test can be ordered to aid the diagnosis and treatment of bacterial, viral, fungal or parasitic skin infections.[16]

### Hair, urine, serum and blood nutrient levels

Testing of these levels may be indicated when presenting clinical manifestations are suggestive of nutrient deficiency or toxicity, when the presenting condition is likely to be caused by nutrient deficiency or toxicity, or when the condition is likely to contribute to the development of nutrient deficiency or toxicity. Nutrient tests that are particularly relevant to integumentary assessment are hair mineral analysis, red blood cell folate, serum vitamin A, serum vitamin C, serum pyridoxine and serum zinc.

### Radioallergosorbent testing (RAST) and enzyme-linked immunosorbent assay (ELISA)

RAST and ELISA quantify the presence of immunoglobulin E (IgE) in client serum. These tests can help identify the allergen responsible for allergic skin diseases, such as atopic dermatitis. Given that RAST and ELISA detect only a limited number of IgE-mediated allergies, the results of these tests can, in some cases, be misleading.

### Radiology tests
### Ultrasound

Ultrasound uses high-frequency sound waves to assess the position, contour, size and texture of tissues, including the skin. More specifically, this non-invasive procedure can provide useful information about the structure and depth of skin lesions, as well as their relationship with underlying tissues.[66]

### Functional tests
### Functional skin integrity testing

These tests, which include the transepidermal water loss (TEWL), sorption–desorption, electrical resistance (ER) and tritiated water flux (TWF) tests, incorporate a number of investigations that collectively evaluate skin barrier function. They provide information about the water barrier, water accumulation and permeability functions of the skin.[67] While the results of these investigations may highlight potential susceptibilities of the skin to infection, inflammation and pathology, evidence suggests that these tests may not be a valid measure of skin barrier function.[68]

### Invasive tests
### Allergy skin test

An allergy skin test detects the presence of IgE antibodies following exposure to diluted allergens, which can be administered either intraepidermally (prick-puncture method) or intradermally. The presence of a skin wheal is a positive sign of an IgE-mediated allergy, particularly to inhaled allergens, and may be useful in identifying the cause of dermatitis and angiooedema.[16]

### Biopsy

A biopsy is the excision of a small sample of tissue and the subsequent microscopic examination of the sample in order to identify cell morphology and tissue abnormalities. A biopsy of a skin lesion can assist in the identification of basal cell carcinoma, cysts, eczema, fibromas, keloids, keratoses, malignant melanoma, squamous cell carcinoma and warts.[18] Through the use of immunofluorescence, a biopsy may also identify the presence of immunological dermal pathology, such as bullous pemphigoid, dermatitis herpetiformis, lupus erythromatosus and pemphigus.[16]

### Miscellaneous tests
#### Atopic patch testing (APT)

An APT is similar to allergy skin testing in that it is also used to detect the presence of IgE-mediated atopic disease. The difference is that the diluted allergen is applied to the skin surface and subsequently occluded for 48–72 hours. A positive patch test, determined by the presence of erythema, infiltration and/or papules, may help to isolate the cause of atopic dermatitis.[69]

#### Woods light examination

This test uses a specially filtered ultraviolet lamp to highlight the presence of certain microbial strains (by way of fluorescence) in order to identify the aetiology of erythrasma. Green fluorescence, for instance, may indicate the presence of *Pseudomonas* spp. or *Microsporum*, while coral pink fluorescence may occur in *Corynebacterium* infection.[70]

## Endocrine system assessment

The endocrine system consists of all glands, tissues and cells that produce hormones or paracrine factors. Examples of these structures include the hypothalamus, pituitary gland, pineal gland, thyroid and parathyroid glands, thymus, heart, pancreas, adrenal glands, GI tract, kidney, gonads and adipose tissue. Although each of these tissues exhibits a range of different effects, they are fundamentally responsible for growth and development, intercellular communication and homeostasis.

Any structural or functional change to these tissues may therefore result in an inability to maintain these roles, leading to the presentation of adverse signs and symptoms. These points should be taken into consideration when conducting a comprehensive assessment of the endocrine system. An outline of the regions pertinent to endocrine system assessment is illustrated in Figure 3.8.

### Health history
#### History of presenting condition

Once the client's primary complaint has been established, determine the location, severity, onset, frequency, duration and quality of the sign or symptom, the existence of radiating symptoms (e.g. neck pain radiating into the jaw or face is suggestive of thyroiditis or thyroid carcinoma),[71] any aggravating or ameliorating factors (such as alcohol, allergic rhinitis, corticosteroids, physical activity, infection, gonadotropin-releasing hormone analogues, illicit drugs, medications, physical and emotional stress, pregnancy, surgery, foods or tobacco) and any concomitant symptoms

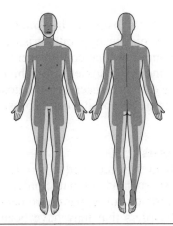

**Figure 3.8:** Endocrine assessment cue card

(including asthenia, change in libido, change in volume, frequency or duration of menstruation, constipation, diarrhoea, fatigue, mood changes, impotence, infertility, insomnia, palpitations, paraesthesias, polydipsia, polyphagia, polyuria, sleep disturbance or weight change).

## Medical history
### Family history
Ascertain whether the client has a genetic predisposition to endocrine disease by assessing whether there is any family history of endocrine illness, including Addison's disease, diabetes mellitus, Cushing's disease, hyperparathyroidism, Graves' disease, phaeochromocytoma or polycystic ovarian syndrome.

### Allergies
Ask if the client has any allergies or intolerances to foods (such as glucose, gluten or lactose), medications (such as chlorpropamide) or environmental substances (such as pesticides and herbicides) that could contribute to the presenting condition or affect clinical management.

### Medications
Determine whether the individual is currently administering or has recently completed any prescribed or over-the-counter herbs, supplements, medications or therapies for an endocrine disorder, including antiprogestin agents, antiandrogen preparations, antithyroid drugs, calcium and bone metabolism preparations, gonadal hormones, haemopoietic agents, insulin, oral hypoglycaemic agents, pituitary hormones or thyroid hormones. Also assess whether the client is receiving any treatments that may mimic endocrine symptoms, such as amiodarone-induced thyrotoxicosis, antipsychotic-induced hyperprolactinaemia, spironolactone-associated gynaecomastia or steroid-induced diabetes mellitus.

### Medical conditions
Ascertain if there are any current or previous medical conditions that involve the pancreas, thyroid, parathyroid, hypothalamus, pituitary, adrenal, gonads and other endocrine glands, such as Addison's disease, adrenal insufficiency, carcinoma, Cushing's

disease, diabetes mellitus, diabetes insipidus, hyperaldosteronism, hyperpituitarism, hyperprolactinaemia, hyperthyroidism, hypopituitarism on hypothyroidism. Explore, too, the existence of other conditions that could generate endocrine-type symptoms or mimic endocrine disease, including anxiety, bronchial carcinoma, chronic fatigue syndrome, depression, eating disorders, haemochromatosis, illicit drug use, liver disease, nutrient deficiency or toxicity, obesity, osteoporosis, psychiatric disorders and renal failure.

### Surgical and investigational procedures

Determine whether the client has received any relevant surgical or investigational procedures in the past (such as adrenalectomy, biopsy, excision of nodules or lesions, oophorectomy, orchidectomy, parathyroidectomy or thyroidectomy) to identify other endocrine disorders that may have been overlooked in the health history.

### Lifestyle history

Identify if there are any factors that may increase the client's risk of endocrine disease or worsen the presenting condition, such as tobacco use (including number and strength of cigarettes inhaled in a day),[72,73] alcohol consumption (including number of standard drinks and type of alcoholic beverage consumed in a day),[74] illicit drug use (including type, route and quantity of drug used per day), diet and fluid intake (such as fibre, fruit and vegetable consumption, gluten, iodine, non-fermented soy products and simple sugar intake),[75,76] quality and duration of sleep (e.g. broken sleep, sleep apnoea),[77] and frequency, duration and type of exercise.[78]

### Socioeconomic background

Establish if there are any socioeconomic factors that may increase the individual's risk of endocrine disease, affect their understanding of the condition or the management of the illness, such as level of educational attainment (i.e. primary, secondary and/or tertiary education), occupation and employment status (i.e. day or nightshift, full or part time, number of jobs, hours worked each week), residential and/or work environment (i.e. whether these environments create significant emotional stress and whether the client is exposed to industrial chemicals or radiation), family environment (i.e. marital status, number and ages of children), religion, ethnicity, race or cultural background (i.e. whether the individual follows strict dietary practices and whether culture, race or ethnic background places the client at increased risk of developing endocrine or metabolic disease) and level of social support (i.e. whether the client lives alone or receives community services).

## Physical examination

### Inspection

Physical examination of the endocrine system begins with careful examination of the integumentary system. This includes inspection of the face (e.g. myxoedema facies of hypothyroidism, moon-shaped facies of Cushing's syndrome, prognathoid mandible, prominent nose and thickened lips of acromegaly), nails (e.g. onycholysis of hyperthyroidism), skin pigmentation (e.g. hypopigmentation in hypopituitarism, hyperpigmentation in Addison's disease, pink purple striae in Cushing's syndrome, acanthosis nigricans in insulin-resistant syndromes), skin lesions (e.g. acne of

Cushing's syndrome), hair distribution and quality (e.g. hirsutism of Cushing's syndrome, loss of pubic and axillary hair in hypoadrenalism) and scarring from endocrine surgery.[12,24]

Other pertinent manifestations of endocrine dysfunction include gynaecomastia (secondary to hypoandrogenism, excess oestrogen, thyrotoxicosis and/or medications), goitre (due to hyperthyroidism or iodine deficiency), proptosis and bilateral eyelid retraction (secondary to hyperthyroidism), tremors (such as the fine peripheral tremor of hyperthyroidism), body shape (including the central adiposity, buffalo hump and thin limbs of Cushing's syndrome, thin extremities, large spade-like hands and kyphosis in acromegaly, obesity of type 2 diabetes mellitus), and virilisation (the manifestation of male secondary sex characteristics in a female, including deepening of the voice and increased muscularity, which may alert to the presence of adrenal hyperplasia or adenoma).[10,12,26] In order to identify possible pituitary or gonadal pathology, the clinician should determine whether secondary sex characteristics correspond with chronological age, including pubic/body hair distribution, breast size and penis size.

## Olfaction
Poor glycaemic control and/or diabetes mellitus may be responsible for a number of characteristic odours, including the sweet odour of hyperglycosuria, the acetone breath of diabetic ketoacidosis and the halitosis of diabetic periodontal disease.[79,80]

## Palpation
The functional status of a client's endocrine system can be further elucidated by examining the client's skin temperature (e.g. increased warmth in acromegaly and hyperthyroidism, coolness in hypothyroidism), pulse rate (e.g. tachycardia in hyperthyroidism, bradycardia in hypothyroidism), skin moisture (e.g. increased sweating in hyperthyroidism, phaeochromocytoma, hypoglycaemia and acromegaly, skin dryness in hypothyroidism and hypoparathyroidism), breasts and gonads (breast, ovarian and testicular atrophy may be a sign of hypopituitarism, conditions such as cryptorchidism, testicular or ovarian carcinoma, orchitis and ovarian cysts may be responsible for gonadal dysfunction), muscle strength (proximal muscle weakness may manifest in hyperthyroidism or Cushing's syndrome) and deep tendon reflexes (a delayed relaxation response of deep tendon reflexes may be evident in hypothyroidism).

More specific signs of endocrine dysfunction include goitre tenderness (which may be indicative of thyroiditis), thyroid thrill (a palpable vibratory sensation indicative of increased thyroid blood flow, which may occur in thyrotoxicosis), Trousseau's sign (the development of a hand contracture within 4 minutes of sphygmomanometer inflation on the upper arm can be indicative of hypocalcaemia/hypoparathyroidism), Chvostek's sign (a transient twitch of the corner of the mouth, triggered by gentle preauricular tapping, may manifest in hypocalcaemia or hypoparathyroidism).[10,12,24]

## Percussion
A change in the percussive tone over the manubrium from resonance to dullness may be indicative of retrosternal goitre, although this is not considered to be a reliable sign.[24] Percussive dullness over the left upper quadrant, on the other hand, may identify some cases of pancreatitis.[81]

## Auscultation

Auscultation does not play a major role in endocrine assessment. The presence of a thyroid bruit (an abnormally harsh sound due to increased blood flow) may support suspicions of hyperthyroidism.[24]

## Additional signs

Clinical data not derived from the abovementioned physical examination, which can provide important information about the aetiology of a presenting condition, as well as the general health and nutritional status of the client, can be derived from the assessment of core body temperature, blood pressure, pulse rate, weight, height, BMI, waist circumference and skinfold thickness.

## Clinical assessment tools

Examples of instruments that can be used to evaluate the severity or effect of endocrine disorders or the effect of treatment on these conditions include the following.

### Chronic thyroid questionnaire (CTQ)

CTQ assesses the physical, emotional, wellbeing and cognitive effects of hypothyroidism on health-related quality of life.

### Diabetes quality of life measure (DQOL)

DQOL measures the effect of diabetes on health-related quality of life in areas such as disease burden, life satisfaction, worries about diabetes and social and/or vocational concerns.

### Menopause rating scale (MRS)

MRS evaluates the effect of psychological, somatovegetative and urogenital symptoms of menopause on health-related quality of life in women.

### Osteoporosis assessment questionnaire (OPAQ)

OPAQ examines the physical, emotional, symptomatic and social effects of osteoporosis on health-related quality of life.

### Polycystic ovary syndrome questionnaire (PCOSQ)

PCOSQ measures the effect of polycystic ovary syndrome on health-related quality of life, specifically, in the areas of emotion, weight, body hair, infertility and menstruation.

## Diagnostics

### Pathology tests

#### Adrenocorticotropic hormone (ACTH), or corticotropin

ACTH is a peptide hormone synthesised by the anterior pituitary. Under the control of hypothalamus-derived corticotropin-releasing hormone, ACTH regulates the release of glucocorticoids from the adrenal cortex. Elevated levels of this hormone may be seen in Addison's disease, congenital adrenal hyperplasia, Cushing's syndrome, depression, ectopic ACTH syndrome, pregnancy, sepsis, stress and type 2 diabetes mellitus. Conditions demonstrating reduced levels of circulating ACTH include adrenal adenoma or carcinoma, adrenocorticol hyperfunction, haemochromatosis, hypopituitarism and secondary adrenocorticol insufficiency.[18]

### Aldosterone

This is a mineralocorticoid that is released by the adrenal cortex for the purpose of maintaining blood sodium and potassium levels. Specifically, aldosterone increases sodium reabsorption by the kidneys, which, in effect, causes osmotic reabsorption of water and the subsequent loss of potassium. These effects lead to a rise in blood volume and blood pressure.[54] Common causes of aldosteronism include adrenocorticol hyperplasia, adrenal adenoma, Cushing's syndrome, diuretics, hyperkalaemia, hyponatraemia, hypovolaemia, laxative abuse, oral contraceptives, pregnancy, renal arterial stenosis and stress. Below normal levels of aldosterone may be found in Addison's disease, antihypertensive or corticosteroid therapy, hypernatraemia, hypokalaemia, pre-eclampsia and renin deficiency.[32]

### Antidiuretic hormone (ADH), or vasopressin

ADH is a peptide hormone synthesised by the hypothalamus and stored in the posterior pituitary gland. The primary role of ADH is to maintain blood osmolarity by increasing water resorption from the kidneys. Acute porphyria, dehydration, hypovolaemia, nephrogenic diabetes insipidus, physical stress, tuberculosis and syndrome of inadequate ADH are all associated with increased circulating levels of ADH. Reduced levels of the hormone may be found in conditions such as hypervolaemia, nephrotic syndrome and neurogenic diabetes insipidus.[34]

### Calcitonin

Calcitonin, a hormone secreted by the C cells of the thyroid gland, serves to reduce calcium concentration in the blood by increasing urinary calcium excretion and decreasing bone resorption. Conditions associated with elevated serum calcitonin include alcoholic cirrhosis, breast, lung, pancreatic or thyroid carcinoma, hypercalcaemia, hyperparathyroidism, thyroiditis and Zollinger-Ellison syndrome.[32]

### Catecholamines, including adrenaline, noradrenaline and dopamine

These are amino acid-derived hormones secreted by the adrenal medulla, brain and sympathetic nerve endings. Bronchodilatation, glucolysis, glycogenolysis, increased force of cardiac contraction, lipolysis, tachycardia and vasoconstriction are just a few of their many adrenergic effects.[54] Abnormally elevated levels of catecholamines within the urine or blood may occur as a result of diabetic acidosis, ganglioblastoma, hypothyroidism, myocardial infarction, neuroblastoma, phaeochromocytoma, shock and strenuous exercise. A fall in circulating catecholamines may be present in conditions such as autonomic nervous system dysfunction, orthostatic hypotension and Parkinson's disease.[18]

### Cortisol

Cortisol is a major glucocorticoid secreted by the adrenal cortex. Glucolysis, glycogenesis, fatty acid and amino acid mobilisation, and anti-inflammatory activity are just some of the key functions of this hormone. Conditions that are associated with a reduction in urinary or serum cortisol include Addison's disease, adrenal hyperplasia, hypopituitarism, hypothyroidism and liver disease. An increase in cortisol levels may be indicative of adrenal tumour, Cushing's syndrome, ectopic ACTH-producing tumours, hyperthyroidism, obesity, pregnancy and stress.[16]

### Follicle-stimulating hormone (FSH)

FSH is a glycoprotein secreted by the anterior pituitary gland. The hormone is primarily responsible for follicle development and oestrogen production in females, and sperm maturation in males.[54] Increased blood levels of FSH can be associated with alcohol abuse, anorchia, hypogonadism, Klinefelter's syndrome, menopause, orchitis, pituitary tumours and Turner's syndrome. Reduced levels of FSH can occur in anorexia nervosa, haemochromatosis, hyperprolactinaemia, pituitary or hypothalamus dysfunction, polycystic ovarian syndrome and pregnancy.[18]

### Glucagon

This hormone, secreted by the alpha cells of the pancreatic islets, plays a key role in maintaining glycaemic control. Specifically, glucagon elevates blood glucose levels by accelerating glycogenolysis and hepatic gluconeogenesis. A fall in blood glycogen levels may occur in chronic pancreatitis, cystic fibrosis, glucagon deficiency, postpancreatectomy and pancreatic cancer. An abnormal increase in glycogen levels may be indicative of acromegaly, acute pancreatitis, Cushing's syndrome, diabetes mellitus, glucagonoma, hypoglycaemia, phaeochromocytoma, renal failure and severe physical stress or trauma.[16]

### Glycated haemoglobin (HbA1c)

HbA1c is one of three components of haemoglobin that combines most strongly with glucose. HbA1c is used as a long-term measure of a client's average glucose level over approximately 100–120 days. Elevated HbA1c levels may be indicative of chronic hyperglycaemia or poorly controlled diabetes mellitus, whereas reduced HbA1c levels may be explained by conditions affecting circulating haemoglobin, such as haemolytic anaemia, haemorrhage or renal failure.[18]

### Growth hormone (GH)

GH is a peptide hormone secreted by the anterior pituitary gland. The key functions of GH are protein synthesis, cellular growth, stem cell division, glycogenolysis and fatty acid mobilisation.[54] Conditions associated with a reduction in circulating GH include adrenocorticol hyperactivity, dwarfism, failure to thrive, hyperglycaemia and pituitary insufficiency. Increased levels of GH may be related to acromegaly, anorexia, diabetes mellitus, gigantism, physical stress and strenuous exercise.[16]

### Hair, urine, serum and blood nutrient levels

These tests may be indicated when presenting clinical manifestations are suggestive of nutrient deficiency or toxicity, when the presenting condition is likely to be caused by nutrient deficiency or toxicity, or when the condition is likely to contribute to the development of nutrient deficiency or toxicity. Nutrient tests that are particularly relevant to endocrine assessment are hair mineral analysis, iron studies, red blood cell folate, serum vitamin A, serum vitamin $B_{12}$, serum vitamin C, serum calcium, serum cholecalciferol, serum chromium, serum magnesium, serum pyridoxine and serum zinc.

## Insulin

Insulin is a peptide hormone secreted by the beta cells of the pancreatic islets and, like glucagon, plays a major role in maintaining glycaemic control. Insulin is responsible for reducing blood glucose levels by accelerating glucose uptake and utilisation as well as glycogenesis,[54] which glucagon is not. Conditions such as diabetes mellitus and hypopituitarism are associated with a reduction in the production and release of insulin. Hyperinsulinaemia may be a consequence of acromegaly, alcohol abuse, Cushing's syndrome, insulinoma, metabolic syndrome and obesity.[32]

## Luteinising hormone (LH)

LH is a glycoprotein secreted by the anterior pituitary gland. In females LH is responsible for ovulation, corpus luteum development and progesterone production. In males LH stimulates the release of testosterone.[54] A reduction in circulating LH levels can occur in anorexia nervosa, hypothalamus dysfunction, malnutrition, pituitary dysfunction and stress. Elevated levels of LH can arise from anorchia, hypogonadism, menopause, Klinefelter's syndrome, pituitary adenoma, polycystic ovarian syndrome and Turner's syndrome.[34]

## Oestrogens, including oestrone (E1) and oestradiol (E2)

Oestrogens are steroid hormones secreted primarily by the ovaries. These hormones play a key role in maintaining female secondary sex characteristics, reproductive organ function, and endometrial growth and repair.[54] A reduction in urine or blood oestrogen may be a sign of anorexia nervosa, failing pregnancy, hypogonadism, hypopituitarism, menopause or Turner's syndrome. By contrast, elevated oestrogen levels may be indicative of hyperthyroidism, liver disease, normal pregnancy or ovarian, testicular or adrenal tumour.[32]

## Oral glucose tolerance test (OGTT)

- *Fasting blood glucose level (FBGL)* is defined as the level of blood glucose after an 8-hour period of fasting. Low levels of fasting blood glucose may be indicative of acute alcohol ingestion, Addison's disease, insulin overdose, insulinoma, hypothyroidism, hypopituitarism, starvation or glucagon deficiency. Elevated FBGL is suggestive of impaired fasting glucose, diabetes mellitus, acute stress reaction, Cushing's syndrome, pancreatitis, strenuous exercise, thyrotoxicosis and thiamine deficiency.[16]
- *Postprandial glucose level (PPG)* is defined as the level of blood glucose 2 hours after a meal or glucose challenge. PPG is another measure of glycaemic control, in particular, a measure of insulin response to glucose challenge. Elevated PPG levels may be indicative of impaired glucose tolerance, diabetes mellitus, acute stress reaction, Cushing's syndrome, excessive glucose intake, pancreatitis, pregnancy, strenuous exercise or thyrotoxicosis. Low PPG levels may be suggestive of Addison's disease, coeliac disease, insulinoma, hypothyroidism, hypopituitarism, starvation or Whipple's disease.[15]

## Progesterone

This is a steroid hormone produced by the ovaries, whose primary function is to prepare the endometrium for implantation and the breasts for lactation.[54] Elevated levels of progesterone in the blood or the metabolite pregnanediol in the urine may suggest the presence of Cushing's syndrome, hydatidiform mole, luteal ovarian cysts, ovulation, pregnancy or ovarian carcinoma. Decreased progesterone levels may be indicative of hypogonadism, ovarian or breast cancer, pre-eclampsia or threatened miscarriage.[16]

### Prolactin
Prolactin is a hormone produced by the anterior pituitary gland. While the main function of this hormone is to promote lactation and, as such, is expected to be elevated in a woman who is pregnant or breastfeeding, blood levels of prolactin can also be abnormally elevated in adrenal insufficiency, amenorrhoea, anorexia nervosa, galactorrhoea, hypothyroidism, liver or renal failure, physical stress, pituitary tumour and polycystic ovarian syndrome.[32]

### Testosterone
Testosterone is a steroid hormone manufactured primarily by the Leydig cells of the testes, with smaller amounts produced by the ovaries and adrenal glands. The maintenance of male secondary sex characteristics and spermatogenesis are key functions of this hormone. A fall in blood testosterone levels may occur in alcohol abuse, cryptorchidism, Down syndrome, hypogonadism, hypopituitarism, Klinefelter's syndrome, liver disease or orchidectomy. Increased testosterone levels may be a sign of adrenocorticol, ovarian or testicular tumours, androgen resistance syndrome, hyperthyroidism or polycystic ovarian syndrome.[18]

### Thyroid function test (TFT)
TFT is a useful measure of thyroid activity and function. Circulating levels of the two thyroid hormones, thyroxine (T4) and triiodothyronine (T3), provide important information about thyroid gland output, while levels of the pituitary-secreted thyroid stimulating hormone (TSH) ascertains the degree of thyroid stimulation. Elevated TSH levels alongside reduced T4 and T3 levels are indicative of hypothyroidism, while the reverse is true for hyperthyroidism. Normal TSH levels with increased or decreased T4 and T3 levels may be indicative of severe illness or medication-induced thyroid dysfunction.[32]

## Radiology tests
### Computed tomography (CT)
CT uses multiple X-ray beams to create cross-sectional images of endocrine structures, including the adrenal glands, ovaries, pancreas and pituitary gland. These images may be useful in detecting the presence of abscesses, adenoma, cysts, haemorrhage, inflammation and tumours.[20]

### Magnetic resonance imaging (MRI)
MRI uses magnetic and radiofrequency energy to generate images of the ovaries, pancreas and pituitary gland in order to identify underlying pathological processes, such as abscesses, cancer, haemorrhage, infarction, inflammation, infection or obstruction.[18]

### Scintigraphy
Scintigraphy measures the level of radionuclide uptake within endocrine tissues, including the adrenal, parathyroid and thyroid glands, in order to assess their size, function, shape and position. Heterogeneous uptake of the radionuclide may suggest

the presence of adenomas, cysts, Graves' disease, fibrosis, hyperplasia, inflammation, nodules, phaeochromocytoma or tumours.[18]

## Ultrasound

Ultrasound uses high-frequency sound waves to assess the position, size, contour and texture of the ovaries, pancreas, parathyroid glands, testes and thyroid gland. Pathological conditions that can be detected by ultrasound include abscesses, cysts, goitre, hydrocoele, hyperplasia, infarction, inflammation, obstruction and tumours.[18]

## Functional tests

### Adrenal hormone profile

This assesses the concentrations of cortisol and DHEA sulfate in the saliva over a 24-hour period. As a surrogate measure of physical and emotional stress, the test may be useful in identifying the cause of affective disorders, chronic fatigue, cardiovascular disease, dysglycaemia, obesity, recurrent infections and sleep disturbance.[82]

### Bone metabolism assessment

This measures bone resorption by quantifying the level of type I bone collagen fragments (i.e. cross-linked N-telopeptide or deoxypyridinoline) within the urine. Elevated levels of these fragments within the urine may be indicative of increased bone resorption, secondary to primary hyperparathyroidism or skeletal pathology.[83]

### Female hormone profile

This profile measures salivary levels of oestradiol, progesterone, testosterone and DHEA over a single 28-day menstrual cycle. Abnormal levels of these hormones at different points in the menstrual cycle and their correlation with pertinent symptoms may identify the cause of altered libido, breast cancer, affective disorders, endometriosis, infertility, menstrual irregularities, polycystic ovary disease and premenstrual syndrome.[55]

### Male hormone profile

This measures the level of DHEA, dihydrotestosterone (DHT), free testosterone, oestradiol, PSA and sex-hormone binding globulin (SHBG) from a single serum sample. An abnormal profile may be useful in identifying the cause of affective disorders, alopecia, altered libido, cardiovascular disease, myasthenia, and prostatic hypertrophy or cancer.[56]

## Invasive tests

### Biopsy

A biopsy is the excision of a small sample of tissue and the subsequent microscopic examination of the sample in order to identify cell morphology and tissue abnormalities. A biopsy of endocrine tissue can aid the detection of cancer, cysts, infection and/or inflammation.[18]

## Miscellaneous tests

### Basal body temperature, or the temperature of the body upon rising

This test is used by some practitioners as a surrogate measure of thyroid function. While experimental studies suggest that hypothyroidism may be associated with a reduction in core body temperature,[84,85] the reliability of this method in human subjects remains uncertain.

## Nervous system assessment

The nervous system is divided into a central and a peripheral system. The central nervous system comprises the cerebrum, cerebellum, diencephalon, brainstem, cranial nerves and spinal cord. The peripheral nervous system incorporates all sensory and motor nerves that connect peripheral receptors, glands and muscles to the central nervous system. Subdivisions of the peripheral system include the sympathetic and parasympathetic pathways.

The key roles of the nervous system are sensory and motor communication, integration, and mental and cognitive function. Clinical manifestations of this system may result when the system is unable to maintain these roles, for instance, when structure or function is impaired. Keep these points in mind when conducting a comprehensive assessment of the nervous system. An outline of the regions pertinent to nervous system assessment is illustrated in Figure 3.9.

### Health history
#### History of presenting condition

Identify the client's primary problem and determine the severity, onset, location, duration, quality and frequency of the sign or symptom, the existence of radiating symptoms (e.g. sciatica pain, which radiates down the buttock and posterior leg and is a sign of peripheral nerve root compression),[26] any aggravating or ameliorating factors (such as acute illness, alcohol, anatomical position, emotional stress, foods, hypoglycaemia, hypoxia, light, mastication, medications, movement, physical activity, pressure, sounds or touch) and any concomitant symptoms (including asthenia, changes in speech, confusion, constipation, coughing, faecal or urinary incontinence, fatigue, headache, hearing loss, irritability, impaired memory, nausea, photophobia, pyrexia, pain, paraesthesias, seizures, sexual dysfunction, visual, auditory, tactile or gustatory hallucinations, vertigo, visual impairment or vomiting).

### Medical history
#### Family history

Establish whether the individual has a genetic predisposition to neurological disease by assessing whether the individual has any family history of neurological dysfunction, including Alzheimer's disease, anxiety, depression, epilepsy, Huntington's

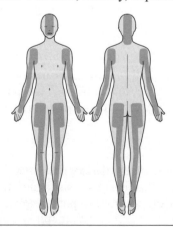

**Figure 3.9:** Nervous system assessment cue card

disease, migraine, motor neuron disease, multiple sclerosis, obsessive-compulsive disorder, Parkinson's disease or schizophrenia.

## Allergies

Determine whether the client has any allergies or sensitivities to environmental substances (such as fragrances or industrial or household chemicals), foods (such as corn, dairy, gluten or soy) or medications (such as anticonvulsants) that could contribute to the presenting complaint or affect clinical management.

## Medications

Find out if the client is presently administering or has recently finished any over-the-counter or prescribed herbs, supplements, medications or therapies for a neurological disorder, including acetylcholinesterase inhibitors, analgesics, anticonvulsants, antidepressants, antipsychotics, anxiolytics, hyperkinetic agents, Parkinsonian agents and sedatives. It should also be noted if the client is receiving any treatments that may generate neurological symptoms (e.g. acyclovir-induced psychosis, antibiotic-induced convulsions, carbamazepine-associated ataxia, or ibuprofen-induced aseptic meningitis).

## Medical conditions

Ascertain whether the client has any current or previous medical conditions that involve the central or peripheral nervous system, including Alzheimer's disease, anxiety, carcinoma, carpal tunnel syndrome, chorea, depression, epilepsy, hydrocephalus, Ménière's disease, meningitis, motor neuron disease, multiple sclerosis, neuropathy, Parkinson's disease, psychiatric disorders, retinopathy, sciatica, sleep disorders, stroke, tinnitus and traumatic injury. The clinician should also identify other conditions that may generate neurological-type symptoms or mimic neurological disease (e.g. caffeine toxicity, diabetes mellitus, heavy metal toxicity, menopause, musculoskeletal disorders, nutrient deficiency or toxicity, sinusitis, syphilis, thyroid disorder, trauma, vascular disease and Wilson's disease).

### Surgical and investigational procedures

Ask whether the client has received any investigational or surgical procedure in the past (e.g. biopsy, carpal tunnel release, cerebral arteriography, clipping of cerebral aneurysm, corpus callosotomy, deep brain stimulation, excision of tumour, lumbar puncture, nerve decompression, nerve repair/reconstruction, temporal lobectomy) to identify other neurological conditions that may have been missed in the health history.

## Lifestyle history

Investigate the presence of other factors that may increase the client's risk of neurological disease or exacerbate the presenting condition, such as tobacco use (including number and strength of cigarettes inhaled in a day),[86] alcohol consumption (including number of standard drinks and type of alcoholic beverage consumed in a day),[87] illicit drug use (including type, route and quantity of drug used per day),[88] diet and fluid intake (such as corn, dairy, wheat, soy consumption, gluten exposure, fruit and vegetable consumption, ketogenic diet, Mediterranean diet),[89,90] quality and duration of sleep (e.g. broken sleep, sleep apnoea)[91,92] and frequency, duration and type of exercise.[93,94]

## Socioeconomic background

Explore if there are any socioeconomic factors that may increase the client's risk of neurological disease, affect their understanding of the condition or the management of the illness, such as occupation and employment status (i.e. day or nightshift, full or part time, number of jobs, hours worked each week), residential and/or work environment (i.e. whether these environments create significant emotional stress, whether the client is exposed to industrial chemicals, irradiation or heavy metals, whether the individual's occupation involves significant stationary or repetitive activity), family environment (i.e. marital status, number and ages of children), religion, ethnicity, race or cultural background (i.e. whether the client follows stringent dietary practices, whether the client's culture, race or ethnic background places the client at increased risk of developing neurological disease), level of social support (i.e. whether the client lives alone or receives community services) and level of educational attainment (i.e. primary, secondary and/or tertiary education).

## Physical examination

### Inspection

As the client enters the consultation room observe the client for anomalies in coordination (e.g. ataxic movements secondary to cerebellar lesions, cerebral palsy or multiple sclerosis), posture (e.g. lateral lean in hemiplegia, stooped posture of Parkinson's disease) and gait (e.g. ataxic gait of cerebellar dysfunction or peripheral neuropathy, shuffled Parkinsonian gait, high-stepping gait of footdrop, waddling gait of proximal myopathy).[10,24,26] A number of cerebellar function tests can then be performed to determine whether any of these manifestations are likely to be the result of cerebellar disease, including the finger-to-nose test, Romberg test, rapid alternating movement test and the heel-to-knee test. Abnormal findings of these tests, including swaying, wobbling, intention tremor and slow or clumsy movements, may be indicative of cerebellar disease.[10,24]

Given these symptoms can also be caused by muscle weakness, it is imperative that muscle mass be examined.[24] A general survey of the major muscle groups for symmetry, muscular atrophy and fasciculations, for instance, may alert to possible motor neuron lesions, Guillian-Barré syndrome, radiculopathy, myasthenia gravis, magnesium or nutrient deficiency and peripheral neuropathy.[9,24] Other types of involuntary movements indicative of neurological function include tremors (e.g. Parkinson's disease), tics (e.g. Tourette syndrome), dyskinesias (e.g. chronic psychoses), chorea (e.g. Huntington's disease), athetosis (e.g. cerebral palsy) and dystonia (e.g. spasmodic torticollis).[9]

The cranial nerve (CN) survey is another important component of the neurological assessment. Lesions to any one of the 12 cranial nerves can result in a number of sensory and motor impairments to the head, neck and special senses. Some of these manifestations include anosmia (CN-I), amaurosis (CN-II), diplopia (CN-III, CN-IV, CN-VI), facial numbness (CN-IV), xerostomia (CN-VII), vertigo (CN-VIII), pharyngeal anaesthesia (CN-IX), dysphagia (CN-X), hoarseness (CN-XI) and tongue wasting (CN-XII).[10,24]

Throughout the neurological assessment, the clinician should also take note of features that might be indicative of impaired mental function. Some of the key observations that could support suspicions of mental illness include the client's appearance (e.g. inappropriate clothing, dishevelled look), attitude (e.g. uncooperative, hostile), affect (e.g. sadness, euphoria), attention span (e.g. easily distracted) and motor behaviour (e.g. pacing, retarded, withdrawn).[95]

## Olfaction

Many psychiatric disorders (including schizophrenia, drug-induced psychosis and dementia) and neurological conditions (including intracranial tumours, head injury and seizures) manifest somatic-type perceptual disturbances that can include delusions and/or hallucinations of halitosis and offensive body odour, even though these conditions may not be detected by the clinician.[96] Unfortunately, the very medications used to treat these conditions can often cause xerostomia and subsequent halitosis.[97] Poorly managed mental and neurological illness may also affect a client's capacity to self-care. This inability to manage one's personal needs can lead to poor personal hygiene and subsequent halitosis and/or offensive body odour.

## Palpation

Palpation is a particularly important component of the nervous system assessment as it adds valuable information about a person's motor and sensory function. The clinician should begin this process by assessing the strength of all major muscle groups. By testing muscle strength first, a clinician may be in a better position to understand the origin of the presenting condition, that is, whether the weakness is the direct result of muscular disease (which often manifests as proximal weakness) or neurological illness (which generally presents as distal weakness).[10] Another method of assessing motor function is to test the client's ability to flex, extend, abduct and adduct the arms, forearms, wrists, fingers, thumbs, hips, knees, ankles and big toes. Any difficulties in performing these movements may signify a change in the integrity of the motor nerve unit, possibly due to neuromuscular junction disease, muscular dystrophy, motor neuron lesions or radiculopathy.[98]

Testing sensory function is somewhat more complex and time-consuming than testing motor function, as different cutaneous receptors need to be stimulated (i.e. thermoreceptors, mechanoreceptors, nociceptors) in order to test the integrity of various spinal sensory pathways. This part of the examination begins with assessment of the client's response to pain (sharp and blunt), temperature (hot and cold), light touch, proprioception and vibration. This enables the practitioner to ascertain the existence, severity and distribution of sensory impairment. When the sensory abnormality does not fit a particular dermatome, peripheral nerve or peripheral neuropathy pattern, investigate a more central cause of the impairment. Parietal lobe disease or a sensory cortex lesion, for instance, may be suspected if an examination of two-point discrimination (the ability to distinguish one stimulus from two in close proximity), stereognosis (the ability to identify a common object in the hand), graphesthesia (the ability to identify numbers drawn on the palm of the hand) and point localisation (the ability to point to the same location touched by the clinician) generate abnormal findings.[9,10,24]

Other signs that may help to support suspicions of neurological disease, specifically, meningeal irritation, include neck rigidity, Brudzinski's sign (the manifestation of hip and knee flexion following neck flexion) and Kernig's sign (the presentation of neck pain or resistance following knee extension and hip flexion). Signs indicative of pyramidal tract disease include Babinski's reflex (plantar flexion of the big toe following stroking of the lateral aspect of the plantar surface of the foot), Oppenheim's sign (dorsiflexion of the big toe following downward pressure on the anterior lower leg) and Hoffman's sign (adduction and flexion of the thumb, and flexion of the fingers following rapid flexion of the middle terminal phalanx).[10] The assessment of infantile automatisms in newborns and younger infants can also alert to the possible presence of neurological disease. The most common of these automatisms are the acoustic blink response, sucking response, rooting response, plantar grasp, palmar grasp, startle reflex and stepping response.[10]

## Percussion
Even though the audiometric properties of conventional percussion play little part in neurological assessment, the technique can be applied in a similar fashion to test deep tendon reflexes. By striking the biceps, triceps, brachioradialis, patellar and Achilles tendons, the clinician is able to gain an insight into the integrity of specific sensorimotor pathways that synapse along different spinal segments.[9] The manifestation of a hyperactive reflex may suggest the presence of hyperthyroidism, spinal cord lesions, electrolyte disturbance or pyramidal tract disease, while diminished reflexes may be a sign of myopathy, hypothyroidism or anterior horn cell disease.[10]

## Auscultation
While the stethoscope has no particular role in nervous system assessment, the open ear does. This is because the content, speed and delivery of a client's speech provides important information about a person's mental function. In schizophrenic disorders, for instance, echolalia, sudden changes in subject matter, paranoid thoughts, delusions and perceptual disturbances may be evident. Delusions of grandeur, impulsivity and/or tachylalia may be a sign of mania.[26] A person with depression, however, may express feelings of helplessness, suicidal ideation, hopelessness, poor self-esteem and social withdrawal.[99] Dysarthria, or poor articulation of speech, may manifest in both psychiatric and neurological illness, including amyotrophic lateral sclerosis, cerebellar disease, delirium, dementia, Guillian-Barré syndrome, mania, multiple sclerosis, myasthenia gravis, Parkinsonism, poliomyelitis and stroke.[100]

Another important indicator of neurological or psychiatric impairment is memory. Changes in memory retention, memory recall and orientation, for instance, may manifest in conditions such as Alzheimer's disease, brain infection or inflammation, brain tumour, depression, head injury, nutrient imbalance or deficiency, Parkinson's disease, stroke and substance abuse.[99]

## Additional signs
Clinical data not derived from the abovementioned physical examination, which can provide important information about the aetiology of a presenting condition, as well as the general health and nutritional status of the client, can be derived from an assessment of core body temperature, blood pressure, pulse rate, BMI, waist circumference and skinfold thickness.

## Clinical assessment tools
Examples of instruments that may be used to evaluate the severity or effect of nervous or mental health disorders or the effect of treatment on these conditions are as follows.

### Hamilton anxiety rating scale (HAM-A)
HAM-A assesses the severity of anxiety, including the overall level of anxiety, and the degree of psychic distress and somatic complaints.

### Hamilton rating scale for depression (HRSD)
HRSD measures the severity of depression by probing clients about depressive symptoms, anxiety, suicide, guilt, sleep disturbances and weight loss.

### McGill pain questionnaire (MPQ)
MPQ describes the quality and intensity of pain by capturing its sensory and affective components.

### Migraine-specific quality of life questionnaire (MSQ)
MSQ measures the effect of migraine on health-related quality of life, in particular, the effect on role restriction, role prevention, and emotional functioning.

### Multiple sclerosis impact scale (MSIS)
MSIS evaluates the physical and psychological effects of multiple sclerosis.

### Quality of life in epilepsy inventory (QOLIE)
QOLIE assesses the effect of epilepsy on quality of life, daily activity, mood, memory and concentration.

## Diagnostics
### Pathology tests
#### C-reactive protein (CRP)
A marker of inflammatory activity, this protein may be produced by the liver in conditions such as acute rheumatic fever, bacterial meningitis, coronary artery disease, cerebrovascular disease, inflammatory bowel disease, non-specific bacterial infection, neuritis, rheumatoid arthritis and systemic lupus erythromatosus.[18]

#### Hair, urine, serum and blood nutrient levels
These tests may be indicated when presenting clinical manifestations are suggestive of nutrient deficiency or toxicity, when the presenting condition is likely to be caused by nutrient deficiency or toxicity, or when the condition is likely to contribute to the development of nutrient deficiency or toxicity. Nutrient tests that are particularly relevant to neurological assessment are hair mineral analysis, serum vitamin $B_{12}$, serum magnesium, serum pyridoxine and serum selenium.

#### Soluble amyloid beta protein precursors (sBAPP)
sBAPP are neurotropic and neuroprotective proteins located within the cerebrospinal fluid (CSF). In conditions such as Alzheimer's disease, beta-amyloid proteins are deposited on the brain in the form of plaques, which subsequently reduces the level of this protein in the CSF.[16]

### Radiology tests
#### Cerebral angiography
Cerebral angiography is an invasive procedure in which a cerebral blood vessel is injected with contrast media and a series of X-ray images is taken. This procedure is used to assess blood flow dynamics and blood vessel defects, thereby aiding the diagnosis of aneurysm, thrombosis, vessel stenosis or occlusion or vascular malformation.[16]

### Computed tomography (CT)

CT uses multiple X-ray beams to generate cross-sectional images of the brain, intracranial tissues and spine. Abnormal neurological findings that may be identified on CT include abscesses, aneurysm, atrophy, cerebral oedema, congenital malformations, cysts, haematoma, hydrocephaly, multiple sclerosis, stroke and tumours.[20]

### Magnetic resonance imaging (MRI)

MRI uses magnetic and radiofrequency energy to generate images of pertinent structures, such as the brain and spinal column. These images can identify relevant neurological pathology, including abscesses, Alzheimer's disease, aneurysms, congenital malformations, cysts, haematomas, herniated discs, multiple sclerosis, nerve compression, Parkinson's disease, stroke and tumours.[18]

### Myelography, or myelogram

A myelography uses X-ray imaging, along with the administration of contrast media into the subarachnoid space of the spinal canal, to facilitate the identification or pertinent pathology. Myelography is particularly useful in detecting ankylosing spondylosis, astrocytoma, cysts, herniated discs, nerve root avulsion, neurofibroma and tumours.[16]

### Positron emission tomography (PET)

PET provides anatomical and functional information about the brain. Following the administration of an inhaled or intravenous radionuclide, areas of radionuclide accumulation (which reflect the level of cellular metabolic activity) are tracked by CT imaging and positron detectors. A reduction in positron emission, and thus cerebral metabolism, can occur in conditions such as Alzheimer's disease, dementia, haemorrhage and stroke. Increased cellular metabolism may be a sign of epilepsy, Huntington's disease, Parkinson's disease or tumours.[16] Other abnormal states that may be detected by PET include aneurysms and Creutzfeldt-Jakob disease.[18]

## Functional tests

### Functional brain mapping

With the assistance of functional MRI or PET imaging, functional brain mapping detects changes in brain metabolism and/or blood flow in response to particular tasks.[101] While this technique may help in localising seizure foci or guiding neurosurgery, its role as a diagnostic tool warrants further investigation.[102]

## Invasive tests

### Lumbar puncture, or spinal tap

This involves the insertion of a sterile needle into the subarachnoid space of the spinal column in order to withdraw CSF for examination. As a diagnostic tool the procedure can be used to assess the presence of demyelinating diseases, encephalitis, haemorrhage, hepatic encephalopathy, meningitis, myelitis, neurosyphilis and tumours.[16]

### Nerve biopsy

This involves the excision of a small sample of nerve tissue and the subsequent microscopic examination of the sample in order to identify cell morphology and tissue abnormalities. Biopsy of nerve tissue can be useful in detecting demyelination, infection, inflammation, nerve dysfunction and neuropathy.[18]

### Miscellaneous tests

#### Electroencephalogram (EEG)

An EEG measures the electrical activity of the brain by placing electrodes on an individual's scalp and connecting them to an electroencephalograph. The abnormal frequency, characteristics and amplitude of these brainwave patterns, either at rest or following stimulation, may indicate the presence and location of epilepsy, abscesses, encephalitis, head injury, intracranial haemorrhage or infarction, narcolepsy or tumours.[16]

#### Nerve conduction studies, or electroneurography

These measure nerve conduction velocity. Two electrodes, proximal and distal, are applied over the nerve of interest, and then a stimulus is applied to the electrodes. The time required for the impulse to travel from the proximal electrode to the distal electrode is measured in metres per second. A significant decrease in the nerve's conduction velocity can indicate peripheral nerve injury or disease, such as carpal tunnel syndrome, diabetic neuropathy, herniated disc disease or myasthenia gravis.[18]

## Musculoskeletal system assessment

The muscular and skeletal systems, which incorporate the bones, muscles, articulations, ligaments, tendons and bursae, are often grouped together as they serve similar functions. Both of these systems are needed, for instance, for tissue support, protection, posture, movement and nutrient storage. The skeletal system also plays an important role in blood cell production, while the muscular system assists in the generation of heat. When musculoskeletal integrity or function deviates from normal, the ability of the system to maintain these roles is adversely affected, which can result in the manifestation of undesirable signs and symptoms. These considerations should be taken into account when conducting a comprehensive assessment of the musculoskeletal system. An outline of the regions pertinent to nervous system assessment is illustrated in Figure 3.10.

### Health history

#### History of presenting condition

After establishing the client's primary problem, determine the quality, duration, frequency, severity, onset and location of the sign or symptom, the existence of radiating symptoms (e.g. neck pain radiating to the occiput or shoulders is

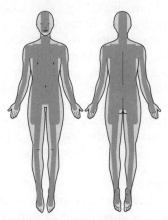

**Figure 3.10:** Musculoskeletal assessment cue card

indicative of cervical spondylosis),[103] any aggravating or ameliorating factors (such as alcohol, anatomical position, cold, emotional stress, exercise, extension, fatigue, flexion, heat, inactivity, massage, medications, movement, palpation, rest, rotation or sleep) and any concomitant symptoms (including arthralgia, asthenia, crepitus, fasciculations, fatigue, immobility, joint instability, malaise, muscle spasms, myalgia, nausea, paraesthesias, pyrexia, reduced range of motion, stiffness or vomiting).

## Medical history
### Family history
Find out whether the client has a genetic predisposition to muscular or skeletal disease by assessing whether there is any family history of musculoskeletal illness, including ankylosing spondylitis, disc herniation, Paget's disease, osteoporosis, rheumatoid arthritis and sciatica.

### Allergies
Establish whether the client has any sensitivities or allergies to foods (such as dairy, food colours or gluten), environmental substances (such as insect bites or stings) or medications (such as minocycline or intramuscular injections) that might contribute to the presenting condition or affect clinical management.

### Medications
Ask the client if they are presently administering or have recently completed any prescribed or over-the-counter medications, herbs, supplements or therapies for a musculoskeletal condition, including analgesics, anti-inflammatories, antirheumatoid agents, antispasmodics, bone metabolism agents, parasympathomimetics, rubefacients and xanthine oxidase inhibitors. Also make note of any other treatments the client is receiving that could generate muscular or skeletal symptoms, including biphosphonate-associated osteonecrosis, corticosteroid-induced osteoporosis, fluoroquinolone-induced arthralgia and statin-induced myopathy.

### Medical conditions
Ask the client if they have any current or previous medical conditions that involve the muscular or skeletal systems, including ankylosing spondylitis, bursitis, contractures, epicondylitis, epiphysitis, fibromyalgia, fractures, gout, neurogenic arthropathy, osteoarthritis, osteomyelitis, osteoporosis, Paget's disease, polymyalgia rheumatica, polymyositis, rheumatoid arthritis, scoliosis, spasmodic torticollis, tendinitis, tenosynovitis or tumours. Also identify other conditions that may generate musculoskeletal-type symptoms or mimic musculoskeletal disease (e.g. chronic fatigue syndrome, endocarditis, endocrine disease, gonorrhoea, heavy metal toxicity, hypothyroidism, nutrient deficiency or toxicity, obesity, peripheral vascular disease, psoriasis, scleroderma, syphilis, systemic lupus erythromatosus or viral illness).

### Surgical and investigational procedures
Ascertain whether the individual has received any relevant investigational or surgical procedures in the past (e.g. amputation, arthroscopy, biopsy, bunionectomy, discectomy, joint replacement, fracture reduction, laminectomy, rotator cuff repair,

spinal fusion, tendon or ligament reconstruction) to identify other musculoskeletal disorders that may have been overlooked in the health history.

## Lifestyle history
Determine whether there are other factors that may increase the client's risk of musculoskeletal disease or worsen the presenting condition, such as tobacco use (including number and strength of cigarettes inhaled in a day),[104,105] alcohol consumption (including number of standard drinks and type of alcoholic beverage consumed in a day),[104,105] illicit drug use (including drug type and frequency of use),[106] diet and fluid intake (such as calcium, food additives, gluten, energy consumption, fruit and vegetable intake, magnesium, omega 3 fatty acids, vitamin D),[107–109] quality and duration of sleep (e.g. broken sleep, long sleep onset latency)[110,111] and frequency, duration and type of exercise.[26,112]

## Socioeconomic background
Identify any socioeconomic factors that may increase the client's risk of musculoskeletal disease, affect their understanding of the condition or the management of the illness, such as occupation and employment status (i.e. day or nightshift, full or part time, number of jobs, hours worked each week), residential and/or work environment (i.e. whether these environments create significant emotional stress, whether the individual's occupation involves significant stationary or repetitive activity), family environment (i.e. marital status, number and ages of children), religion, ethnicity, race or cultural background (i.e. whether the client follows strict dietary practices and whether the client's culture, race or ethnic background place the client at increased risk of developing musculoskeletal disease), level of social support (i.e. whether the client lives alone or receives community services) and level of educational attainment (i.e. primary, secondary and/or tertiary education).

## Physical examination
### Inspection
Visual inspection of the musculoskeletal system begins when the client enters the consultation room. Visual inspection includes observation of the client's gait (for signs of limb or foot drag, non-weight bearing or spasticity), posture (for signs of kyphosis, gibbus, list, scoliosis, lordosis and unequal limb length) and body language (for indications of musculoskeletal discomfort and compensation). When the individual is unclothed and appropriately draped, the clinician may also be able to assess the presence of swelling (as a sign of joint effusion, synovitis, gout, arthritic bony overgrowth or bursitis), erythema (as a sign of septic or gouty arthritis), deformity (such as postural defects, dislocation, fractures, hallux valgus and bowlegs), scars (from possible musculoskeletal surgery or trauma), gouty tophi (from hyperuricaemia and/or gout), nodules (such as non-tender, subcutaneous nodules of rheumatoid arthritis), impaired chest expansion (from rib fractures, scoliosis or ankylosing spondylosis) and callosus (from abnormal gait or posture).[9,24,26]

A general survey of the major muscle groups for symmetry, tone, muscular atrophy and fasciculations also may alert to possible arthroses, motor neuron lesions, radiculopathy, myasthenia gravis, magnesium or nutrient deficiency and peripheral neuropathy.[9,24] Also examine passive range of motion (ROM) of all major articulations, including the spine, shoulders, elbows, wrists, metacarpophalangeal joints, hips, knees, ankles and metatarsophalangeal joints. Any reduction in joint ROM may be indicative of trauma (such as ligament or rotator cuff injury) or underlying disease, including ankylosing spondylosis, arthritis, bursitis and tenosynovitis.[9]

### Olfaction

There is no particular role for olfaction in the musculoskeletal assessment.

### Palpation

Palpation is a necessary technique in musculoskeletal assessment as it helps to identify the aetiology or severity of the presenting complaint. The detection of heat and palpable tenderness, for instance, may indicate the presence of an infectious or inflammatory process, such as bursitis, tendinitis, synovitis, tenosynovitis or septic or gouty arthritis.[9] The identification of palpable crepitus and friction rubs (as described below), as well as swelling (as outlined above), may also help to support such diagnoses. Palpation is also useful in assessing the integrity and strength of pertinent muscle groups, tendons and ligaments, as well as the active ROM of relevant articulations. During this assessment, the client's ability to flex, extend, abduct and adduct the arms, forearms, wrists, fingers, thumbs, hips, knees, ankles and big toes is examined. A reduction in muscle strength and/or difficulties in performing these movements may alert to the presence of localised inflammatory disease (e.g. arthritis, tenosynovitis), neurological illness (e.g. motor neuron lesions, radiculopathy) or systemic disease (e.g. muscular dystrophy, myopathy, polymyositis).[9,98]

### Percussion

Even though percussion can be useful in distinguishing muscle from bone and determining the presence of tenderness, palpation is generally sufficient for these purposes. A more specific application of percussion is the assessment of Tinel's sign. This test can be applied to one of three locations: the median nerve over the carpal tunnel, the posterior tibial nerve behind the medial malleolus or the deep peroneal nerve anterior to the ankle. A positive Tinel's sign, defined by the presence of tingling or paraesthesias distal to the percussed nerve, may be indicative of carpal tunnel syndrome or neuroma of the deep peroneal or posterior tibial nerves.[113]

### Auscultation

Listening for the presence of crepitus (a grating or grinding noise) can identify areas of bone or articular dysfunction, such as fractures, arthritis or cartilage injury.[113] Friction rubs (the snapping sound of tendon slipping over bone) on the hand may allude to the presence of tendinitis, tenosynovitis or tendinosis.[26,113]

### Additional signs

Clinical data not derived from the abovementioned physical examination, which can provide important information about the aetiology of a presenting condition, as well as the general health and nutritional status of the client, can be derived from the assessment of core body temperature, weight, height, BMI, waist circumference and skinfold thickness. For infants, occipitofrontal head circumference can also be assessed.

### Clinical assessment tools

Examples of instruments that may be used to evaluate the severity or effect of musculoskeletal complaints, or the effect of treatment on these conditions, are outlined below.

### Aberdeen back pain scale (ABPS)
ABPS assesses the frequency, onset, ameliorating or aggravating factors, radiation and concomitant symptoms of back pain, as well as the effect of back pain on daily activities, work, sleep, sexual activity and leisure.

### Arthritis impact measurement scales (AIMS2)
AIMS2 measures the effect of arthritis on physical activity, social function, activities of daily living and work.

### Fibromyalgia impact questionnaire (FIQ)
FIQ assesses the effect of fibromyalgia on daily activities, work and wellbeing, as well as the severity of symptoms.

### Foot function index (FFI)
FFI evaluates the level of pain and disability associated with non-specific foot pathology.

### Osteoporosis assessment questionnaire (OPAQ)
OPAQ examines the physical, emotional, symptomatic and social effects of osteoporosis on health-related quality of life.

## Diagnostics
### Pathology tests
#### Antinuclear antibodies (ANA)
ANA are autoantibodies targeted at the nucleus of affected cells. The formation of these ANA cell nucleus immune complexes results in autoimmune tissue damage. The presence of these antibodies in the blood can be associated with conditions such as liver disease, mixed connective tissue disease, polymyositis, rheumatoid arthritis, scleroderma, Sjögren's disease and systemic lupus erythromatosus.[16]

#### C-reactive protein (CRP)
CRP is a marker of inflammatory activity. The protein may be produced by the liver in conditions such as acute rheumatic fever, coronary artery disease, inflammatory bowel disease, non-specific bacterial infection, rheumatoid arthritis and systemic lupus erythromatosus.[18]

#### Creatinine
Creatinine is a product of creatine metabolism, an amino acid stored predominantly in skeletal muscle. If renal and dietary factors can be eliminated, serum creatinine can be a useful indicator of muscle integrity. Above normal levels of creatinine may result from, for instance, acromegaly, hyperthyroidism, gigantism, muscle tremors, myositis, rhabdomyolysis and strenuous exercise, while reduced levels may be present in debility, liver disease, muscular dystrophy and myasthenia gravis.[18]

#### Hair, urine, serum and blood nutrient levels
These tests may be indicated when presenting clinical manifestations are suggestive of nutrient deficiency or toxicity, when the presenting condition is likely to be caused by nutrient deficiency or toxicity or when the condition is likely to contribute to the development of nutrient deficiency or toxicity. Nutrient tests that are particularly

relevant to musculoskeletal assessment are hair mineral analysis, serum vitamin C, serum calcium, serum cholecalciferol and serum magnesium.

### Rheumatoid factor (RF)

RF is a reactive immunoglobulin M (IgM) antibody. The reactive antibody forms immune complexes with abnormal immunoglobulin G (IgG) in the synovial membranes, leading to a cascade of events that result in joint destruction. High RF titres are indicative of rheumatoid arthritis, whereas moderately elevated titres suggest the presence of chronic hepatitis, dermatomyositis, infectious mononucleosis, scleroderma, Sjögren's syndrome, subacute bacterial endocarditis or systemic lupus erythromatosus.[16]

### Uric acid

Uric acid is an end product of purine catabolism. If renal dysfunction can be excluded, hyperuricaemia and uricosuria may be indicative of gout, high purine intake, lactic acidosis, leukaemia, metastatic cancer and multiple myeloma. Low serum and urinary uric acid levels may suggest the presence of liver disease, low-purine diet or Wilson's disease.[18]

## Radiology tests
### Bone densitometry

This test measures bone mineral density (BMD) of specific bony sites, including the spine, wrist, hip and calcaneus, in order to diagnose osteoporosis or osteopenia. This can be assessed by using one of a number of different imaging techniques, including dual-energy X-ray absorptiometry (DEXA), CT or ultrasound. The BMD is subsequently calculated by dividing the amount of photons not absorbed by the bone by the surface area of the bone.[16]

### Computed tomography (CT)

CT uses multiple X-ray beams to create cross-sectional images of tissues, such as skeletal muscle and bone. These images may detect a number of pathological conditions of the musculoskeletal system, including cysts, congenital malformations, herniated discs, spondylosis and tumours.[20]

### Magnetic resonance imaging (MRI)

MRI uses magnetic and radiofrequency energy to produce images of relevant structures, such as skeletal muscle, joints and bone. Musculoskeletal disorders that may be detected by MRI include arthritis, bone marrow disease, fractures, herniated discs, meniscal tears, osteomyelitis, osteonecrosis, spondylosis, synovitis and tumours.[18]

### Plain film X-ray

This test uses electromagnetic radiation to generate images of the articular cartilage, bone and surrounding soft tissue. These radiographs can aid the diagnosis of arthritis, bony spurs, fractures, osteomyelitis, joint dislocation, joint effusion, osteopenia, osteoporosis, Paget's disease or tumours.[20]

### Ultrasound

Ultrasound uses high-frequency sound waves to evaluate the size, texture, position and contour of organs and tissues, including skeletal muscle, tendons, ligaments, bone, joint spaces and articular cartilage. This non-invasive procedure may be useful in detecting arthritis, arthropathy, cysts, haematomas, muscle, tendon or ligament trauma, myositis, osteoporosis, synovitis and tumours.[114]

## Functional tests
### Bone metabolism assessment
This test measures bone resorption by quantifying the level of type I bone collagen fragments (i.e. cross-linked N-telopeptide or deoxypyridinoline) within the urine. Elevated levels of these fragments within the urine may be indicative of increased bone resorption, secondary to arthritic disease, connective tissue disorders, metastatic or alcoholic bone disease, osteomalacia, osteoporosis or Paget's disease.[83]

## Invasive tests
### Arthrocentesis, or joint aspiration
This involves the insertion of a sterile needle into a joint space for the purpose of removing fluid. As a diagnostic tool, the procedure can be used to examine the presence of gout, neoplasms, osteoarthritis, rheumatoid arthritis, septic arthritis, synovitis and systemic lupus erythromatosus.[16]

### Arthroscopy
An arthroscopy provides direct visualisation of the joint and related structures (including ligaments, tendons, cartilage and muscle) through the use of a fiberoptic arthroscope. Arthroscopy can be used to determine the presence of arthritis, chondromalacia, cysts, gout, joint degeneration, osteochondritis, subluxation, synovitis and trauma.[20]

### Biopsy
This involves the excision of a small sample of tissue, and the subsequent microscopic examination of the sample to identify cell morphology and tissue abnormalities. A biopsy of muscle or skeletal tissue may assist in the diagnosis of cancer, infection, inflammation, myasthenia gravis, myopathy and polymyositis.[18]

## Miscellaneous tests
### Electromyography (EMG)
An EMG involves the insertion of percutaneous electrodes into selected muscle groups in order to assess the level of muscle activity at rest, as well as voluntary contraction and electrical stimulation. A reduction in the amplitude of the electrical waveforms is suggestive of muscular dystrophies, myasthenia gravis, myopathies and polymyositis. The presence of fasciculations and fibrillations can be indicative of nerve disease or spastic myotonic muscle disease.[16]

### Quantitative sensory testing (QST)
QST provides a systematic measure of sensory thresholds, compared with the more qualitative method of bedside sensory testing. The procedure involves the application of different stimuli (including heat, cold, light touch, vibration, brushing, pinprick and blunt pressure) at different levels of intensity. The intensity, spatial and temporal characteristics of the stimuli are controlled by automated devices and analysed alongside client response times. By precisely measuring the magnitude of sensory deficits, QST can quantify the level of allodynia, hyperalgesia and sensory neuropathies, although validity and reliability studies are still needed.[115]

## Summary

Clinical assessment is a fundamental component of the DeFCAM as it informs every stage of the process. The approach to clinical assessment is a key determinant of clinical practice outcomes. For that reason, the adoption of a comprehensive and systematic approach to assessment may help to improve the quality of client care by providing assurance that data pertinent to the formulation of decisions that affect client outcomes are not omitted. The CAM assessment process is an example of such an approach, in that it incorporates the health history, physical examination and relevant diagnostics. The translation of these assessment data into CAM diagnoses is conducted using diagnostic reasoning, which the following chapter will discuss in detail.

### Learning activities

1 Describe the principles of clinical assessment. Discuss how each of these principles affects the overall clinical process.
2 Compare and contrast subjective and objective data. List five examples of subjective and five examples of objective data that may be collected during a clinical assessment.
3 Compare and contrast the three stages of the CAM assessment process. Focusing only on the field of CAM you practise, what additional elements of each stage would you need to include? Why?
4 Using the criteria listed in Table 3.2, rewrite the four incomplete presenting complaint statements provided below; ensure that each statement is clear, concise, objective and complete (incorporate knowledge from your own experience and education where information is lacking):
   a. an 87-year-old woman with a continuous, moderate dull ache to the left shoulder, secondary to osteoarthritis
   b. a 43-year-old woman with a 3-year history of a harsh productive cough with yellow sputum, which is worse on rising and improved with smoking
   c. a 55-year-old male with severe sharp, shooting pain down the right buttock and right posterior upper leg, accompanied by mild foot numbness and muscle weakness
   d. a 4-year-old girl with erythemic, dry, scaly, pruritic lesions to both cheeks (both 50 mm in diameter), which manifest intermittently and last for 5–10 days at a time.
5 For each of the symptoms presented below, list (and justify) five clinical assessment techniques or tests that could be used or accessed by your discipline, which would be most helpful in understanding the cause of the presenting condition:
   a. dyspnoea
   b. lumbago
   c. skin rash
   d. dysmenorrhoea
   e. diarrhoea.

# References

1. Reilly JJ et al (2008) Objective measurement of physical activity and sedentary behaviour: review with new data. Archives of Disease in Childhood, 93(7): 614–19.
2. Shulman LM et al (2006) Subjective report versus objective measurement of activities of daily living in Parkinson's disease. Movement Disorders, 21(6): 794–9.
3. Melman A. Fogarty J. Hafron J. (2005) Can self-administered questionnaires supplant objective testing of erectile function? A comparison between the international index of erectile function and objective studies. International Journal of Impotence Research, 18: 126–9.
4. Al-Shahrani M. Lovatsis D. (2005) Do subjective symptoms of obstructive voiding correlate with postvoid residual urine volume in women? International Urogynecology Journal, 16(1): 12–14.
5. Leach MJ. (2005) Rapport: a key to treatment success. Complementary Therapies in Clinical Practice, 11(4): 262–5.
6. Australian Traditional Medicine Society. (2008) Annual report 2007/08. Sydney: Australian Traditional Medicine Society.
7. Bensoussan A. Myers SP. (1996) Towards a safer choice. The practice of traditional Chinese medicine in Australia. Sydney: Faculty of Health, University of Western Sydney.
8. New South Wales Health Care Complaints Commission. (2007) Annual report 2006/07. Sydney: New South Wales Health Care Complaints Commission.
9. Bickley LS. Szilagyi PG. (2007) Bates' guide to physical examination and history taking. 9th ed. Philadelphia: Lippincott, Williams & Wilkins.
10. Swartz MH. (2009) Textbook of physical diagnosis: history and examination. 6th ed. Philadelphia: Saunders.
11. Mozaffarian D. Wilson PWF. Kannel W. (2008) Beyond established and novel risk factors: lifestyle risk factors for cardiovascular disease. Circulation, 117(23): 3031–8.
12. Epstein O et al (2008) Clinical examination. 4th ed. Edinburgh: Mosby.
13. Dunder K et al (2004) Evaluation of a scoring scheme, including proinsulin and the apolipoprotein B/apolipoprotein A1 ratio, for the risk of acute coronary events in middle-aged men. American Heart Journal, 148: 596–601.
14. Khan U et al (2007) Asymmetric dimethylarginine in cerebral small vessel disease. Stroke, 38: 411–13.
15. National Heart Foundation of Australia (NHFA). Cardiac Society of Australia and New Zealand (CSANZ). (2005) Position statement on lipid management—2005. Heart Lung and Circulation, 14: 275–291.
16. Pagana KD. Pagana TJ. (2008) Mosby's diagnostic and laboratory test reference. 9th ed. St Louis: Elsevier Mosby.
17. van Guldener C. Nanayakkara WB. Stehouwer CDA. (2007) Homocysteine and asymmetric dimethylarginine (ADMA): biochemically linked but differently related to vascular disease in chronic kidney disease. Clinical Chemistry and Laboratory Medicine, 45(12): 1683–7.
18. Van Leeuwen AM. Poelhuis-Leth DJ. (2009) Davis's comprehensive handbook of laboratory and diagnostic tests with nursing implications. 3rd ed. Philadelphia: FA Davis Company.
19. Hadaegh F et al (2006) Association of total cholesterol versus other serum lipid parameters with the short-term prediction of cardiovascular outcomes: Tehran Lipid and Glucose Study. European Journal of Cardiovascular Prevention and Rehabilitation, 13: 571–7.
20. Fischbach FT. Dunning MB. (2008) A manual of laboratory and diagnostic tests. 8th ed. Philadelphia: Lippincott Williams & Wilkins.
21. Fernandez A et al (2009) Relation of corneal arcus to cardiovascular disease (from the Framingham Heart Study Data Set). American Journal of Cardiology, 103(1): 64–6.
22. Reilly K et al (2008) Risk factors for chronic obstructive pulmonary disease mortality in Chinese adults. American Journal of Epidemiology, 167(8): 998–1004.
23. Celik F. Topcu F. (2006) Nutritional risk factors for the development of chronic obstructive pulmonary disease (COPD) in male smokers. Clinical Nutrition, 25(6): 955–61.
24. Talley NJ. O'Connor S. (2006) Clinical examination: a systematic guide to physical diagnosis 5th ed. Sydney: Churchill Livingstone.
25. Tatjana PG. Om PS. (2006) Clinical atlas of interstitial lung disease. London: Springer.
26. Porter R, Kaplan J, Beers M, editors. (2007) The Merck manual. Rahway: Merck Research Laboratories.
27. Thomas GA. Rhodes J. Ingram JR. (2005) Mechanisms of disease: nicotine: a review of its actions in the context of gastrointestinal disease. Nature Clinical Practice Gastroenterology and Hepatology, 2(11): 536–44.
28. Taylor B. Rehm J. (2005) Moderate alcohol consumption and diseases of the gastrointestinal system: a review of pathophysiological processes. Digestive Diseases, 23(3–4): 177–80.
29. Lock K et al (2005) The global burden of disease attributable to low consumption of fruit and vegetables: implications for the global strategy on diet. Bulletin of the World Health Organization, 83(2): 100–8.
30. Vege SS et al (2004) Functional gastrointestinal disorders among people with sleep disturbances: a population-based study. Mayo Clinic Proceedings, 79: 1501–6.
31. Ravi N et al (2005) Effect of physical exercise on esophageal motility in patients with esophageal disease. Diseases of the Esophagus, 18(6): 374–7.
32. Nicoll D. McPhee SJ. Pignone M. (2007) Pocket guide to diagnostic tests. 5th ed. New York: McGraw-Hill Professional.
33. Saad RJ. Chey WD. (2007) Breath tests for gastrointestinal disease: the real deal or just a lot of hot air? Gastroenterology, 133(6): 1763–6.
34. Wallach JB. (2007) Interpretation of diagnostic tests. 8th ed. Philadelphia: Lippincott Williams & Wilkins.
35. Liska D. Lyon M. Jones DS. (2006) Detoxification and biotransformational imbalances. EXPLORE: Journal of Science and Healing, 2(2): 122–40
36. Genova Diagnostics. (2008) Comprehensive digestive stool analysis. Asheville: Genova Diagnostics.
37. Genova Diagnostics. (2008) Intestinal permeability test. Asheville: Genova Diagnostics.
38. Subak LL et al (2009) Weight loss to treat urinary incontinence in overweight and obese women. New England Journal of Medicine, 360(5): 481–90.

39. Murta-Nascimento C et al (2007) Epidemiology of urinary bladder cancer: from tumor development to patient's death. World Journal of Urology, 25(3): 285–95.

40. Daviglus M et al (2005) Relation of nutrient intake to microalbuminuria in nondiabetic middle-aged men and women: International Population Study on Macronutrients and Blood Pressure (INTERMAP). American Journal of Kidney Diseases, 45(2): 256–66.

41. Faulx MD et al (2007) Obstructive sleep apnea is associated with increased urinary albumin excretion. Sleep, 30(7): 923–9.

42. Rohrmann S et al (2005) Association of cigarette smoking, alcohol consumption and physical activity with lower urinary tract symptoms in older American men: findings from the third National Health And Nutrition Examination Survey. BJU International, 96(1): 77–82.

43. Meyer TW. Hostetter TH. (2007) Uremia. New England Journal of Medicine, 357(13): 1316–25.

44. Springhouse. (2005) Professional guide to assessment. Philadelphia: Lippincott, Williams & Wilkins.

45. Baert AL. (2008) Encyclopedia of diagnostic imaging. Berlin: Springer.

46. Leyendecker JR. Barnes CE. Zagoria RJ. (2008) MR urography: techniques and clinical applications. RadioGraphics, 28: 23–46.

47. Ainbinder SW. Ramin SM. DeCherney AH. (2007) Sexually transmitted diseases and pelvic infections. In: Current diagnosis and treatment: obstetrics and gynecology. 10th ed. DeCherney AH et al, editors. New York: McGraw-Hill Professional.

48. Shah M. DeSilva A. (2008) The male genitalia: a clinician's guide to skin problems and sexually transmitted infections. Oxford: Radcliffe Publishing.

49. He J et al (2007) Cigarette smoking and erectile dysfunction among Chinese men without clinical vascular disease. American Journal of Epidemiology, 166(7): 803–9.

50. Homan GF. Davies M. Norman R. (2007) The impact of lifestyle factors on reproductive performance in the general population and those undergoing infertility treatment: a review. Human Reproduction Update, 13(3): 209–23.

51. Rostad B. Schei B. Sundby J. (2006) Fertility in Norwegian women: results from a population-based health survey. Scandinavian Journal of Public Health, 34(1): 5–10.

52. Fjerbaek A. Knudsen U. (2007) Endometriosis, dysmenorrhea and diet: What is the evidence? European Journal of Obstetrics and Gynecology and Reproductive Biology, 132 (2): 140–7.

53. Zias N et al (2009) Obstructive sleep apnea and erectile dysfunction: still a neglected risk factor? Sleep and Breathing, 13(1): 3–10.

54. Martini FH. Ober WC. Garrison CW. Welch K. Hutchings RT. (2006) Fundamentals of anatomy and physiology. 7th ed. San Francisco: Pearson Education.

55. Genova Diagnostics. (2008) Rhythm. Asheville: Genova Diagnostics.

56. Genova Diagnostics. (2008) Male hormones plus. Asheville: Genova Diagnostics.

57. Grimes DA et al (2005) Fertility awareness-based methods for contraception: systematic review of randomized controlled trials. Contraception, 72(2): 85–90.

58. Straten MV et al (2001) Tobacco use and skin disease. Southern Medical Journal, 94(6): 561–8.

59. Behnam SM. Behnam SE. Koo JY. (2005) Alcohol as a risk factor for plaque-type psoriasis. Cutis, 76(3): 181–5.

60. Kirby B et al (2008) Alcohol consumption and psychological distress in patients with psoriasis. British Journal of Dermatology, 158(1): 138–40.

61. Kelsay K. (2006) Management of sleep disturbance associated with atopic dermatitis. Journal of Allergy and Clinical Immunology, 118(1): 198–201.

62. Emery CF et al (2005) Exercise accelerates wound healing among healthy older adults: a preliminary investigation. Journals of Gerontology Series A-Biological Sciences and Medical Sciences, 60(11): 1432–6.

63. Lyon CC. Smith AJ. (2001) Infections. In: Abdominal stomas and their skin disorders: an atlas of diagnosis and management. Lyon CC, Smith AJ, editors. London: Martin Dunitz.

64. Cogen AL. Nizet V. Gallo RL. (2008) Skin microbiota: a source of disease or defence? British Journal of Dermatology, 158(3): 442–55.

65. Lambert TJ. Wells MJ. Wisniewski KW. (2006) Subcutaneous emphysema resulting from liquid nitrogen spray. Journal of the American Academy of Dermatology, 55(5, Suppl 1): S95–6.

66. Wortsman XC et al (2004) Real-time spatial compound ultrasound imaging of skin. Skin Research and Technology, 10(1): 23–31.

67. Heylings JR. Clowes HM. Hughes L. (2001) Comparison of tissue sources for the skin integrity function test (SIFT). Toxicology In Vitro, 15(4–5): 597–600.

68. Chilcott RP et al (2002) Transepidermal water loss does not correlate with skin barrier function in vitro. Journal of Investigative Dermatology, 118: 871–5.

69. Mehl A et al (2006) The atopy patch test in the diagnostic workup of suspected food-related symptoms in children. Journal of Allergy and Clinical Immunology, 118(4): 923–9.

70. Wargon O. (2005) Tinea of the skin, hair and nails. In: Dermatology. 2nd ed. Marks R, editor. Sydney: Australasian Medical Publishing Company.

71. British Association of Endocrine Surgeons (2006) Guidelines for the surgical management of endocrine disease and training requirements for endocrine surgery. London: British Association of Endocrine Surgeons.

72. Bartalena L et al (2007) Environment and thyroid autoimmunity. In: The thyroid and autoimmunity. Wiersinga WM et al, editors. Stuttgart: Thieme.

73. Kapoor D. Jones TH. (2005) Smoking and hormones in health and endocrine disorders. European Journal of Endocrinology, 152(4): 491–9.

74. Hendriks HFJ. (2007) Moderate alcohol consumption and insulin sensitivity: observations and possible mechanisms. Annals of Epidemiology, 17(5, Suppl 1): S40–42.

75. Steyn NP et al (2004) Diet, nutrition and the prevention of type 2 diabetes. Public Health Nutrition, 7: 147–65.

76. Vanderpump MPJ et al (2008) Thyroid disease: the facts. 4th ed. Oxford: Oxford University Press.

77. Liu PY et al (2007) Sleep apnea and neuroendocrine function. Sleep Medicine Clinics, 2(2): 225–36.

78. Coker RH. Kjaer M. (2005) Glucoregulation during exercise: the role of the neuroendocrine system. Sports Medicine, 35(7): 575–83.

79. Galassetti PR et al (2005) Breath ethanol and acetone as indicators of serum glucose levels: an initial report. Diabetes Technology and Therapeutics, 7(1): 115–23.

80. Southerland JH. Taylor GW. Offenbacher S. (2005) Diabetes and periodontal infection: making the connection. Clinical Diabetes, 23: 171–8.
81. Kapadia CR. Taylor C. Crawford JM. (2003) An atlas of gastroenterology: a guide to diagnosis and differential diagnosis. Lancaster: Parthenon Publishing.
82. ARL Pathology. (2008) Adrenal hormone profile. Melbourne: ARL Functional Pathology.
83. Genova Diagnostics. (2008) Bone resorption assessment. Asheville: Genova Diagnostics.
84. Mori M et al (1989) Hypothyroidism enhances carbachol-induced hypothermia in the rat. Research Communications in Chemical Pathology and Pharmacology, 65(1): 97–104.
85. Wikstrom L et al (1998) Abnormal heart rate and body temperature in mice lacking thyroid hormone receptor alpha 1. EMBO Journal, 17(2): 455–61.
86. Swan GE. Lessov-Schlagger CN. (2007) The effects of tobacco smoke and nicotine on cognition and the brain. Neuropsychology Review, 17(3): 259–73.
87. Dickinson BD et al (2004) The neurocognitive effects of alcohol on adolescents and college students. Preventive Medicine, 40(1): 23–32.
88. Davies RD. Thurstone C. Woyewodzic K. (2004) Substance use disorders and neurologic illness. Current Treatment Options in Neurology, 6(5): 421–32.
89. Gasior M. Rogawski MA. Hartman AL. (2006) Neuroprotective and disease-modifying effects of the ketogenic diet. Behavioural Pharmacology, 17(5–6): 431–9.
90. Scarmeas N et al (2007) Mediterranean diet and Alzheimer disease mortality. Neurology, 69: 1084–93.
91. Gau SSF et al (2007) Association between sleep problems and symptoms of attention-deficit/hyperactivity disorder in young adults. Sleep, 30(2): 195–201.
92. Yantis MA. Neatherlin J. (2005) Obstructive sleep apnea in neurological patients. Journal of Neuroscience Nursing, 37(3): 150–5.
93. Fisher BE et al (2008) The effect of exercise training in improving motor performance and corticomotor excitability in people with early Parkinson's disease. Archives of Physical Medicine and Rehabilitation, 89(7): 1221–9.
94. Oken BS et al (2004) Randomized controlled trial of yoga and exercise in multiple sclerosis. Neurology, 62: 2058–64.
95. Rhoads J. (2006) Advanced health assessment and diagnostic reasoning. Philadelphia: Lippincott, Williams & Wilkins.
96. Fatemi SH. Clayton PJ. Sartorius N. (2008) The medical basis of psychiatry. 3rd ed. Totowa: Humana Press.
97. Reisfield GM. Rosielle DA. Wilson GR. (2009) Xerostomia. 2nd ed. #182. Journal of Palliative Medicine, 12(2): 189–90.
98. Hauser SL et al (2006) Harrison's neurology in clinical medicine. New York: McGraw-Hill.
99. Salloway S. Harrington C. Jacobson S. (2006) Psychiatric evaluation of the neurological patient. In: Psychiatry for neurologists. Jeste DV, Friedman JH, editors. New York: Springer.
100. Jeste DV, Friedman JH, editors. (2006) Psychiatry for neurologists. New York: Springer.
101. Kriegeskorte N. Goebel R. Bandettini P. (2006) Information-based functional brain mapping. Proceedings of the National Academy of Science USA, 103(10): 3863–8.
102. McEvoy AW. Trivedi BM. Kitchen ND. (2004) Stereotactic surgery for epilepsy. In: The treatment of epilepsy. 2nd ed. Shorvon SD et al, editors. Oxford: Blackwell Science.
103. Abbed KM. Coumans JV. (2007) Cervical radiculopathy: pathophysiology, presentation, and clinical evaluation. Neurosurgery, 60(1, Suppl 1): S28–34.
104. Kim M. Chung Y. Sung C. (2007) Negative effects of alcohol consumption and tobacco use on bone formation markers in young Korean adult males. Nutrition Research, 27(2): 104–8.
105. Smith DR et al (2006) A detailed analysis of musculoskeletal disorder risk factors among Japanese nurses. Journal of Safety Research, 37(2): 195–200.
106. Cush JJ. Kavanaugh A. Stein CM. (2005) Rheumatology: diagnosis and therapeutics. 2nd ed. Philadelphia: Lippincott, Williams & Wilkins.
107. Kozanoglu E. Basaran S. Goncu MK. (2005) Proximal myopathy as an unusual presenting feature of celiac disease. Clinical Rheumatology, 24(1): 76–8.
108. Sharkey PF et al (2007) Diet, nutrition, obesity and their role in arthritis. Seminars in Arthroplasty, 18(2): 117–21.
109. van de Laar MA. van der Korst JK. (1992) Food intolerance in rheumatoid arthritis. I. A double blind, controlled trial of the clinical effects of elimination of milk allergens and azo dyes. Annals of the Rheumatic Diseases, 51(3): 298–302.
110. Meltzer LJ. Logan DE. Mindell JA. (2005) Sleep patterns in female adolescents with chronic musculoskeletal pain. Behavioural Sleep Medicine, 3(4): 193–208.
111. Okura K et al (2008) Comparison of sleep variables between chronic widespread musculoskeletal pain, insomnia, periodic leg movements syndrome and control subjects in a clinical sleep medicine practice. Sleep Medicine, 9(4): 352–61.
112. Cassisi G et al (2008) Symptoms and signs in fibromyalgia syndrome. Reumatismo, 60(Suppl 1): S15–24.
113. Magee DJ. (2007) Orthopedic physical assessment. 5th ed. Philadelphia: Elsevier.
114. Campbell SE. Adler R. Sofka CM. (2005) Ultrasound of muscle abnormalities. Ultrasound Quarterly, 21(2): 87–94.
115. Hansson P. Backonja M. Bouhassira D. (2007) Usefulness and limitations of quantitative sensory testing: clinical and research application in neuropathic pain states. Pain, 129(3): 256–9.

# 4
# Diagnosis

## Chapter overview

Clinical diagnoses play a pivotal role in the DeFCAM, but, more importantly, help to improve client outcomes by informing CAM practitioners about the potential cause of a presenting condition, as well as an appropriate course of treatment. In order to formulate plausible diagnoses a clinician needs to understand the process of diagnostic reasoning, including knowledge of the many reasoning styles that can guide clinical judgement. Given that many of these reasoning approaches are complex and often difficult to comprehend, and furthermore, lack relevance to CAM practice, there is clearly a demand for a CAM diagnostic reasoning approach. Details of this approach and the associated formation of CAM diagnoses are described in further detail throughout this chapter.

## Learning objectives

The content of this chapter will assist the reader to:
- understand the purpose of clinical diagnosis
- recognise the factors that affect diagnostic accuracy
- outline the process of deductive and inductive reasoning
- identify the range of diagnostic reasoning models used in clinical practice
- describe the CAM diagnostic reasoning approach
- recognise the purpose, structure and components of CAM diagnoses.

## Chapter outline

- Introduction
- Defining diagnosis
- Rationale for diagnosis
- Factors affecting diagnostic accuracy
- The process of diagnostic reasoning
- CAM diagnostic reasoning process
- CAM diagnosis
- Summary

## Introduction

A diverse range of clinicians practise CAM across the globe, each with varying levels of education and disparate methods of practice. While noticeable differences in service delivery are expected between CAM disciplines, there is no reason why CAM practitioners cannot practise consistently within each specialisation. A method to improve practice consistency within the field of CAM is DeFCAM (in particular, the application of diagnostic reasoning and the formulation of CAM diagnoses). The purpose and rationale for using CAM diagnoses in clinical practice is elucidated throughout this chapter, followed by examples of how these diagnoses can be structured and documented in order to ameliorate client care, enhance clinical outcomes and facilitate the professionalisation of CAM. First though, it is important to understand what the term 'diagnosis' represents.

## Defining diagnosis

A diagnosis is a statement that identifies the nature or cause of a given phenomenon.[1] What this definition highlights is that diagnosis is not a term limited to the healthcare sector, but a phrase used in any industry, including the automotive, engineering and computing sectors. One factor distinguishing a diagnosis made by a health professional to one formulated by a non-health-related discipline is the human element. Even though this element is shared by the health occupations, each healthcare profession interprets diagnosis differently. A medical diagnosis, for instance, is the identification of a specific disease or pathological condition based on a presenting pattern of signs and symptoms. By contrast, a nursing diagnosis is a statement that defines a human response to an actual or potential health problem that nurses can recognise and treat. A nutrition diagnosis is a 'food and nutrition professional's identification and labelling of an existing nutrition problem that the food and nutrition professional is responsible for treating independently'.[2] The key point that emerges from each of these definitions is that diagnoses are profession-specific, that is, each profession has a particular knowledge base and skill set to competently formulate and treat specific types of diagnoses. In other words, while a nurse may be qualified to generate and treat nursing diagnoses, in most cases they would not be able to competently formulate or treat nutritional or medical diagnoses. Put simply, nurses make nursing diagnoses, dieticians make nutrition diagnoses.

So what does this mean for CAM practitioners? What this suggests is that although CAM practitioners may possess the knowledge and skills to interpret medical, nursing or nutrition diagnoses (understand, for example, what diabetes mellitus, fluid volume deficit or energy deficit represents), they are only qualified to make CAM diagnoses that fall within the scope of their practice. Given that 'CAM diagnosis' is a relatively new term, the phrase warrants a definition. A CAM diagnosis is defined as a client-centred statement that identifies an actual or potential health problem and the aetiology of the condition that CAM practitioners can formulate and treat.

## Rationale for diagnosis

There are many arguments for and against the formulation of clinical diagnoses. One opposing viewpoint is that medical diagnoses inappropriately label clients, creating a state in which the condition defines the individual, such as 'the asthmatic' or 'the arthritic'. The negative connotations associated with the label may, as a result, adversely affect the psychological wellbeing of a client and dampen an individual's motivation towards improving health. Another concern that may have adverse, even fatal, consequences for the client is the formulation of premature or incorrect diagnoses. In this situation a misdiagnosis can direct a CAM practitioner towards an unsuitable course of treatment that could not only unnecessarily delay client progress, but potentially worsen the individual's state of health. If, for example, a client presenting with cephalgia is treated for tension headache, but in fact has an intracranial lesion, then the lesion may go unchecked for some time. This could have significant repercussions for the client in terms of quality and duration of life.

From an affirmative position, clinical diagnoses may help to focus a practitioner's attention towards the cause of a client complaint. This argument supports one of the philosophical principles of CAM, that is, addressing the aetiology of the presenting condition. Through a better understanding of the cause of an illness, a clinical diagnosis can assist the clinician to create a more specific and pertinent treatment plan and, in effect, hasten the attainment of positive client outcomes. The treatment approach for an individual presenting with general fatigue, for instance, would be comparatively less specific, less individualised and potentially less effective than a plan for a client diagnosed with hypothyroidism and, as such, would inevitably hinder clinical progress. As well as the benefits to the client and CAM practitioner, clinical diagnoses can also help to improve interprofessional communication by providing a common language that is understood by most CAM and orthodox practitioners.

## Factors affecting diagnostic accuracy

Other than the benefits mentioned above, clinical diagnosis also provides a clear and transparent link between assessment and treatment. It is not surprising, therefore, that misdiagnosis can lead to delayed or inappropriate clinical management and/or unnecessary disease progression that result in an increased risk of client morbidity and/or mortality. Even though the rate of misdiagnosis is uncertain in most countries due to the paucity of valid and reliable data, a German study of 100 randomly selected patients who died in hospital in 1999–2000 sheds some light; it reported a rate of misdiagnosis of eleven per cent.[3] The global impact of misdiagnosis on all-cause morbidity and mortality has also been poorly investigated, although the social consequences are somewhat clearer, with more than twenty-one per cent of new public and private sector medical indemnity claims made in Australia in 2005–06 attributed to diagnostic error.[4] Recognising and addressing the many determinants of diagnostic accuracy may help to minimise the risk of adverse events, as well as the subsequent risk of litigation against CAM practitioners.

Several intrinsic and extrinsic factors can influence diagnostic accuracy. These variables fall into one of five categories, including professional, environmental, personal, intellectual and client elements. In relation to professional factors, these include codes of practice, legal and ethical forces, and scope of practice. A clinician who practises outside their scope of practice, for example, may not have the necessary skills, resources or competency to either detect or accurately diagnose certain conditions. This could, in effect, increase a client's risk of harm.

Personal factors relate to practitioner self-confidence, beliefs, preferences, stress coping strategies and short-term memory capacity.[5] The effect on clinical performance of alcohol, illicit drugs and/or excessive fatigue is a good case in point. A practitioner directly affected by these elements may, for instance, have difficulty retaining and processing information, which could lead to higher rates of diagnostic error and potentially delay client progress.

Another important intrinsic factor is intellectual attributes. This component incorporates critical thinking skills, experience, content knowledge, use of evidence-based practice and diagnostic skills. A practitioner who lacks any one of these attributes could, in all likelihood, have difficulty collecting pertinent information, recognising pathognomonic clusters of data and/or formulating differential diagnoses, which could result in misdiagnosis.

Among the extrinsic influences of diagnostic accuracy are the environmental elements. These refer to the availability of diagnostic resources, type of clinical setting, time constraints and interruptions or distractions. Resource access is a particular concern for most CAM practitioners, as many do not have access to subsidised investigations or have the skills or competencies required to perform these tests (at least not in Australia). Without access to certain investigations, or access to clinicians who have the capacity to perform these tests, some practitioners may have difficulty in establishing a diagnosis or determining the possible causes of the presenting complaint.

Client-derived factors encompass elements such as client compliance, cognitive or intellectual capacity, health literacy, income and ability to communicate. All of these factors, with the exception of income, affect the quality of interpersonal communication, which in turn influences the quality of the assessment and, consequently, the accuracy of the diagnosis. Since many of these intrinsic and extrinsic factors are modifiable, CAM practitioners have the capacity to significantly improve diagnostic accuracy and client outcomes through the adoption of relatively straightforward measures, such as further education, reflective practice and interprofessional collaboration.

Adding to these factors are a number of elements that may further increase the risk of misdiagnosis in CAM practice, determinants that include limited access to diagnostic tools, variability of professional educational standards and limited interprofessional communication.[6] The effect of training and education on diagnostic competency, in particular, has been recently highlighted in a survey of 617 Australian CAM practitioners. The study found that most clinicians used Western and CAM diagnostic techniques that they had received training in, except for the interpretation of pathological and radiological tests, of which one-third of practitioners had not received any training, even though they interpreted these tests in clinical practice.[7] This is of concern, as adequate training is needed to develop sufficient competency in diagnostic skills[8] in order to reduce the risk of misinterpretation and misdiagnosis.

Training in a variety of diagnostic tests has also been shown to be positively related to practitioner confidence in identifying clients requiring referral ($p<0.05$),[7] which again highlights the probable association between inadequate education and increased risk of client harm. Thus, given that thirty-four per cent of patients were reported by Grace et al[7] to have occasionally or never been assessed by a doctor prior to a CAM consultation, and that many CAM practitioners may not have the necessary skills, tools, confidence or competency to accurately diagnose or refer, suggests that some groups of clients may be at greater risk of being misdiagnosed and of receiving delayed or inappropriate treatment.

## The process of diagnostic reasoning

Diagnostic reasoning, which is a 'dynamic thinking process that … leads to a diagnosis that best explains the symptoms and clinical evidence in a given clinical situation',[9] may help clinicians to bridge the gap between assessment and diagnosis. Given that assessment and diagnosis are closely linked, however, with both steps informing each other, it is important to acknowledge that diagnostic reasoning is not a process limited to the third phase of DeFCAM, but it is another essential component of clinical assessment.

Guiding CAM practitioners through the process of diagnostic reasoning needs to take into account a number of important elements. Experience, for instance, is one factor that can influence the adopted style of diagnostic reasoning, as well as the quality of client outcomes. Even so, expertise takes time to acquire and, depending on the opportunities that present to the practitioner, experience may not necessarily lead to the development of an effective or efficient reasoning process. This is because a theoretical foundation needs to inform the process. Therefore, a factor that may greatly improve the outcomes of diagnostic reasoning, and one that does not discriminate between novice and expert clinicians, is the adoption of an appropriate critical thinking framework.

Apart from assisting CAM practitioners to better understand how healthcare professionals with different levels of expertise formulate clinical diagnoses, diagnostic reasoning models enable practitioners to recognise how to acquire, combine and process information to improve diagnostic accuracy,[10,11] and thereby to solve clinical problems. In fact, Groves et al[11] have shown that clinicians who follow a clear and streamlined diagnostic reasoning process and who interpret data correctly demonstrate greater diagnostic accuracy than practitioners who adopt a less efficient reasoning approach. The vast number of diagnostic reasoning models available to educators and practitioners of CAM (Table 4.1), as well as the frequent use of jargon within these frameworks, may make the selection of an appropriate model difficult.

| **Table 4.1:** Examples of diagnostic reasoning models | |
|---|---|
| Bowen (2006) process[12] | Data acquisition, problem representation, hypothesis generation, illness script selection, and final diagnosis |
| Clinical reasoning process (Groves et al 2003)[11] | Identify relevant information, data interpretation, data integration, hypothesis generation, hypothesis testing, and working diagnosis |
| Clinical thinking process (Bates 1995)[13] | Identify abnormal findings, cluster data, localise findings, interpret data, generate hypotheses, test hypotheses, and define problem |
| Diagnostic strategy (Murtagh 2007)[14] | Determine probability diagnosis, potentially serious disorders, possible pitfalls, masquerading conditions, and patient hidden agendas |
| Hermeneutical model (Ritter 2003)[15] | Pattern recognition, similarity recognition, common-sense understanding, skilled know-how, senses of salience, deliberative rationality, data gathering, and cue interpretation |
| Hypothesis-driven strategy (Szaflarski 1997)[16] | Problem identification, hypothesis generation, hypothesis evaluation, hypothesis analysis, hypothesis assembly, and final diagnosis |
| Information processing model (Ritter 2003)[15] | Data collection, further cue acquisition, formulation of possible solutions, problem identification, hypothesis generation, cue interpretation, and hypothesis evaluation |
| Nagelkerk (2001) process[17] | Formulate competing diagnoses, order diagnostics, and select a diagnosis |
| Nursing diagnostic model (Perry 2008)[18] | Data validation, data clustering, data interpretation, identification of client needs, and formulation of nursing diagnosis |
| Participative decision-making model (Ballard-Reisch 1990)[19] | The diagnostic phase of the model consists of two stages – information gathering, and information interpretation |
| Zunkel et al (2004) model[9] | Data collection, data synthesis, and hypothesis formation |

In order to simplify matters, diagnostic reasoning frameworks can be categorised into two main styles, that is, models based on inductive or deductive reasoning. Inductive reasoning, which guides the Hermeneutical, nursing diagnostic and Zunkel et al[9] models, is a bottom-up reasoning approach by which specific data are developed into generalisations. As illustrated in Figure 4.1, the approach refers to the processing of specific symptoms and observations acquired during clinical assessment into meaningful clusters of information. These clusters are then continuously grouped into larger and more meaningful chunks of data until an appropriate diagnosis or range of differential diagnoses are generated. In clinical terms, this style of reasoning may progress as follows: succeeding the completion of a client assessment, specific symptoms such as pyrexia and malaise can be clustered together to represent any number of infectious or oncological disorders. When another cluster of data is added to the equation, such as dysuria and increased urine odour, the new chunk of information portrays greater meaning. In this example, the two clusters of data suggest that a urological condition may be present. Additional information from a urinalysis and urine culture can then be used to either support or dismiss a diagnosis of symptomatic bacteriuria.

Deductive reasoning is by contrast a top-down method of reasoning whereby generalisations are narrowed down to specific conclusions, as illustrated in Figure 4.2. Models informed by deductive reasoning include the Murtagh[14] diagnostic strategy, hypothesis-driven strategy and Nagelkerk[17] process (see Table 4.1). When using this style of reasoning, a clinician formulates one or more hypotheses, or tentative diagnoses, and through critical enquiry – 'if–then' statements and emerging clinical data – tests whether the proposed diagnoses are probable or unlikely. This process of enquiry and the acquisition of additional data continues until a single plausible diagnosis is generated. The clinical application of deductive reasoning is exemplified as follows: a clinician assessing a client with fatigue may construct a range of hypotheses, including malnutrition, hypothyroidism and anaemia. The absence of pallor and shortness of breath, as well as a normal haemoglobin level, would eliminate anaemia as a possible diagnosis. Likewise, the consumption of a well-balanced, nutrient-dense diet, together with a normal comprehensive digestive stool analysis, would reduce the likelihood of malnutrition. The elimination of these alternative

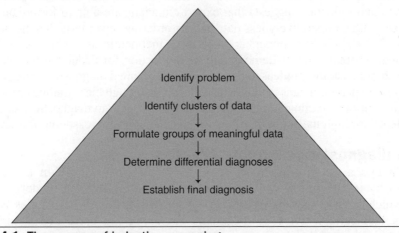

**Figure 4.1:** The process of inductive reasoning

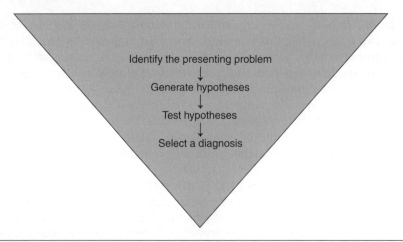

**Figure 4.2:** The process of deductive reasoning

hypotheses and the presence of weight gain, depression and an elevated level of serum thyroid-stimulating hormone would point towards hypothyroidism as a highly probable diagnosis.

Some models, such as the clinical reasoning process, information processing model and clinical thinking process (see Table 4.1), use a mixed inductive–deductive reasoning approach. In these models, inductive reasoning is used to formulate differential diagnoses, from which a specific diagnosis is generated through deductive reasoning. Different variations to this approach are also evident.

As previously discussed, there are numerous deductive and inductive reasoning models that can potentially guide CAM practitioners through the process of diagnostic reasoning. However, there are noticeable inter- and intraprofessional differences in the types of models adopted in clinical practice. One of the key determinants of reasoning style is a clinician's level of expertise.

Many studies have explored the diagnostic reasoning styles of novice and expert clinicians, with medical students, dentists, medical specialists and nurses being the few professional groups examined. What these studies reveal is that there are distinct differences in the way novice and expert clinicians acquire, organise, process and interpret data. Evidence suggests that expert clinicians are able to formulate correct diagnoses with comparatively less data and by ordering fewer tests than novice practitioners.[20,21] Expert practitioners are also more inclined to use inductive or forward reasoning, whereas novices demonstrate a predilection for deductive reasoning.[15,16] Improved organisation of ideas and evidence of a planned diagnostic strategy further distinguish expert clinicians from novices.[20,21] Even though these findings may be discouraging for novice clinicians, it is possible that the path to diagnostic success may be hastened through the adoption of an organised diagnostic reasoning framework.

## CAM diagnostic reasoning process

Even though a CAM practitioner may derive a conclusion about a presenting problem by using one of many structured diagnostic reasoning models, it is not clear which process may be best suited to CAM practice. What studies do highlight is that certain styles of diagnostic reasoning are correlated with greater diagnostic accuracy.[21,22] In fact, after examining the clinical reasoning styles of twenty final-year 'clinical clerks' and twenty expert gastroenterologists, Coderre et al[22] found the odds of diagnostic success when using inductive reasoning were 5.1 times greater (p<0.0001) than the odds of success with deductive reasoning, which was independent of expertise and clinical presentation. Comparable findings from a study examining the diagnostic reasoning approaches of beginner, competent and expert dentists[21] adds to this body of evidence.

Even though there is some indication that frameworks adopting an inductive reasoning style may be most beneficial for clients and practitioners, and therefore to CAM practice, some of these models are poorly defined and, furthermore, make an assumption that practitioners already possess adequate skills in diagnostic reasoning. Hence, some of these models may not be useful to novice clinicians. Many existing frameworks also fail to take into consideration the myriad factors that influence CAM practitioner reasoning, including CAM philosophy, experience, skill, knowledge, intuition, the clinical environment, and client–clinician culture, beliefs, values and preferences. Another legitimate concern is that the process of diagnostic reasoning has been oversimplified in studies to date, as the style of reasoning used in clinical practice is likely to vary according to the complexity of the problem and the level of practitioner expertise.[10] In some cases, multiple reasoning processes may be used simultaneously.[15] A diagnostic reasoning model that uses a mixed inductive–deductive approach with a predominant focus on inductive reasoning that is also descriptive, user-friendly and applicable to CAM practitioners with diverse levels of expertise is needed. It is for these reasons that the CAM diagnostic reasoning approach was developed.

The CAM diagnostic reasoning approach consists of a central eight-stage inductive reasoning framework that sits alongside a three-phase deductive reasoning process. Informing the model (in no particular sequence) are six key influential factors of diagnostic reasoning, which are illustrated in Figure 4.3. Though the model appears to follow clinical assessment and precede the planning phase of DeFCAM, it needs to be acknowledged that the model is an integral component of clinical assessment, and thus both the assessment and diagnostic phases of DeF-CAM should be viewed as interlinked, with assessment informing diagnosis and vice versa.

The first stage of the diagnostic reasoning approach is the identification of a presenting problem or problems, such as cough or pyrexia. A fundamental requirement of this step is to ensure that the problem is reported from a client's perspective, not only because of the need to maintain a client-centred approach, but also because the identified problem is a pivotal component of CAM diagnoses, as highlighted later in this chapter.

Once a problem has been clearly identified, all aetiological factors that may potentially contribute to the development of the problem need to be considered to ensure that the key principle of CAM is not overlooked, that is, the cause of the complaint needs to be addressed. Given the nature of some complaints this list may be considerably large and may include a combination of nutritional, lifestyle, environmental, physiological, infectious, energetic, structural, psychogenic, iatrogenic and/or metabolic causes, to name but a few. It is also at this turning point in the process where a practitioner may either continue to follow an inductive reasoning approach, choose to follow a deductive reasoning style and generate hypotheses, or adopt a mixed inductive–deductive reasoning style.

If a clinician decides to follow a path of deductive reasoning, they will continue to gather additional data in order to support or refute hypotheses until a final plausible diagnosis can be established. A CAM practitioner may then validate the selected diagnosis through a final evaluation of clinical data. If an inductive reasoning approach is followed, a clinician would need to gather enough information from the health history so that clusters of meaningful data can be generated. At this stage, a clinician would group together different combinations of often unconnected signs and symptoms to form clusters of information that may be indicative of different pathological states. Cough and pyrexia, for example, when clustered together can indicate the presence of a respiratory tract infection, yet, when cough and heartburn are grouped together, this may be suggestive of gastro-oesophageal reflux disease. These clusters of information can then be ranked according to conditions that are 'most probable', 'possible' and 'unlikely'. The collection of additional data from the physical assessment, and pathological, functional or radiological tests, and the generation of much larger chunks of information, enables the clinician to then formulate and rank a number of differential CAM diagnoses. Acquiring pertinent data to support or refute these diagnoses and integrating these findings with previously collected information enables the practitioner to isolate the most plausible CAM diagnosis.

## CAM diagnosis

As highlighted earlier in this chapter, CAM diagnoses are client-centred statements that isolate actual or potential health problems and the aetiology of the problems that CAM practitioners can construct and manage. It is important that clinicians understand the structure and purpose of these statements, as they form an integral part of the CAM diagnostic reasoning approach. In order to appreciate the configuration

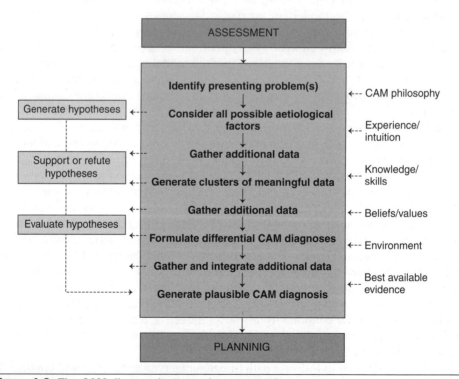

**Figure 4.3:** The CAM diagnostic reasoning approach

of CAM diagnoses, it is useful to first examine the formula of other structured, profession-specific diagnoses, such as those used in nursing and dietetics.

Nursing diagnoses are three-part statements that consist of a possible, potential or actual problem, an aetiology and defining characteristics. For an individual with dehydration, a nurse may formulate the following nursing diagnosis: fluid volume deficit, related to vomiting and diarrhoea, manifested by poor skin turgor and increased pulse rate. Not dissimilar to nursing diagnoses are nutrition diagnoses, which also consist of a three-part statement, including an altered, impaired, ineffective, risk of, increased, decreased, acute or chronic problem, an aetiology and associated signs and symptoms.[23] An example of a nutrition diagnosis is as follows: decreased energy intake related to anorexia, as evidenced by a BMI of 17.4 $kg/m^2$ and a daily energy intake 4000 kJ less than recommended for age, gender and activity level. A key benefit of both of these approaches is that they help the clinician to focus on the cause of the presenting problem, which is compatible with the principles of CAM practice; in particular, the need to attend to the underlying aetiology of the condition.

One of the limitations of nursing and nutrition diagnoses that are not congruent with the principles of CAM practice is the problem statement. The fundamental issue with these statements is that they are clinician-centred, in that they serve to meet the wants of the practitioner over the needs of the client. Although a practitioner-centred approach, such as increasing fluid intake to address a fluid volume deficit, is likely to make a clinician's decision about treatment easier, this approach detracts from what the client perceives as being most important to them, for example, the vomiting and diarrhoea. Given that individuals who perceive their care to be client-centred demonstrate comparatively better clinical outcomes and require fewer diagnostic tests and referrals than those who perceive their care not to be client-centred[24] provides some justification for the need to adopt a client-centred approach. Other benefits, such as increased client responsibility, treatment satisfaction, quality of life and treatment compliance,[25] add further support to the argument for client-centred care. One way to reinforce a client-centred approach in CAM practice is through clinical language, documentation and decision making, which DeFCAM and CAM diagnoses facilitate.

The development of CAM diagnoses emerged from a need to improve communication and documentation in CAM practice, as well as to improve efficiency, transparency and consistency of care. The need to improve client outcomes and to foster the professionalisation of CAM while remaining cognisant of the core principles of CAM (i.e. identifying the underlying cause of the presenting condition, preventing illness), provided further justification for the creation of CAM diagnoses. In order to meet these needs CAM diagnoses had to be clear, concise, objective, accurate and specific (see Table 4.2). These statements also needed to integrate the benefits of nursing and nutrition diagnoses noted above, yet had to be client-centred and relevant to CAM practice. The four-part structure of CAM diagnoses that has emerged is as follows.

Client-centred problem … (qualifier) … *secondary to* (secondary cause(s)) … *related to* (primary cause(s))

At the forefront of the CAM diagnosis is the client-centred problem, which is not only an integral part of the diagnostic reasoning process, but also helps to define the outcome measures of the planning and evaluation stages of client care. It is imperative then that a client identifies this problem as their most important concern because the problem identified will have major implications for the overall plan of care. A qualifier should accompany this problem in order to identify whether the complaint is actual or potential. This part of the CAM diagnosis enables practitioners to be more transparent and explicit about their involvement in preventative healthcare, which again supports the principles of CAM practice. The second half of the diagnosis focuses on the causes of the client's complaint. The first of these are the secondary causes. This component identifies the medical diagnosis (e.g. diabetes mellitus, hypothyroidism, osteoarthritis), which serves to improve interprofessional communication, as well as understanding of the pathophysiological basis of the presenting complaint. The factors that are most likely to contribute to the development of the medical diagnosis and client problem are then recorded as primary causes (e.g. nutritional deficiency, vertebral subluxation, excess yang, kapha imbalance). These causes are expected to vary within and between professions due to differences in practitioner knowledge, skill, expertise, beliefs, resources, philosophy and diagnostic approaches. Specific examples of CAM diagnoses that may be observed in CAM practice are listed in Table 4.3.

| Table 4.2: Essential requirements of a CAM diagnosis | |
|---|---|
| Accurate | Clear |
| Client-centred | Concise |
| Derived from assessment data | Integrates the biomedical perspective |
| Mindful of CAM principles | Objective |
| Rules out alternative diagnoses | Specific |

**Table 4.3: Examples of CAM diagnoses**[*]

**ACNE (actual)**, *related to* altered immune function, endocrine imbalance, high glycaemic load diet, nutritional imbalance, pitta imbalance, poor hygiene practices.

**ANXIETY (actual)**, *related to* emotional stress, excess yang, life-changing event, hyperthyroidism, lactic acidosis, nutritional imbalance.

**ARTHRALGIA (actual)**, *secondary to* osteoarthritis, *related to* elevated proteolytic enzyme activity, impaired cartilage formation, increased proinflammatory cytokine levels, joint misalignment, poor posture.

**COLON CANCER (potential)**, *related to* cigarette smoking, inadequate frequency or duration of physical activity, inflammatory bowel disease, insufficient fibre intake, obesity.

**CONSTIPATION (actual)**, *related to* chronic yin xu, decreased mobility, inadequate water intake, insufficient fibre intake, laxative abuse.

**CORONARY HEART DISEASE (potential)**, *related to* cigarette smoking, hypercholesterolaemia, hypertension, obesity, sedentary lifestyle.

**COUGH (actual)**, *secondary to* bronchitis, *related to* altered immune function, cigarette smoking, environmental irritants, excess yang, kapha imbalance, gastro-oesophageal reflux, impaired lung function.

**DIARRHOEA (actual)**, *secondary to* irritable bowel syndrome, *related to* antibiotic therapy, emotional stress, food intolerance, intestinal dysbiosis, pitta imbalance.

**DYSMENORRHOEA (actual)**, *related to* elevated oestrogen levels, elevated prostaglandin levels, emotional stress, nutritional imbalance, progesterone deficiency.

**Table 4.3:** Examples of CAM diagnoses*—*continued*

**DYSPEPSIA (actual)**, *secondary to* gastric ulceration, *related to* anti-inflammatory medication, caffeine, cigarette smoking, food intolerance, *Helicobacter pylori* infection, impaired gastric mucosal integrity, obesity, pitta imbalance.

**DYSURIA (actual)**, *secondary to* urinary tract infection, *related to* altered immune function, excess yang, impaired uroepithelial tissue integrity, inadequate water intake, poor hygiene practices, vaginal dysbiosis.

**EARACHE (actual)**, *secondary to* chronic otitis media, *related to* altered immune function, environmental allergy, food intolerance, impaired mucous membrane integrity, nutritional imbalance.

**ERECTILE DYSFUNCTION (potential)**, *related to* anxiety, neuropathy, nutritional imbalance, poor glycaemic control, vascular disease.

**FATIGUE (actual)**, *related to* altered immune function, depression, emotional stress, hypothyroidism, kapha imbalance, neurotransmitter imbalance, nutritional imbalance.

**FLAT AFFECT (actual)**, *secondary to* depression, *related to* chronic yang xu, emotional stress, hypothyroidism, insufficient sleep, life-changing event, neurotransmitter imbalance, nutritional imbalance.

**HEADACHE (actual)**, *related to* dehydration, emotional stress, food intolerance, hypertension, physical stress or trauma, poor posture, vertebral subluxation.

**HYPERCHOLESTEROLAEMIA (actual)**, *related to* cigarette smoking, excessive saturated fat consumption, obesity, oxidative stress, poor glycaemic control.

**HYPERGLYCAEMIA (potential)**, *secondary to* type 2 diabetes mellitus, *related to* high glycaemic load diet, insufficient physical activity, insulin resistance, nutritional imbalance, obesity.

**HYPERTENSION (potential)**, *related to* cigarette smoking, emotional stress, excessive sodium intake, excessive saturated fat consumption, obesity, poor glycaemic control.

**INSOMNIA (actual)**, *related to* adverse environmental conditions, anxiety, chronic yin xu, emotional stress, hormonal fluctuations, medications, melatonin deficiency, nutritional imbalance.

**LEG ULCERATION (potential)**, *secondary to* venous insufficiency, *related to* elevated proinflammatory cytokine levels, impaired capillary permeability, impaired venous integrity, increased proteolytic enzyme activity, oxidative stress.

**MYALGIA (actual)**, *secondary to* fibromyalgia, *related to* abnormal sleep pattern, deconditioned muscles, emotional stress, impaired immune function, serotonin imbalance.

**NASAL CONGESTION (actual)** *secondary to* chronic sinusitis, *related to* emotional stress, environmental allergy, food intolerance, impaired immune function, kapha imbalance, poor mucous membrane integrity.

**NAUSEA (actual)**, *related to* emotional stress, food intolerance, kapha imbalance, medication, pregnancy, vertebral subluxation.

**NEPHROPATHY (potential)**, *secondary to* type 2 diabetes mellitus, *related to* cigarette smoking, hypertension, insulin resistance, poor glycaemic control.

**NOCTURIA (actual)**, *secondary to* benign prostatic hypertrophy, *related to* chronic yang xu, elevated dihydrotestosterone, elevated oestrogen.

**OBESITY/OVERWEIGHT (actual)**, *related to* increased energy intake, decreased energy expenditure, hypothyroidism, insulin resistance, sedentary lifestyle.

**PARESTHESIAS (actual)**, *related to* heavy metal exposure, hypothyroidism, nerve entrapment, nutritional deficiency, poor glycaemic control.

**PRURITUS (actual)**, *secondary to* eczema, *related to* elevated proinflammatory cytokine levels, emotional stress, environmental irritants, food intolerance, intestinal dysbiosis.

**RETINOPATHY (potential)**, *secondary to* diabetes mellitus, *related to* cigarette smoking, dyslipidaemia, hypertension, insulin resistance, pitta imbalance, poor glycaemic control.

**RHINORRHOEA (actual)**, *secondary to* allergic rhinitis, *related to* environmental allergy, elevated proinflammatory cytokine levels, food intolerance, kapha imbalance, nutritional imbalance, poor mucous membrane integrity.

*Continued*

> **Table 4.3: Examples of CAM diagnoses*—*continued*
>
> **SKIN LESION (actual)**, *secondary to* psoriasis, *related to* bowel toxaemia, elevated proinflammatory cytokine levels, impaired liver function, incomplete protein digestion, reduced cyclic adenosine monophosphate activity.
>
> **STROKE (cerebrovascular accident) (potential)**, *related to* cigarette smoking, hypercholesterolaemia, hypertension, obesity.
>
> **TINNITUS (actual)**, *related to* anaemia, atherosclerosis, emotional stress, excessive noise exposure, medication.
>
> **URTICARIA (actual)**, *related to* contact allergy, elevated proinflammatory cytokine levels, emotional stress, food intolerance, medications.
>
> **WHEEZE (actual)**, *secondary to* asthma, *related to* environmental irritants, food intolerance, kapha imbalance, nutritional imbalance, oxidative stress, sedentary lifestyle.

*The diagnoses listed are examples only and should not be considered an exhaustive list. The phrasing of these diagnoses will also vary according to an individual's presenting complaint.

The CAM diagnostic reasoning approach and the formulation of CAM diagnoses endeavour to improve the quality of care provided by CAM practitioners. A case example of how these approaches might be implemented in clinical practice is illustrated in Box 4.1.

---

### Box 4.1: Application of the CAM diagnostic reasoning approach and the formulation of CAM diagnoses

#### Presenting case

A 27-year-old married woman presents to her CAM practitioner reporting a 6-week history of mild diarrhoea. The client has two children under the age of 5 years and works full time as a paramedic.

#### Diagnostic reasoning

#### Identify presenting problem

The problem of primary concern to the client is diarrhoea.

#### Consider all possible aetiological factors

Diarrhoea can be caused by a number of intrinsic and extrinsic factors, including iatrogenic (i.e. radiation-, antibiotic-, laxative-induced diarrhoea), infective (i.e. bacterial, viral, fungal or protozoal infection), inflammatory (i.e. ulcerative colitis, Crohn's disease), endocrine (i.e. hyperthyroidism), pancreatic (i.e. pancreatitis), gastric (i.e. dumping syndrome), psychogenic (i.e. anxiety), dietary (i.e. food intolerance), neoplastic (i.e. colon cancer) or non-specific causes (i.e. irritable bowel disease, faecal impaction, dysbiosis).

#### Gather additional data

The client reports that the loose bowel actions commenced 6 weeks ago while completing a 4-week course of amoxycillin for acute bronchitis. The bowel actions are brown, loose but non-watery, slightly malodorous and easy to pass; there are no signs of blood, mucous or fat in or on the faeces. There is increased flatus, abdominal bloating and mild and intermittent left lower quadrant (LLQ) abdominal discomfort, but no signs of nausea, vomiting, anorexia or tenesmus. The aforementioned signs are ameliorated by defaecation, yet no known exacerbating factors are identified.

The client has no known allergies or sensitivities, no surgical history and does not smoke tobacco. A cyclic history of dysmenorrhoea is reported, for which the client self-administers paracetamol with good effect. The only other medication used by the client is a daily vitamin B complex supplement. A typical daily diet for the client includes the following.

- *Breakfast*: Special K® cereal with low-fat milk.
- *Morning tea*: K-Time muffin bar®.
- *Lunch*: white salad roll with 200 mL orange juice when working, a cup of instant soup with white bread when not.
- *Afternoon tea*: Black tea with milk.
- *Dinner*: chicken burger with white roll, cottage pie, chicken Kiev with peas, potato and corn.
- *Fluid intake*: 500–750 mL diluted apple juice a day.
- *Takeaway*: twice a week, which includes battered fish and chips, or pasta.
- *Alcohol*: 2 glasses of white wine a week.

## Generate clusters of meaningful data

From the health history provided, the following clusters of meaningful data can be generated.

### Most probable conditions

- Flatus + LLQ discomfort + bloating + diarrhoea = food/lactose intolerance.
- Flatus + LLQ discomfort + bloating + diarrhoea = irritable bowel syndrome.
- Recent antibiotic use + flatus + diarrhoea = antibiotic-associated diarrhoea.
- Recent antibiotic use + LLQ discomfort + diarrhoea = antibiotic-associated colitis.

### Possible conditions

- Psychosocial demands + LLQ discomfort + diarrhoea = psychogenic diarrhoea.
- Abdominal discomfort + bloating + diarrhoea = coeliac disease.
- LLQ discomfort + diarrhoea = diverticular disease.
- Abdominal discomfort + diarrhoea = neoplasia.

### Unlikely conditions

- Dumping syndrome is unlikely as there is no history of gastric surgery.
- Inflammatory bowel disease is doubtful due to absence of blood or mucous in the faeces.
- Infective gastroenteritis is not likely as there is no nausea or vomiting.
- Faecal impaction is doubtful due to the absence of rectal pain, straining and tenesmus.

### Gather additional data

On clinical examination, the client is found to be afebrile (36.4°C), normotensive (114/64) and of normal weight (BMI = 23.8 kg/m$^2$). Body weight has remained stable for the past 12 months. Abdominal examination reveals no visible signs of scarring or herniation. The abdomen is flat, soft and non-tender, bowel sounds are normoactive and there is no percussable dullness or palpable masses. The client states that she enjoys her work and the company of her family, and does not feel noticeably stressed or anxious in these environments.

### Formulate differential CAM diagnoses

The young age of the client, and the absence of anxiety, weight loss, fever, abdominal protuberances, masses, distension, tenderness and dullness, reduces the likelihood that psychogenic diarrhoea, diverticular disease, neoplasia, inflammatory bowel disease, coeliac disease or irritable bowel syndrome are responsible. A diagnosis of irritable bowel syndrome is also inappropriate as the symptoms have been present for less than 3 months. The differential CAM diagnosis for this client is therefore: diarrhoea (actual) *related to* food intolerance, lactose intolerance, and/or intestinal dysbiosis.

### Gather and integrate additional data

To support or refute these diagnoses, further testing is required. Functional profiles, such as an intestinal permeability assessment or comprehensive digestive stool analysis may support suspicions of intestinal dysbiosis, whereas an elimination diet may determine the presence of a food intolerance. The client agrees to completing a 1-week elimination diet and food diary, and then to return for review. When she does, the elimination diet and food diary indicate that there are no dietary factors exacerbating the diarrhoea; thus, food intolerance is unlikely to be the cause of the diarrhoea.

### Generate plausible CAM diagnosis

Through the elimination of all probable and possible causes, the most plausible CAM diagnosis for this case would be

- diarrhoea (actual), *secondary to* antibiotic-associated diarrhoea, *related to* intestinal dysbiosis.

## Summary

CAM diagnoses and the CAM diagnostic reasoning approach are integral components of DeFCAM. Apart from providing a link between assessment and planning, these processes assist clinicians in identifying the aetiology of the presenting problem at the same time as maintaining a client-centred approach that is compatible with the principles of CAM. Adding to this is the capacity to improve CAM communication, documentation and clinical practice and, in effect, client outcomes. It is through the generation of plausible CAM diagnoses and the achievement of these benefits that a CAM practitioner is then able to begin to adequately prepare an individual's plan of care.

## Learning activities

1 List all extrinsic and intrinsic factors that affect your ability to formulate an accurate diagnosis. Highlight which of these determinants are modifiable and what strategies you could put in place to resolve these factors.

2 Compare and contrast the different models of diagnostic reasoning that are used in clinical practice.

3 From the following list of symptoms – abdominal discomfort, anxiety, cough, diarrhoea, dyspnoea, fatigue, fever, nausea, pallor and vomiting – match 10 separate clusters of data with 10 probable medical conditions. Nausea, vomiting and diarrhoea (a three-symptom cluster), for example, could be indicative of gastroenteritis.

4 Using the CAM diagnostic reasoning approach as a decision-making framework, describe how a presentation of fatigue could proceed into a single plausible CAM diagnosis.

5 Construct a CAM differential diagnosis for each of the following cases:
   a. a 20-year-old woman wanting to manage stress more effectively in order to prepare for a final-year university exam
   b. a 17-year-old boy complaining of pruritic psoriatic plaques to the abdomen and lower back
   c. a 43-year-old man complaining of chronic lumbago from an old workplace lifting injury
   d. a 57-year-old woman with hand stiffness and pain due to rheumatoid arthritis
   e. a 35-year-old woman with a family history of colon cancer who wishes to reduce the risk of developing the disease.

# References

1. Parker PM, editor. (2008) Webster's online dictionary. Fontainebleau: INSEAD.
2. Bueche J et al (2008) Nutrition care process and model part I: the 2008 update. Journal of the American Dietetic Association, 108(7): 1113–17.
3. Kirsch W. Shapiro F. Folsch UR. (2004) Healthcare quality: Misdiagnosis at a university hospital in five medical eras. Journal of Public Health, 12(3): 154–61.
4. Australian Institute of Health and Welfare (2007) Public and private sector medical indemnity claims in Australia 2005–06: a summary. Canberra: Australian Institute of Health and Welfare.
5. Anderson L. (1998) Exploring the diagnostic reasoning process to improve advanced physical assessments. Perspectives, 22(1): 17–22.
6. Bensoussan A et al (2006) Risks associated with the practice of naturopathy and Western herbal medicine. In: The practice and regulatory requirements of naturopathy and Western herbal medicine. Lin V et al, editors. Melbourne: School of Public Health, La Trobe University.
7. Grace S. Vemulpad S. Beirman R. (2006) Training in and use of diagnostic techniques among CAM practitioners: an Australian study. Journal of Alternative and Complementary Medicine, 12(7): 695–700.
8. Seely D. Mills E. (2006) Diagnostic accuracy among the allied health professions: commentary on Grace et al. Journal of Alternative and Complementary Medicine 12(7): 701–2.
9. Zunkel G et al (2004) Enhancing diagnostic reasoning skills in nurse practitioner students: a teaching tool. Nurse Educator, 29(4): 161–5.
10. Forde R. (1998) Competing conceptions of diagnostic reasoning: is there a way out? Theoretical Medicine and Bioethics, 19: 59–72.
11. Groves M. O'Rourke P. Alexander H. (2003) The clinical reasoning characteristics of diagnostic experts. Medical Teacher, 25(3): 308–13.
12. Bowen JL. (2006) Educational strategies to promote clinical diagnostic reasoning. New England Journal of Medicine, 355(21): 2217–25.
13. Bates B. (1995) A guide to clinical thinking. Philadelphia: JB Lippincott.
14. Murtagh J. (2007) A safe diagnostic strategy. In: General practice. 4th ed. Murtagh J, editor. Sydney: McGraw Hill Medical.
15. Ritter BJ. (2003) An analysis of expert nurse practitioners' diagnostic reasoning. Journal of the American Academy of Nurse Practitioners, 15(3): 137–41.

16. Szaflarski NL. (1997) Diagnostic reasoning in acute and critical care. AACN Clinical Issues, 8(3): 291–302.

17. Nagelkerk J. (2001) Clinical decision-making in primary care. In: Diagnostic reasoning: case analysis in primary care practice. Nagelkerk J, editor. Philadelphia: WB Saunders.

18. Perry AG. (2008) Nursing diagnosis. In: Potter and Perry's fundamentals of nursing. 3rd ed. Crisp J, Taylor C, editors. Sydney: Elsevier.

19. Ballard-Reisch DS. (1990) A model of participative decision making for physician-patient interaction. Health Communication, 2(2): 91–104.

20. Bloch R et al (2003) The role of strategy and redundancy in diagnostic reasoning. BMC Medical Education, 3(1). Accessed at <www.pubmedcentral.nih.gov/articlerender.fcgi?artid=149359>, 28 January 2009.

21. Crespo K. Torres J. Recio M. (2004) Reasoning process characteristics in the diagnostic skills of beginner, competent, and expert dentists. Journal of Dental Education, 68(12): 1235–44.

22. Coderre S et al (2003) Diagnostic reasoning strategies and diagnostic success. Medical Education, 37: 695–703.

23. Lacey K. Pritchett E. (2003) Nutrition care process and model: ADA adopts road map to quality care and outcomes management. Journal of the American Dietetic Association, 103(8): 1061–72.

24. Stewart M et al (2000) The impact of patient-centered care on outcomes. Journal of Family Practice, 49(9): 796–804.

25. Harkness J. (2005) Patient involvement: a vital principle for patient-centred healthcare. World Hospital Health Services, 41(2): 12–16, 40–3.

# 5
# Planning

## Chapter overview
Many factors contribute to the successful achievement of clinical outcomes, including client–practitioner rapport, comprehensive client assessment, accurate differential diagnoses, evidence-based care and the objective evaluation of client progress. One element that is of equal importance to these factors is the planning of client care. This chapter will highlight the importance of care planning and emphasise how the use of a clear, systematic planning framework can help to deliver a more transparent and consistent approach to client care that can greatly improve individual health and wellbeing by hastening the achievement of clinical outcomes.

## Learning objectives
The content of this chapter will assist the reader to:
· define the planning phase of client care
· state the reasons for planning client care
· outline the shortfalls of the planning process
· discuss the key criteria for setting goals
· describe the two-stage planning process.

## Chapter outline
· Introduction
· Planning defined
· Rationale for planning
· Concerns about planning
· The planning process
· Summary

## Introduction

The healthcare system is a complex bureaucracy, driven not only by policy, budgets and changing technology, but also by the needs of many key stakeholders. Some authorities argue that the existing system of healthcare is not designed to effectively meet the needs and expectations of all stakeholders, particularly the needs of consumers, and that major reform is needed.[1] The areas requiring particular attention relate to service access, efficiency, continuity of care, client participation in care and the coordination of health services.[1,2] It is argued that all of these issues could be improved through the effective planning of care, of which more individualised, participative and coordinated treatment could be delivered over universalistic, problem-based, clinician-centred care. In fact, a goal-centred model of care is more likely to facilitate an interdisciplinary, client-centred approach, unlike problem-oriented or disease-oriented care, which place greater emphasis on physician control and measures of success.[3] A client-centred approach is also more closely aligned with the core principles of CAM.

Despite the advantages of planning, it is claimed that few clinicians document clear goals in clinical practice, involve clients in the management of their care or fully understand individual concerns, beliefs and preferences. The reasons why practitioners might not engage in the planning of client care may relate to time limitations, system restraints, a lack of skill in developing client-centred goals or lack of awareness of the importance of goal setting.[1,4,5] This is not surprising given that there is a lack of explicit instruction in and consensus on the process of care planning in the literature. To address these issues, this chapter proffers a clear, systematic framework for planning client care, taking into consideration the justification and concerns about the process, with a view to delivering a consistent and unequivocal approach to care planning in CAM practice, to enhance client care, improve clinical outcomes and ameliorate clinic, team and organisational efficiency.

## Planning defined

The planning phase of client care, which immediately follows clinical assessment and CAM diagnosis but precedes treatment and client review, is a projected course of action aimed at strategically addressing a client's presenting problem. A key component of care planning is goal setting, which is fundamental in assisting the client and CAM practitioner in identifying and prioritising strategies that may prevent, reduce or resolve individual problems, or that facilitate or augment client function. These goals, or expected outcomes, also provide an endpoint towards which client care is directed by identifying a desirable psychological, social, physiological or cognitive state that is to be achieved.[6] Planning is therefore an essential part of delivering healthcare and, as such, is an integral component of DeFCAM.

## Rationale for planning

Care planning and goal setting generate several benefits for clients, CAM practitioners and institutions. Fundamentally, planning improves the organisation of client care by establishing common treatment objectives[4] that pave a path towards a desired clinical outcome.[7] These objectives provide an activity with a sense of purpose, relevance, clarity and control,[8] which in turn improve continuity of care. As demonstrated in a number of studies, continuity of care can lead to improvements in client and clinician satisfaction, clinical outcomes and reduced episodes of care.[1] Adequate planning is fundamental to improving continuity of care, as well as delivering a more consistent approach to care and, as such, would be conducive to interdisciplinary practice. The effective delivery of an integrative health service is a good case in point. If, for example, every individual practitioner in a healthcare team developed goals of care in isolation, then client care would almost certainly be fragmented and with probable overlap or omissions in care; it would be less efficient also. An integrative healthcare team that develops mutually derived goals, on the other hand, would be relatively more efficient and the care more consistent, as clinicians would be working towards common goals of care. This approach also could be associated with improvements in the coordination of client care, as well as enhanced communication between team members[1,4] (see chapter 6 for a more detailed discussion of the benefits of interdisciplinary and integrative healthcare). Thus, by directing attention towards relevant activities and away from irrelevant actions,[9] planning minimises the effect that external and internal factors have on achieving a goal by directing all efforts and resources towards a common goal.

As well as improvements in organisational efficiency, planning also ameliorates practitioner performance by motivating the clinician and integrative healthcare team to perform, by facilitating positive changes in practitioner behaviour, by increasing clinician accountability and autonomy and by rewarding the practitioner and client through the achievement of goals.[1,4,5,10–12] CAM practitioners who set goals may also experience less emotional distress and demonstrate improvements in concentration, self-confidence and self-motivation.[5] These improvements in clinician performance and morale, together with the increased level of client–practitioner interaction associated with goal setting, can significantly enhance the quality of client care.

Planning care and setting goals is particularly important in enabling the effective evaluation of clinical outcomes,[4,13] as goals provide well-defined, measurable endpoints of care. The purposeful appraisal of client goals may promptly identify delays in the achievement of expected outcomes and thus effectively determine if a treatment needs to be modified or altered to better meet client needs.[14] Other than providing assurance that client needs have been effectively met, care planning, when used in conjunction with client review, can also provide a means for evaluating the performance of clinicians,[6,15] the efficacy of selected interventions, the effect of the therapy on client outcomes and, thus, the efficiency of a clinic or institution. In other words, care planning could be used as an effective auditing or quality management tool.[15]

One clinical outcome that is positively correlated with goal attainment is quality of life. In a case series study using a within-subjects, repeated measures design, in which 47 patients with chronic fatigue syndrome were required to set three to five individualised goals for a 4-month support and education program, goal attainment was found to be the only predictor of quality of life. This was independent of sociodemographic characteristics, comorbid psychiatric diagnosis, and fatigue and symptom severity.[16] Although other confounding factors, such as available support structures, may have contributed to these findings, the positive association between goal attainment and health-related quality of life continues to be supported across several diverse client populations, including individuals post-myocardial infarction[17] and those following pelvic floor dysfunction surgery.[18]

In a community psychiatric nursing service in Sussex, the nursing process was incorporated into departmental documentation with a view to delivering a more organised service. After the integration of the nursing process, it was noted that the turnover rate of patients increased. The reason for this was that the nursing process, in particular the clearly documented treatment objectives, enabled nurses to clearly identify when a client's problem had resolved and when nursing care was no longer required. The service also observed after the integration of the process an improvement in staff morale and performance, the quality of nursing care and the professionalism of staff.[19] Although the findings of this system evaluation are anecdotal, the integration of the nursing process into perioperative assessment forms within a Cincinnati paediatric burns unit resulted in similar changes, including subjective improvements in staff satisfaction, service efficiency and client care delivery.[6]

Similar improvements in healthcare service delivery have also been observed in spinal rehabilitation, an area that is particularly relevant to practitioners of manipulative therapies. An evaluation of existing practice in a Canadian spinal cord rehabilitation centre, for instance, identified several discrepancies in clinical documentation, a lack of client participation in the planning of care, a lack of interdisciplinary action and the adoption of a discipline-driven, problem-based approach to client care following a series of semistructured interviews.[20] These concerns prompted the integration of a Donabedian structure–process–outcome goal-setting framework into all relevant client and interdisciplinary documentation. Despite initial resistance and scepticism towards the changing approach to client care, the difficulty in establishing target dates for each goal and the effort to actively involve clients in the setting and prioritisation of goals, the 12-month evaluation of the new framework (by way of team meeting audits) revealed some positive outcomes for clinicians and clients. By demonstrating a shift towards a more goal-oriented, team-driven approach to client care, staff reported an improvement in the structure and organisation of meetings, increased accountability for the documented actions aligned to each goal and greater clarity over team expectations.[20] Clients, through increased participation in the rehabilitation process, demonstrated increased accountability towards achieving goals.

Several clinical studies add further support to the positive correlation between the adoption of goal planning and improved client outcomes, including clients with knee injury,[21] cerebral palsy,[22] sports injury,[23,24] rheumatoid arthritis,[25] brain injury,[26] spinal cord injury[27] and individuals requiring dietary changes.[28,29] While these improvements occurred in orthodox clinical environments, it is envisaged that similar changes to client outcomes would occur in CAM practice, although further research in this area is needed to verify this claim.

## Concerns about planning

To this point, the careful planning of client care appears to be a simple and effective strategy that can improve healthcare outcomes. Yet not all authorities share this point of view. Some argue that planning is an innate, unconscious activity that many practitioners already perform[8] and that a prescribed planning framework is not necessary for delivering superior client care. However, it is uncertain whether this innate process of planning is administered in a systematic, rationalised and client-centred manner. Given the evidence presented above, it is unlikely that this is the case. To ensure that care is planned in a manner that is purposeful, justified and systematically administered, several key concerns need to be addressed.

The planning of care and the formulation of goals in a participatory manner require a rise in clinician workload and an increase in the time allocated to documentation.[4,27] In view of the increasing demand for CAM services,[30] the probable constraints on practitioner time and the need to deliver a financially viable service, it may be difficult for some CAM practitioners to effectively plan client care. Some clinicians may also view the planning of care as restrictive and intrusive to the therapeutic relationship,[31] though this is only likely if a paternalistic approach to goal setting, in which client collaboration and respect are not usually considered, is adopted.

A qualitative exploratory study of practising nurses across five contrasting hospital wards in Northern Ireland corroborated concerns, through the use of participant observation, focus groups and diaries, that the process of creating and maintaining care plans may be an unnecessary burden on the provision of care. One ward did view care plans favourably. Apart from the fact that care plans were more effectively integrated into practice in the exceptional ward, this positive perception of care plans may have been attributed to the different approach to care planning, where care plans were not only more individualised, but were also created by staff in collaboration with the client.[32] This participatory approach to care planning, as highlighted below, is not only pivotal in facilitating client rapport and alleviating anxiety, but in the long-term may also contribute to fewer follow-up consultations, greater patient cost savings and a more competitive health service by expediting the achievement of desired clinical outcomes. Given the time and resources that can be saved though goal setting,[31] and the many immediate and long-term benefits associated with the planning of care, it would be undesirable if goal setting were depreciated by CAM practitioners or, at worst, completely disregarded.

Planning client care in order to effectively develop mutually derived goals also requires effective communication between the client and CAM practitioner.[4] Although greater interaction between a client and clinician demands additional time, which may already be constrained, not taking the time to listen to the client and, in effect, not providing an environment that fosters rapport, may compromise the quality of a client's assessment and the accuracy of the diagnosis and, subsequently, adversely affect the outcome of the prescribed treatment.

Some authorities also argue that planning is limited by the capabilities of the individual and as a result cannot be applied to all clients. Atkinson,[31] for example, points out that individuals with acute psychotic illness, serious ill health, aphasia, cognitive or sensory impairments and clients from non-English-speaking backgrounds may not be suitable for setting mutually derived goals because client motivation and understanding are fundamental requirements for goal attainment.[33] Nevertheless, these limitations can be easily resolved through the provision of alternative and innovative communication aids and the involvement of family and significant others,[31] which provides some assurance that care is planned around client needs, capacity and preference.

## The planning process

As previously highlighted, DeFCAM provides a systematic approach to the planning and implementation of client care; however, before treatment goals can be developed and a care plan established, client problems need to be prioritised. The choice about which diagnosis to address foremost should be determined by the level of risk that the problem poses to the client, with conditions demonstrating a higher risk of harm demanding a higher priority of care.[34,35] Of course, in keeping with client-centred care, the prioritisation of problems should also take into account client preference and readiness to change. Once diagnoses have been prioritised, the most important diagnosis then can be used to formulate the goals of treatment.

According to Wright,[13] treatment goals must be SMART – **s**pecific, **m**easurable, **a**chievable, **r**ealistic and **t**ime-specific – but to achieve this, each goal must address only one problem and one outcome.[5,34,35] Even though SMART is a useful aid for setting goals, it ignores other essential criteria for goal setting, including the need for goals to be client-centred, adequately documented and mutually derived. A summary of the necessary criteria for setting goals and expected outcomes is illustrated in Figure 5.1. It is also necessary to examine some of these criteria in further detail to highlight the importance of these factors in the planning process.

To begin with, goal setting should be participative or mutually derived in that the client should be actively involved, as this is more likely to motivate the client to set higher goals and to achieve these targets.[5,33] This may be because the client is more likely to take some ownership of and responsibility towards achieving these goals.[4] This is particularly pertinent to CAM practice, as many CAM therapies demand a relatively greater degree of behavioural change from clients (i.e. dietary modification, lifestyle change, mind–body therapy) than that expected from orthodox medicine, where compliance is primarily limited to medication administration. Given that client actions are central to treatment success, it is also important that goals are client-centred, individualised and written from the client's perspective, not from the clinician's standpoint, so that goals are meaningful and relevant to the client.[15] A comparison between client-centred goals and practitioner-centred goals is illustrated in Table 5.1.

A participative approach to care planning provides some assurance that goals are achievable and realistic for the client, although studies comparing practitioner-assigned

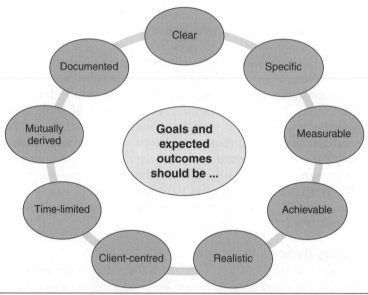

**Figure 5.1:** Essential criteria for setting goals and expected outcomes

| Table 5.1: Comparing client-centred goals with practitioner-centred goals | | |
|---|---|---|
| **CAM diagnosis** | **Client-centred goal** | **Practitioner-centred goal** |
| **ADL dependence (actual), secondary to rheumatoid arthritis**… | The client will demonstrate greater independence with ADLs. | Joint pain will be adequately controlled. |
| **Dysuria (actual), secondary to symptomatic bacteriuria**… | The client will be free from dysuria. | Bacteriuria will be absent. |
| **Flat affect (actual), secondary to hypothyroidism**… | The client will report an improvement in affect. | Serum thyroxine levels will remain within normal range. |
| **Poor exercise tolerance (actual), secondary to asthma**… | The client will report an improvement in exercise tolerance. | Peak expiratory flow rate will be maintained within the age-adjusted range. |
| **Lethargy (actual) secondary to type 2 diabetes mellitus**… | The client will be less lethargic. | Glycosylated haemoglobin (HbA1c) will be under 7.0%. |

Note: ADL = activities of daily living

goals with participative-set goals in the 1970s and 1980s have yielded inconsistent results in relation to client performance.[9,36] Factors contributing to these disparate findings may relate to variations in study duration, settings, interventions, degree of participant input and level of subject support and follow-up. More recent findings are beginning to shift the scales of evidence in favour of a client-centred approach.

In one poorly defined study of 27 patients with urinary incontinence, patients who were actively involved in the setting of their treatment goals were more likely to report successful outcomes.[37] Another qualitative study, which interviewed 18 neurological rehabilitation patients, discovered that collaborative goal setting may also increase client motivation, perceptions of control and freedom in decision making.[37,38] While some may argue that these qualitative studies are unable to establish a cause and effect relationship between goal setting and clinical outcomes, findings from well-designed controlled studies can.

Adding support to these studies are findings from a randomised controlled trial of 77 rehabilitation patients that found participative goal setting, when compared to physiotherapist-directed care, resulted in higher ratings on quality of care scales and better clinical outcomes for range of motion, strength and balance at discharge.[39] Evidence indicates, then, that a more paternalistic approach to care planning may attenuate the progression towards goal-attainment, reduce individual autonomy and promote a sense of helplessness among clients.[10]

Despite the rationale for adopting a participative approach to goal setting, studies indicate that some clinicians may still be using a paternalistic approach. In a postal survey of 202 representative members of the British society of rehabilitation medicine, for example, only forty-two per cent of respondents indicated that they used a participative approach to goal setting, less than forty per cent fully involved patients in the setting of goals and less than thirty per cent involved patients in the evaluation of set goals.[40] The authors claimed that this paternalistic approach may have stemmed from a lack of resources and to insufficient practitioner skill and knowledge of effective goal setting. Some clinicians may have also believed that they were acting in the person's best interests when setting goals without client input, but several studies across different populations indicate that there is significant disagreement between treatment goals set by practitioners and those set by clients and family members.[41,42] It is likely that many clinicians will benefit from being informed about the process and outcomes of effective care planning and the need to involve clients in goal setting. A list of potential questions that could facilitate the identification of client-centred goals and further CAM practitioner progress through the planning process is listed in Table 5.2.

Apart from being client-centred, goals should also be clear and specific, as this is likely to eliminate confusion and potential misinterpretation among clients and CAM practitioners. It is also important that goals are measurable, as this is necessary in determining whether the client has achieved or is working towards their goal and to what extent the client has progressed towards this defined endpoint. In addition to being clear, specific and measurable, goals should also be time-limited or date-stamped. These dates (dd/mm/yyyy), which generally reflect the date of the next appointment, provide motivation for the client and clinician to work towards the goal,[13] reduce ambiguity about the achievement of an expected outcome[5,9] and identify when further intervention is needed.

Treatment goals must also take into consideration the cost of treatment, available resources, staffing, client age, environment, values, beliefs, culture and social status, and the cognitive, physical and emotional capacity of the client.[31,43] If, for example,

> **Table 5.2:** Questions to assist clients and CAM practitioners in identifying appropriate treatment goals
>
> **Overall concerns**
> - What are your main health concerns at present?
> - Which of these issues concerns you the most? Why?
> - How does this health concern affect you physically, socially, emotionally and financially?
> - How would you like to see this health concern improve over the next few days, weeks or months?
>
> **Presenting condition**
> - In relation to your presenting condition, what is your main concern? Why?
> - How does this health concern affect you physically, socially, emotionally and financially?
> - How would you like to see this health concern improve in the short term and in the long term?

an individual does not have the functional capacity to perform key tasks, is not motivated or ready to try a new treatment, cannot afford to purchase the treatment or does not accept or understand the existence or consequences of their illness, they are less likely to achieve their treatment goal. Put simply, goals should be achievable in that available resources, practitioner skill and client ability and desire should enable the target to be achieved.

Effective assimilation of these criteria into the planning of client care can be facilitated using the following two-stage process. The first step of this process involves the construction of general goals that are the overall desired outcomes of care,[7] taking into account the factors that can influence treatment success, yet not explicitly stating how the goals will be achieved. These general goals can be centred around the following themes: safety, independence, social and family relationships, personal health (including physical, emotional, mental and spiritual), economic stability and autonomy.[7] An example of a general goal for a client with impaired mobility secondary to osteoarthritis may be that 'The client will walk independently without mobility aids'.

The second step of the planning process is the expected outcomes, or explicit goals. These outcomes direct clinical care by specifically indicating how and when the general goals of treatment might be achieved. As illustrated in several studies to date,[44,45] it is important that long-term and short-term outcomes are included, as long-term objectives alone are less likely to lead to improved clinical outcomes. An episode of care is therefore likely to encompass multiple goals and expected outcomes, with many of these endpoints emerging and resolving at different points in time.

As do goals, expected outcomes should also be client-centred so that endpoints remain pertinent to individual needs. To achieve client-centredness, expected outcomes need to be directly related to the presenting complaint and planned goals. These endpoints also need to focus on addressing the goals of care. To ensure that outcomes can be effectively evaluated, endpoints also need to be measurable, time-limited and include a client behaviour and criterion of acceptable behaviour.[46] An example of an expected outcome for an individual with dehydration is as follows: 'The client (client-centred) will drink (behaviour) 1500 mL of water a day (realistic, measurable criterion) by dd/mm/yyyy (time-limited)'. Further examples of the two-stage planning process, in particular how goals and expected outcomes interface with CAM diagnoses, are presented in Table 5.3.

**Table 5.3:** Examples of the two-stage planning process, including a general goal and expected outcomes (EO)

### Acne

| | |
|---|---|
| CAM diagnosis | Acne (actual), *related to* altered immune-function, high glycaemic load diet and nutritional imbalance |
| Goal | Client will be free from acneiform lesions |
| EO | 1 Client will demonstrate a 50% decrease in the number of acneiform lesions by dd/mm/yyyy.<br>2 Client will exhibit a 50% reduction in the severity of acneiform lesions by dd/mm/yyyy (as measured by the proportion of inflamed lesions to total number of lesions). |

### Arthralgia

| | |
|---|---|
| CAM diagnosis | Arthralgia (actual), *secondary to* osteoarthritis, *related to* elevated proteolytic enzyme activity, impaired cartilage formation and increased proinflammatory cytokine levels |
| Goal | Client will experience an improvement in joint pain |
| EO | 1 Client will report a 50% reduction in the severity of joint pain by dd/mm/yyyy (as measured by numerical pain score).<br>2 Client will demonstrate a 50% decrease in the frequency of joint pain by dd/mm/yyyy (as measured by symptom diary). |

### Cerebrovascular accident (CVA)

| | |
|---|---|
| CAM diagnosis | Cerebrovascular accident (potential), *related to* hypercholesterolaemia and hypertension |
| Goal | Client will not experience a cerebrovascular accident (CVA) |
| EO | 1 Client will not demonstrate any signs of transient ischaemic attack (TIA) over the next 12 months (by dd/mm/yyyy).<br>2 Client's resting blood pressure will fall below 130/80 mmHg by dd/mm/yyyy.<br>3 Client's fasting total cholesterol level will drop below 5.0 mmol/L by dd/mm/yyyy. |

### Constipation

| | |
|---|---|
| CAM diagnosis | Constipation (actual), *related to* inadequate fluid intake, sedentary lifestyle and insufficient fibre intake |
| Goal | Client will demonstrate an improvement in bowel activity |
| EO | 1 Client's bowel actions will be soft and formed by dd/mm/yyyy (ranging between types 3 and 4 on the Bristol stool chart).<br>2 Client will have one bowel action daily by dd/mm/yyyy. |

### Cough

| | |
|---|---|
| CAM diagnosis | Productive cough (actual), *secondary to* lower respiratory tract infection, *related to* altered immune function |
| Goal | Client will be free from a productive cough |
| EO | 1 Client will report a 50% decrease in the frequency of coughing by dd/mm/yyyy (determined by the average number of coughing episodes per hour).<br>2 Client will report a 100% reduction in the volume of expectorated sputum by dd/mm/yyyy (ascertained by the estimated volume of sputum per cough in millilitres). |

*Continued*

**Table 5.3:** Examples of the two-stage planning process, including a general goal and expected outcomes (EO)—*continued*

### Diabetes mellitus

| | |
|---|---|
| **CAM diagnosis** | **Hyperglycaemia (potential),** *secondary to* **type 2 diabetes mellitus,** *related to* **high glycaemic load diet, sedentary lifestyle and insulin resistance** |
| **Goal** | Client will experience few episodes of hyperglycaemia |
| **EO** | 1  Client's fasting blood glucose level will remain between 4.0 and 6.0 mmol/L by dd/mm/yyyy.<br>2  Client's glycated haemoglobin (HbA1c) will be below 7% by dd/mm/yyyy. |

### Diarrhoea

| | |
|---|---|
| **CAM diagnosis** | **Chronic diarrhoea (actual),** *secondary to* **irritable bowel syndrome,** *related to* **intestinal dysbiosis** |
| **Goal** | Client will demonstrate reduced episodes of diarrhoea |
| **EO** | 1  Client's bowel actions will be formed by dd/mm/yyyy (ranging between types 3 and 5 on the Bristol stool chart).<br>2  Client will have one bowel action daily by dd/mm/yyyy. |

### Dysmenorrhoea

| | |
|---|---|
| **CAM diagnosis** | **Dysmenorrhoea (actual),** *related to* **elevated oestrogen levels, elevated prostaglandin levels and progesterone deficiency** |
| **Goal** | Client will demonstrate an improvement in menstrual pain |
| **EO** | 1  Client will report a 30% reduction in the duration (i.e. number of hours/days) of dysmenorrhoea by dd/mm/yyyy.<br>2  Client will report a 50% decrease in the severity of dysmenorrhoea by dd/mm/yyyy (measured by numerical pain score). |

### Dysuria

| | |
|---|---|
| **CAM diagnosis** | **Dysuria (actual),** *secondary to* **urinary tract infection,** *related to* **inadequate fluid intake and immune dysfunction** |
| **Goal** | Client will be free from dysuria |
| **EO** | 1  Client will report a 100% reduction in micturition-associated pain by dd/mm/yyyy (measured by numerical pain score).<br>2  Client will remain free from recurrent episodes of cystitis over the next 6 months (by dd/mm/yyyy). |

### Headache

| | |
|---|---|
| **CAM diagnosis** | **Headache (actual),** *related to* **poor posture and spinal misalignment** |
| **Goal** | Client will be free from recurrent headaches |
| **EO** | 1  Client will report a 50% reduction in the severity of head pain by dd/mm/yyyy (measured by numerical pain score).<br>2  Client will report a 50% reduction in the frequency of headaches by dd/mm/yyyy (based on the number of client diary entries). |

### HIV infection

| | |
|---|---|
| **CAM diagnosis** | **HIV infection (actual),** *related to* **unprotected sex with HIV-infected partner** |
| **Goal** | Client will not develop AIDS |
| **EO** | 1  Client will remain free from opportunistic infection over the next 12 months (to dd/mm/yyyy).<br>2  Client's viral load will remain under 500 copies/mL over the next 12 months (to dd/mm/yyyy). |

**Table 5.3:** Examples of the two-stage planning process, including a general goal and expected outcomes (EO)—*continued*

**Hypertension**

| | |
|---|---|
| CAM diagnosis | Hypertension (actual), *related to* excessive sodium intake and excessive saturated fat consumption |
| Goal | Client will demonstrate a reduction in blood pressure |
| EO | 1  Client will demonstrate a 10 mmHg drop in systolic blood pressure by dd/mm/yyyy.<br>2  Client will demonstrate a 5 mmHg drop in diastolic blood pressure by dd/mm/yyyy. |

**Obesity**

| | |
|---|---|
| CAM diagnosis | Obesity (actual), *related to* increased energy intake, decreased energy expenditure and insulin resistance |
| Goal | Client will demonstrate a reduction in body weight |
| EO | 1  Client will demonstrate a 5 kg drop in body weight by dd/mm/yyyy.<br>2  Client will demonstrate a 2 kg/m$^2$ drop in BMI by dd/mm/yyyy.<br>3  Client will demonstrate a 5 cm reduction in waist circumference by dd/mm/yyyy. |

**Retinopathy**

| | |
|---|---|
| CAM diagnosis | Diabetic retinopathy (potential), *secondary to* diabetes mellitus, *related to* poor glycaemic control |
| Goal | Client will not demonstrate any signs of diabetic retinopathy |
| EO | 1  Client will not report any abnormal visual symptoms within the next 2 years (by dd/mm/yyyy).<br>2  Client will not manifest any retinopathic changes at their next ophthalmology review (on dd/mm/yyyy). |

**Sinus congestion**

| | |
|---|---|
| CAM diagnosis | Sinus congestion and pain (actual), *secondary to* chronic sinusitis, *related to* food intolerance and poor mucous membrane integrity |
| Goal | Client will be free from sinus congestion and pain |
| EO | 1  Client will be free from sinus congestion by dd/mm/yyyy.<br>2  Client will report a 50% reduction in sinus pain by dd/mm/yyyy (measured by numerical pain score).<br>3  Client will report a 50% reduction in sinus tenderness by dd/mm/yyyy (measured by numerical pain score). |

## Summary

The careful planning of client care generates immediate and long-term benefits for clients, CAM practitioners, the integrative healthcare team, administrators and the healthcare system, including improvements in communication, clinician performance, clinic and organisational efficiency, client quality of life and clinical outcomes. However, care planning is not an innate, unconscious activity but one that is systematic and rationalised and requires an appropriate level of skill to plan at a competent level. This chapter has highlighted that the use of a clear, systematic planning framework that integrates goals and expected outcomes that are client-centred, mutually derived, specific, measurable, achievable, realistic and time-limited may help to deliver a transparent and consistent approach to client care and in doing so greatly improve client health and wellbeing by hastening the achievement of clinical outcomes. In the chapter that follows, the application of client care is discussed, particularly the role of evidence-based practice as a component of clinical care.

---

### Learning activities

1 Why is the planning of care important to CAM practice?

2 How can the shortfalls of planning be addressed in clinical practice?

3 Describe the key criteria for setting goals and expected outcomes, including a rationale for their inclusion.

4 What methods can a CAM practitioner adopt to ensure that goals and expected outcomes are client-centred?

5 What factors determine whether goals and/or expected outcomes are achievable and realistic?

6 What is the two-stage planning process?

7 Using the key criteria identified in question 3, formulate one general goal and two expected outcomes for each of the following CAM diagnoses:

   a. wheeze (actual), *secondary to* asthma, *related* to food intolerance

   b. coronary heart disease (potential), *related to* sedentary lifestyle and obesity

   c. lumbago (actual), *related to* muscle strain injury

   d. anxiety (actual), *related to* emotional stress.

---

# References

1. Bergeson S. Dean J. (2006) A systems approach to patient-centered care. Journal of the American Medical Association, 296(23): 2848–51.

2. Leach MJ. (2006) Integrative healthcare: a need for change? Journal of Complementary and Integrative Medicine, 3(1): 1–11.

3. Mold J. Blake G. Becker L. (1991) Goal-oriented medical care. Family Medicine, 23: 46–51.

4. Holliday R. (2004) Goal-setting: just how client-oriented are we? Therapy Weekly, 30(37): 8–11.

5. Kraus J. (2006) The importance of goal setting. Podiatry Management, 25(4): 121–5.

6. Mesmer R. (1997) Patient-focused perioperative documentation: an outcome management approach. Seminars in Perioperative Nursing, 6(4): 223–32.

7. Bradley E et al (1999). Goal-setting in clinical medicine. Social Science and Medicine, 49: 267–78.

8. Hinderer S. (1996) Practically perfect planning. Seminars in Perioperative Nursing, 5(3): 157–64.

9. Locke E. Latham G. (2002) Building a practically useful theory of goal setting and task motivation. American Psychologist, 57(9): 705–17.

10. McGillan P. (1990) Assessment and care planning increase autonomy of practice. Provider, 16(6): 37–8.

11. Playford ED et al (2000) Goal-setting in rehabilitation: report of a workshop to explore professionals' perceptions of goal-setting. Clinical Rehabilitation, 14: 491–6.

12. Wade DT. (1998) Evidence relating to goal planning in rehabilitation. Clinical Rehabilitation, 12: 273–5.

13. Wright K. (2005) Care planning: an easy guide for nurses. Nursing and Residential Care, 7(2): 71–3.

14. Leach MJ. (2007) Revisiting the evaluation of clinical practice. International Journal of Nursing Practice, 13(2): 70–4.

15. Wallen M. Doyle S. (1996) Performance indicators in paediatrics: the role of standardized assessments and goal setting. Australian Occupational Therapy Journal, 43: 172–7.

16. Query M. Taylor R. (2005) Linkages between goal attainment and quality of life for individuals with chronic fatigue syndrome. Occupational Therapy in Health Care, 19(4): 3–22.

17. Boersma S et al (2006) Goal processes in relation to goal attainment: predicting health-related quality of life in myocardial infarction patients. Journal of Health Psychology, 11(6): 927–41.

18. Hullfish K. Bovbjerg V. Steers W. (2004) Patient-centered goals for pelvic floor dysfunction surgery: long-term follow-up. American Journal of Obstetrics and Gynecology, 191(1): 201–5.

19. Manchester J. (1983). A framework for planning. Nursing Mirror, 156(15): 34–6.

20. Heenan C. Piotrowski U. (2000) Creation of a client goal-setting framework. SCI Nursing, 17(4): 153–61.

21. Theodorakis Y et al (1996) The effect of personal goals, self-efficacy, and self-satisfaction on injury rehabilitation. Journal of Sports Rehabilitation, 5: 214–23.

22. Bower E et al (1996) A randomised controlled trial of different intensities of physiotherapy and different goal-setting procedures in 44 children with cerebral palsy. Developmental Medicine and Child Neurology, 38(3): 226–37.

23. Evans L. Hardy L. (2002) Injury rehabilitation: a goal-setting intervention study. Research Quarterly for Exercise and Sport, 73(3): 310–19.

24. Theodorakis Y et al (1997) Examining psychological factors during injury rehabilitation. Journal of Sports Rehabilitation, 6: 355–63.

25. Stenstrom C. (1994) Home exercise in rheumatoid arthritis functional class II: goal setting versus pain attention. Journal of Rheumatology, 21(4): 627–34.

26. Gauggel S. Leinberger R. Richardt M. (2001) Goal setting and reaction time performance in brain-damaged patients. Journal of Clinical and Experimental Neuropsychology, 23(3): 351–61.

27. Macleod GM. Macleod L. (1996) Evaluation of client and staff satisfaction with a goal planning project implemented with people with spinal cord injuries. Spinal Cord, 34(9): 525–30.

28. Berry M et al (1989) Work-site health promotion: the effects of a goal-setting program on nutrition-related behaviors. Journal of the American Dietetic Association, 89(7): 914–20, 923.

29. Cullen K et al (2004) Goal setting is differentially related to change in fruit, juice, and vegetable consumption among fourth-grade children. Health Education and Behavior, 31(2): 258–69.

30. MacLennan AH. Myers SP. Taylor AW. (2006) The continuing use of complementary and alternative medicine in South Australia: costs and beliefs in 2004. Medical Journal of Australia, 184(1): 27–31.

31. Atkinson J. (2004) Goal setting in rehabilitation: costs, benefits and challenges. Therapy Weekly, 30(46): 10–13.

32. Mason C. (1999) Guide to practice or 'load of rubbish'? The influence of care plans on nursing practice in five clinical areas in Northern Ireland. Journal of Advanced Nursing, 29(2): 380–7.

33. Barclay L. (2002) Exploring the factors that influence the goal setting process for occupational therapy intervention with an individual with spinal cord injury. Australian Occupational Therapy Journal, 49: 3–13.

34. Crisp J. Taylor C. (2008) Potter and Perry's fundamentals of nursing. 3rd ed. Sydney: Elsevier Australia.

35. Harkreader H. (2007) Fundamentals of nursing: caring and clinical judgement. 3rd ed. Philadelphia: WB Saunders.

36. Alexy B. (1985) Goal setting and health risk reduction. Nursing Research, 34: 283–8.

37. Roe B et al (1996) An evaluation of health service interventions by primary healthcare teams and continence advisory services on patient outcomes related to incontinence. Oxford: Health Services Research Unit, Oxford University.

38. Conneeley A. (2004) Interdisciplinary collaborative goal planning in a post-acute neurological setting: a qualitative study. British Journal of Occupational Therapy, 67(6): 248–55.

39. Arnetz J et al (2004) Active patient involvement in the establishment of physical therapy goals: effects on treatment outcome and quality of care. Advances in Physiotherapy, 6(2): 50–69.

40. Holliday R. Antoun M. Playford E. (2005) A survey of goal-setting methods used in rehabilitation. Neurorehabilitation and Neural Repair, 19(3): 227–32.

41. Glazier S et al (2004) Taking the next steps in goal ascertainment: a prospective study of patient, team, and family perspectives using a comprehensive standardised menu in a geriatric assessment and treatment unit. Journal of the American Geriatric Society, 52: 284–9.

42. Marteau T et al (1987) Goals of treatment in diabetes: a comparison of doctors and parents of children with diabetes. Journal of Behavioral Medicine, 10(1): 33–48.

43. Berman A et al (2008) Kozier and Erb's fundamentals of nursing: concepts, process, and practice. 8th ed. Upper Saddle River: Prentice Hall.

44. Bandura A. Simon KM. (1977) The role of proximal intentions in self-regulation of refractory behaviour. Cognitive Therapy and Research, 1(3): 177–93.

45. Bar-Eli M. Hartman I. Levy-Kolker N. (1994) Using goal setting to improve physical performance of adolescents with behaviour disorders: the effect of goal proximity. Adapted Physical Activity Quarterly, 11: 86–97.

46. Murray ME. Atkinson LD. (2000) Understanding the nursing process in a changing care environment. 6th ed. New York: McGraw-Hill.

# 6
# Application – Evidence-based practice

## Chapter overview

A major consideration when selecting interventions for CAM practice is the application of evidence-based practice (EBP). This chapter will focus on the EBP framework as a means of improving clinical practice, while the exploration of specific CAM interventions will be covered in chapter 9. This shift towards EBP will enable CAM professionals to move from a culture of delivering care based on tradition, intuition and authority to a situation in which decisions are guided and justified by the best available evidence. In spite of these advantages, many practitioners remain cautious about embracing the model. Part of this opposition is due to a misunderstanding of EBP, which this chapter aims to address.

## Learning objectives

The content of this chapter will assist the reader to:
- define the term evidence
- outline the hierarchy and strength of evidence
- describe the stages of the EBP paradigm
- recognise the elements that impact on evidence-based decision making
- recognise the merits and limitations of integrating EBP into CAM practice.

## Chapter outline

- Introduction
- Defining evidence
- The EBP framework
- Rationale for EBP
- Criticisms of EBP
- Summary

## Introduction

Over the past few decades, terms such as 'evidence-based practice', 'evidence-based medicine', 'evidence-based nursing' and 'evidence-based nutrition' have become commonplace in the international literature. The more inclusive term, 'evidence-based practice' (EBP), has been defined as the selection of clinical interventions for specific client problems that have been '(a) evaluated by well designed clinical research studies, (b) published in peer review journals, and (c) consistently found to be effective or efficacious on consensus review'.[1] As will be explained throughout this chapter, EBP is not just about locating interventions that are supported by findings from randomised controlled trials; EBP is a formal problem-solving framework[2] that facilitates 'the conscientious, explicit, and judicious use of current best evidence in making decisions about the care of individual patients'.[3] Apart from the implications for clinical practice, the capacity of EBP to link study findings to a profession's body of knowledge also indicates that EBP is a useful theoretical framework for research and may therefore provide an effective solution to the research–practice divide[4-6] and an important impetus to the professionalisation of CAM.

The concept of EBP is not new. In fact, its origins may be traced back to ancient Chinese medicine.[7] That said, notions about quality of evidence and best practice are relatively recent. Archibald Cochrane, a Scottish medical epidemiologist, conceived the concept of best practice in the early 1970s,[8,9] but it was not until after Cochrane's death in the late 1980s that medicine began to demonstrate an interest in the EBP paradigm with the establishment of the Cochrane collaboration.[8,10] Since then, professional interest in EBP has grown.[2,11–13] This shift towards EBP has enabled health professionals to move from a culture of delivering care based on tradition, intuition, authority, clinical experience and pathophysiologic rationale to a situation in which decisions are guided and justified by the best available evidence.[2,5,9,12,14] EBP also limits practitioner and consumer dependence on evidence provided by privileged people, authorities and industry by bestowing clinicians with a framework to critically evaluate claims. Even so, there remains some debate over the definition of evidence in the EBP model.

## Defining evidence

Evidence is a fundamental concept of the EBP paradigm, although there is little agreement between practitioners, academics and professional bodies as to the meaning of evidence. Indeed, the insufficient definition of evidence and the different methodological positions of clinicians and academics may all contribute to these discrepant viewpoints. From the broadest sense, evidence is defined as 'any empirical observation about the apparent relation between events'.[2] While this definition suggests that most forms of knowledge could be considered evidence,[14] it is also asserted[14] that the evidence used to guide practice should be 'subjected to historic or scientific evaluation'. Given the long history of use of many CAM interventions, such as herbal medicine, acupuncture and yoga, this would suggest that traditional CAM evidence has a place in EBP. However, not all evidence is considered the same. These differences in the quality of information are known as the 'hierarchy of evidence'.

As shown in Table 6.1, decisions based on findings from randomised controlled trials (RCTs) may be more sound than those guided by case series results. When

| Table 6.1: The hierarchy of evidence | |
|---|---|
| Level I | Systematic reviews |
| Level II | Well-designed randomised controlled trials |
| Level III-1 | Pseudorandomised controlled trials |
| Level III-2 | Comparative studies with concurrent controls, such as cohort studies, case-control studies or interrupted time series studies |
| Level III-3 | Comparative studies without concurrent controls, such as a historical control study, two or more single-arm studies or interrupted time series without a parallel control group |
| Level IV | Case series with post-test or pre-test/post-test outcomes; uncontrolled open label study |
| Level V | Expert opinion or panel consensus |
| Level VI | Traditional evidence |

Adapted from National Health and Medical Research Council (NHMRC 1999)[15] and the Centre for Evidence-based Medicine 2001[16]

findings from controlled trials are unavailable or insufficient, however, decisions should be guided by the next best available evidence. This is particularly relevant to the field of CAM, as many of the interventions used in CAM practice are supported only by lower levels of evidence, such as traditional evidence, and less so by evidence from RCTs and systematic reviews.

The hierarchy of evidence can also be used to identify research findings that supersede and/or invalidate previously accepted treatments and replace them with interventions that are safer, efficacious and cost-effective.[2,5] Basing clinical decisions on the level of evidence is only part of the equation though, as these decisions also need to take into account the strength of the evidence (Table 6.2), specifically, the quality, quantity, consistency, clinical impact and generalisability of the research, as well as the applicability of the findings to the relevant healthcare setting (e.g. if the frequency, intensity, technique, form or dose of the intervention, or the blend of interventions, as administered under experimental conditions, is applicable to CAM practice).[17,18] Of course, determining the grade of evidence may not always be straightforward, as the defining criteria of each grade may not always apply (i.e. the evidence may be generalisable, consistent and of high quality (grade A), but the

| | **Table 6.2:** Strength of evidence | |
|---|---|---|
| **Grade** | **Strength of evidence** | **Definition** |
| A | Excellent | **Evidence:** multiple level I or II studies with low risk of bias<br>**Consistency:** all studies are consistent<br>**Clinical impact:** very large<br>**Generalisability:** the client matches the population studied<br>**Applicability:** findings are directly applicable to the CAM practice setting |
| B | Good | **Evidence:** one or two level II studies with low risk of bias, or multiple level III studies with low risk of bias<br>**Consistency:** most studies are consistent<br>**Clinical impact:** considerable<br>**Generalisability:** the client is similar to the population studied<br>**Applicability:** findings are applicable to the CAM practice setting with few caveats |
| C | Satisfactory | **Evidence:** level I or II studies with moderate risk of bias, or level III studies with low risk of bias<br>**Consistency:** there is some inconsistency<br>**Clinical impact:** modest<br>**Generalisability:** the client is different from the population studied, but the relationship between the two is clinically sensible<br>**Applicability:** findings are probably applicable to the CAM practice setting with several caveats |
| D | Poor | **Evidence:** level IV studies, level V or VI evidence, or level I to III studies with high risk of bias<br>**Consistency:** evidence is inconsistent<br>**Clinical impact:** small<br>**Generalisability:** the client is different from the population studied, and the relationship between the two is not clinically sensible<br>**Applicability:** findings are not applicable to the CAM practice setting |

Adapted from NHMRC 2009[18]

techniques used are not applicable to CAM practice (grade D)). In this situation, the practitioner will need to make a decision about where the bulk of the criteria lies. For this example, it could be ranked conservatively as grade B evidence, or more favourably as grade A evidence.

Another important determinant of evidence-based decision making is the direction of the evidence. This construct establishes whether the body of evidence favours the intervention (positive evidence), the placebo and/or comparative agent (negative evidence) or neither treatment (neutral evidence) (see Table 6.3). When the direction, hierarchy or level and strength of evidence are all taken into consideration, there is a more critical and judicious use of evidence. So, rather than accepting level I or level II evidence on face value alone, these elements stress the need to also identify whether the strength of the evidence is adequate (i.e. level A or B, or possibly C) and the direction of the evidence is positive (+) before integrating the evidence into CAM practice.

## The EBP framework

The EBP model consists of a series of steps that assist the CAM practitioner in finding an answer to a clinical problem, and then applying that solution to clinical practice (see Figure 6.1). The five-stage process begins with the identification of a clinical problem and the subsequent formation of a structured and answerable question.[4,9] In order to be client-centred and relevant to the presenting case, this question needs to incorporate four key components, including the patient, interventions, condition and outcome (otherwise known as the PICO statement). Collectively, these four elements enable a practitioner to narrow down a search to a specific treatment or range of treatments that are likely to produce a precise clinical effect in a certain type of patient with a specific symptom or disease. An example of an answerable clinical question or PICO statement is: 'What interventions, techniques, therapies (i.e. herbs, nutritional supplements, mind–body techniques, manipulative therapies, lifestyle changes) (interventions) would reduce arthralgia (outcome) in a 60-year-old woman (patient) with osteoarthritis of the hands (condition)?

Following the formulation of a suitable PICO statement, the literature is then searched for the best available evidence to answer the proposed question.[4,9] This is often carried out using electronic bibliographic databases, such as Medline, the cumulative index for nursing and allied health literature (CINAHL), alternative and complementary medicine (AMED), CAM on PubMED, and the Cochrane Library. When suitable clinical evidence cannot be located, level V and level VI evidence may need to be sourced from relevant textbooks and desktop references.

| Table 6.3: Direction of evidence | |
|---|---|
| + | Positive evidence – intervention is more effective than the placebo or comparative agent |
| o | Neutral evidence – intervention is as effective or no different than the placebo or comparative agent |
| – | Negative evidence – intervention is less effective than the placebo or comparative agent |

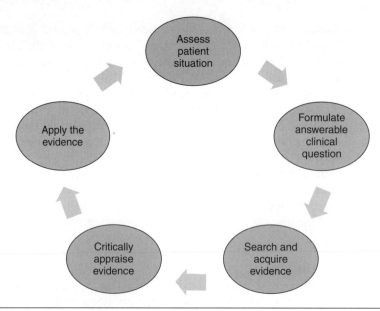

**Figure 6.1:** The EBP paradigm Modified from Dawes et al 2005[4]

Once the best available evidence has been retrieved, it is then critically appraised for its validity, quality, applicability and generalisability.[4,19] A method frequently used by researchers to assess the quality of study findings is to evaluate the factors known to minimise the risk of bias, such as random assignment of treatment, concealment of treatment allocation, suitable control or comparator groups, valid and reliable instrumentation, intention-to-treat analysis and appropriate quality assurance procedures. If the study findings are deemed to be valid, reliable and applicable to the client case, and the treatment is considered appropriate according to clinical expertise, CAM philosophy and available resources,[19] then the best available evidence may be integrated into clinical practice.

Client preferences, psychosocial needs, values, beliefs and expectations form another important component of this decision-making process.[2,19] These preferences may include an aversion or inclination towards certain modalities or methods of administration, or relate to financial, cultural, personal and/or religious constraints. Put simply, effective decision making in CAM depends on the provision of professional expertise, clinical evidence, economic justification and consumer perspective, as well as due consideration of CAM philosophy. Figure 6.2 illustrates how these five components may be integrated into the evidence-based decision-making framework, and Table 6.4 demonstrates how this process can be applied to CAM practice.

## Rationale for EBP

There are many benefits to CAM practitioners, consumers and the healthcare system should they adopt the EBP model. EBP gives rise, for example, to a more transparent clinical decision-making process.[20] While practitioners may not welcome this increased level of scrutiny, greater accountability over decision making is likely to benefit consumers. So, as client expectations increase and practitioners become more accountable for their actions,[9,21] the traditional sourcing of inconsistent and

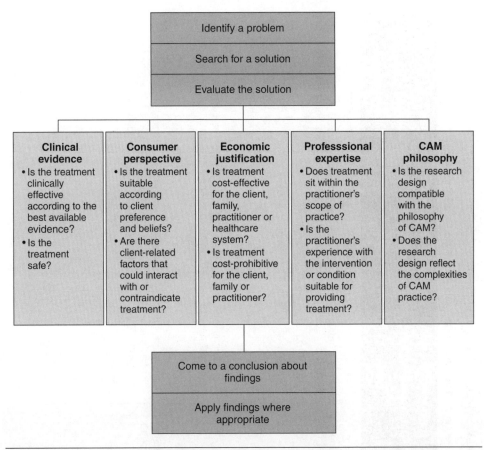

**Figure 6.2:** The evidence-based decision-making framework

incomplete information from peers, manufacturers and historical texts may become outdated.[2,22] EBP therefore challenges existing procedures and facilitates the integration of new and effective interventions into clinical practice. Yet unless practitioners are adequately informed and motivated about EBP, and unless resources are made available for staff to access evidence-based material, clinicians may have difficulty in adopting an EBP approach.[4,23]

According to findings from a recent nationwide survey of system-based CAM practitioners in Australia,[24] these concerns are pertinent to the field of CAM. Of the 126 of 351 randomly selected naturopaths, Western herbalists, homeopaths and traditional Chinese medicine practitioners who responded to the survey, most agreed that access to the internet, free online databases and full-text journal articles would facilitate EBP uptake. Attention to major obstacles of EBP uptake, such as the lack of evidence, skills and industry support, was also important. While the small response rate limits the generalisability of these findings, the sample was considered representative of Australian CAM practitioners. What this study suggests is that even though CAM practitioners may be supportive of EBP, education and training are needed to further improve clinician understanding and application of it.

**Table 6.4: Application of the evidence-based decision-making framework to CAM practice**

| Identify problem | What mind–body therapy would reduce anxiety in a 71-year-old woman with generalised anxiety disorder? | | | | |
|---|---|---|---|---|---|
| **Search for a solution** | **Perform literature search** | Key terms: 'generalised anxiety disorder', 'anxiety', 'anxious' Databases: MEDLINE; CAM on PubMED; the Cochrane Library | | | |
| **Evaluate solutions** | | **Relaxation therapy** | **Tai chi** | **Yoga** | **Flotation therapy** |
| **Clinical effectiveness** | Is the treatment clinically effective? | Yes<br>Level: I (systematic review of 19 RCTs)<br>Strength: A<br>Direction: + | Yes<br>Level: II (multiple RCTs)<br>Strength: C<br>Direction: + | Yes<br>Level: I (systematic review of 6 RCTs)<br>Strength: C<br>Direction: + | Uncertain<br>Level: N/A (no pertinent evidence located)<br>Strength: N/A<br>Direction: N/A |
| | Is the treatment safe? | Yes | Yes | Yes | Uncertain |
| **Consumer perspective** | Is the treatment suitable according to client preference? | Yes | No<br>The client is unable to attend classes | No<br>The client is unable to attend classes | No<br>The client is unable to attend the flotation centre |
| | Are there factors that could interact with the treatment? | Yes<br>Anxiety may affect client adherence to treatment | Yes<br>Anxiety may affect client adherence to treatment | Yes<br>Anxiety may affect client adherence to treatment | Yes<br>Anxiety may affect client adherence to treatment |
| **Economic justification** | Is the treatment cost-effective for the client and CAM practitioner? | Yes | Yes | Yes | Uncertain |
| | Is the treatment cost-prohibitive for the client and CAM practitioner? | No | No | No | No |

| | | | | |
|---|---|---|---|---|
| **Professional expertise** | Does the treatment sit within the CAM practitioner's scope of practice? | Yes | Yes | Yes | Yes |
| | Is the treatment appropriate given the CAM practitioner's experience? | Yes | Yes | Yes | Yes |
| **CAM philosophy** | Is the research compatible with CAM philosophy? | No  Studies used a standardised approach | No  Studies used a standardised approach | No  Studies used a standardised approach | N/A  There is a paucity of research in this area |
| | Does the research reflect the complexities of CAM practice? | No  Studies were decontextualised | No  Studies were decontextualised | No  Studies were decontextualised | No  There is a paucity of research in this area |
| **Conclusion** | Excluding flotation therapy, all mind–body therapies were found to be safe, clinically effective, cost-effective and appropriate to the CAM practitioner's level of expertise. No intervention was investigated using a methodology compatible with CAM philosophy. Relaxation therapy was superior to yoga and tai chi in terms of the strength of evidence and with regard to client preference. Thus, there is adequate justification to incorporate relaxation therapy (i.e. meditation) into the CAM treatment plan for this 71-year-old woman with generalised anxiety disorder. | | | | |

Note: N/A = not applicable.

EBP also plays an important role in improving the quality of care, and reducing the costs of treatment, risk of clinical error and client mortality through improved decision making.[9,12,14,25,26] Although these cost savings may be attributed to the elimination of unnecessary and ineffective interventions, as well as superfluous follow-up care, the provision of high-quality evidence may not necessarily equate to cost reductions. Instead, the cost-effectiveness of alternative interventions should be evaluated using cost–benefit analyses (CBA) and, in the absence of such data, be assessed on a case-by-case basis. If, for example, a CAM practitioner is undecided about which treatment to prescribe for a client, the client has no treatment preference, and the two treatments of choice demonstrate similar benefit (i.e. low risk of harm, ease of administration, similar degree of improvement in clinical outcomes), then it would be in the client's best interest to consider the relative costs of the two interventions. If, say, 1 month of treatment with intervention A costs $45, and for intervention B, $29, then preference should be given to intervention B, as this treatment would bear the greatest cost–benefit to the client.

The disparate practices across clinics, institutions and health professions are another concern in healthcare,[27–31] with the need for more consistent approaches to client problems being long overdue. To address the inconsistencies in clinical practice, CAM practitioners should be encouraged to adopt an EBP approach.[2,22] Failure to use EBP may delay the integration of innovative treatments into clinical care,[5] which could contribute to adverse client outcomes.[12]

Failing to deliver EBP may also reduce the credibility of the CAM profession[14] and, in turn, isolate members of the profession from the multidisciplinary team. In other words, practitioners choosing to ignore EBP may lack adequate justification to continue or change clinical practices.[5,14,32,33] EBP may improve multidisciplinarity[6] and consistency of clinical care, but may also more effectively meet the healthcare needs of individuals.[14] Despite the benefits to CAM practitioners and consumers, EBP is not without limitations.

## Criticisms of EBP

There are many critics of EBP, but as yet these arguments hold little coherence or strength.[20] Some of the resistance in accepting EBP has been attributed to the underlying positivist philosophy of EBP, with concerns that a reductionist approach oversimplifies or inadequately addresses complex client situations[6,25] and the complexities of CAM practice. There is also an assumption that hard science is the only evidence accepted in the model.[25,34,35] The belief that EBP relies only on evidence from RCTs is a common misconception. While an RCT is particularly useful for evaluating the effects of single or multiple interventions, it can be less effective in answering questions about client attitudes, preferences, experiences, prognosis and diagnosis.[9,36] Thus, the criticism towards EBP may not necessarily be directed at the model per se, but towards the type of evidence accepted. A major challenge is for practitioners to recognise that other types of data, such as qualitative findings, are accepted forms of evidence in the EBP model. Of course, the type of evidence adopted should be the best available evidence and, furthermore, should be dictated by the type of question being asked.[10] A question about clinical effectiveness, for example, would be best answered using data from pragmatic RCTs, a query relating to typical responders of CAM treatment would be best addressed using findings from case studies, and a question about client expectations or preferences could be appropriately answered using results from surveys or qualitative investigations.

There is related concern that the evidence derived from RCTs and systematic reviews (which are highly favoured in EBP) may not be applicable to CAM practice. One argument is that the reductionist design of these studies is incompatible with the philosophies of CAM practice,[37] including the principles of holism, client centredness and individualised care. Even though holism is still frequently ignored in these study designs, some attention has been given to individualised care, with a number of RCTs and systematic reviews now beginning to compare the effectiveness of individualised CAM treatments to standardised care and/or placebo treatment.[38–40]

Another point of concern relates to the decontextualised nature of these study designs, particularly the lack of attention afforded to the contextual or indirect effects of treatment (i.e. the effects of the clinical environment, client preference and expectation, and the client–clinician interface). Whole systems research, which considers all aspects of the treatment approach (including those previously stated),[41] attempts to address many of these shortfalls of reductionist scientific studies by gaining important insight into the complexities of real-life CAM practice. While this emerging research design serves to make clinical research more relevant to CAM practice, it does not dismiss altogether the value of RCTs and systematic reviews in EBP.

Some authorities have raised concerns that EBP may produce dehumanised, routine care[14,42] by ignoring clinical expertise and client preference.[25,43] Yet as well as respecting client choice,[21] EBP also requires research findings to be considered alongside clinical expertise.[26,33] As a result EBP is client-centred,[22] individualised[5] and accommodating of practitioner and client needs. In fact, if a clinician failed to acknowledge a client's preference for a particular treatment when integrating evidence into clinical practice, the practitioner would fall short in their professional obligation to respect client wishes, which would almost certainly compromise client–practitioner rapport, treatment compliance and clinical outcomes.

The paucity of high-quality, coherent and consistent scientific evidence in complementary and alternative medicine may explain why some clinicians have difficulty engaging in EBP.[5,9,36] Although systematic reviews have attempted to resolve this problem (albeit in a reductionist and decontextualised manner), clinical experience and traditional evidence are still relied upon in areas where data are absent or ambiguous.[11,36] EBP uses the best available evidence to guide decisions and does not just rely on data from clinical trials.[9,36] In fact, if CAM practitioners used only therapies or techniques that were based on rigorous level I and level II evidence, CAM practice would be considerably limited.

Other barriers to adopting EBP are a lack of motivation, disagreement with findings, lack of autonomy, and inadequate research and critical appraisal skills.[5,12,23,24,36] The lack of time, resources and authority to make changes are also major obstacles to the introduction of EBP.[5,9,23,24,36] Then again, the delivery of EBP may eliminate the time, costs and resources allocated to harmful or ineffective treatments[10,21,26] and, in effect, improve the future demand on clinician time.

Another potential barrier to the integration of EBP, and one that warrants urgent attention, is the lack of evidence for EBP, specifically, the paucity of data linking EBP uptake to improvements in clinical outcomes.[32,44] Until such data emerge, and given the theoretical rationale for EBP, there is no reason why CAM practitioners should not base clinical practice decisions on the best available evidence.

## Summary

Even though some health professionals are cautious about embracing EBP, these practitioners need to be assured that EBP simply provides a useful and 'scientific framework within which to identify and answer priority questions about the effectiveness of … healthcare'.[45] As well as guiding clinical practice, the EBP paradigm also helps to close the research–practice divide. Integrating findings into clinical practice may eventuate only if practitioners undergo further education and if high-quality evidence on the clinical efficacy, cost–benefit and feasibility of CAM interventions (including evidence from pragmatic RCTs and whole systems research) and EBP are made available to clinicians. A greater uptake of clinical evidence within CAM practice may also help to advance the CAM profession by facilitating consistent and quality care, multidisciplinarity and the integration of CAM services into the mainstream healthcare sector. This concept of integrative healthcare is explored in greater depth in the following chapter.

### Learning activities

1 What is your understanding of the term 'evidence'?
2 Construct a hierarchy of evidence table to reflect your preference for the different types or levels of evidence used in your discipline. How does this table compare to Table 6.1? Explain why you have chosen to rank the evidence in this manner.
3 What do you believe are the main barriers to the uptake of EBP within your discipline? How do you think these obstacles could be addressed?
4 Debate whether EBP should be used by practitioners within your discipline.
5 Using the EBP paradigm illustrated in Figure 6.1, formulate an answerable clinical question, and then retrieve and critically appraise the evidence in order to identify a suitable intervention (pertinent to your field of practice) for each of the following situations:
   a. a 24-year-old woman with chronic diarrhoea secondary to Crohn's disease
   b. a 7-year-old boy with dull right earache secondary to otitis media
   c. a 43-year-old woman with recurrent headache related to emotional stress
   d. a 68-year-old man with bilateral hand and wrist arthralgia secondary to rheumatoid arthritis
   e. a 55-year-old man with productive cough secondary to chronic bronchitis.

# References

1. Rosenthal RN. (2006) Overview of evidence-based practices. In: Foundations of evidence-based social work practice. Roberts AR, Yeager K, editors. New York: Oxford University Press.
2. Montori V. Guyatt G. (2008) Progress in evidence-based medicine. Journal of the American Medical Association, 300(15): 1814–16.
3. Sackett D et al (1996) Evidence based medicine: what it is and what it isn't. British Medical Journal, 312(7023): 71–2.
4. Dawes M et al (2005) Sicily statement on evidence-based practice. BMC Medical Education, 5: 1–7.
5. Pape T. (2003) Evidence-based nursing practice: to infinity and beyond. Journal of Continuing Education in Nursing, 34(4): 154–61.
6. Trinder L. (2000) A critical appraisal of evidence-based practice. In: Evidence-based practice: a critical appraisal. Trinder L, Reynolds S, editors. Oxford: Blackwell Science.
7. Sackett DL et al (2000) Evidence based medicine: how to practice and teach EBM. 2nd ed. Edinburgh: Churchill Livingstone.
8. Hill G. (2000) Archie Cochrane and his legacy. An internal challenge to physicians' autonomy? Journal of Clinical Epidemiology, 53(12): 1189–92.
9. McKenna H. Ashton S. Keeney S. (2004) Barriers to evidence based practice in primary care: a review of the literature. International Journal of Nursing Studies, 41: 369–78.
10. Reynolds S. (2000) The anatomy of evidence-based practice: principles and methods. In: Evidence-based practice: a critical appraisal. Trinder L, Reynolds S, editors. Oxford: Blackwell Science.
11. Leung G. (2001) Evidence-based practice revisited. Asia Pacific Journal of Public Health, 13(2): 116–21.
12. Tod A. Palfreyman S. Burke L. (2004) Evidence-based practice is a time of opportunity for nursing. British Journal of Nursing, 13(4): 211–16.
13. Wyatt G. (2003) From research to clinical practice. Evidence-based practice and research methodologies: challenges and implications for the nursing profession. Clinical Journal of Oncology Nursing, 7(3): 337–8.
14. Romyn D et al (2003) The notion of evidence in evidence-based practice by the nursing philosophy working group. Journal of Professional Nursing, 19(4): 184–8.
15. National Health and Medical Research Council (NHMRC). (1999) A guide to the development, implementation and evaluation of clinical practice guidelines. Canberra: NHMRC.
16. Centre for Evidence-Based Medicine. (2001) Oxford centre for evidence-based medicine levels of evidence. Oxford: Centre for Evidence-Based Medicine.
17. Newman MG. Weyant R. Hujoel P. (2007) JEBDP improves grading system and adopts strength of recommendation taxonomy grading (SORT) for guidelines and systematic reviews. Journal of Evidence Based Dental Practice, 7(4): 147–50.
18. National Health and Medical Research Council (NHMRC). (2009) NHMRC additional levels of evidence and grades for recommendations for developers of guidelines – Stage 2 consultation. Canberra: NHMRC.
19. Scales CD et al (2007) Evidence based clinical practice: a primer for urologists. Journal of Urology, 178(3): 775–82.
20. Leach MJ. (2006) Evidence-based practice: A framework for clinical practice and research design. International Journal of Nursing Practice, 12(5): 248–51.
21. Klardie K et al (2004) Integrating the principles of evidence-based practice into clinical practice. Journal of the American Academy of Nurse Practitioners, 16(3): 98–105.
22. Baxter R. Baxter H. (2002) Clinical governance. Journal of Wound Care, 11(1): 7–9.
23. Grol R. Wensing M. (2004) What drives change? Barriers to and incentives for achieving evidence-based practice. Medical Journal of Australia, 180: S57–60.
24. Leach MJ. Gillham D. (2009) Attitude and use of evidence-based practice among complementary medicine practitioners: a descriptive survey. Alternative Therapies in Health and Medicine, 15(3): S149–50.
25. Williams D. Garner J. (2002) The case against 'the evidence': a different perspective on evidence-based medicine. British Journal of Psychiatry, 180: 8–12.
26. Dickersin K. Straus SE. Bero LA. (2007) Evidence based medicine: increasing, not dictating, choice. British Medical Journal, 334(Suppl.1): S10.
27. Ahmed TF et al (2006) Chronic laryngitis associated with gastroesophageal reflux: prospective assessment of differences in practice patterns between gastroenterologists and ENT physicians. American Journal of gastroenterology, 101(3): 470–8.
28. Janson S. Weiss K. (2004) A national survey of asthma knowledge and practices among specialists and primary care physicians. Journal of Asthma, 41(3): 343–8.
29. Jefford M et al (2007) Different professionals' knowledge and perceptions of the management of people with pancreatic cancer. Asia–Pacific Journal of Clinical Oncology, 3(1): 44–51.
30. Novak KL. Chapman GE. (2002) Oncologists' and naturopaths' nutrition beliefs and practices. Cancer Practice, 9(3): 141–6.
31. Yeh KW et al (2006) Survey of asthma care in Taiwan: a comparison of asthma specialists and general practitioners. Annals of Allergy, Asthma and Immunology, 96(4): 593–9.
32. Goodman KW. (2004) Ethics and evidence-based medicine: fallibility and responsibility in clinical science. Cambridge: Cambridge University Press.
33. Zeitz K. McCutcheon H. (2003) Evidence-based practice: to be or not to be, this is the question! International Journal of Nursing Practice, 9(5): 272–9.
34. Bhandari M. Giannoudis PV. (2006) Evidence-based medicine: What it is and what it is not. Injury, 37(4): 302–306.
35. Walker K. (2003) Why evidence-based practice now? A polemic. Nursing Inquiry, 10(3): 145–55.
36. Straus S. McAlister F. (2000) Evidence-based medicine: a commentary on common criticisms. Canadian Medical Association Journal, 163(7): 837–41.
37. Fonnebo V et al (2007) Researching complementary and alternative treatments – the gatekeepers are not at home. BMC Medical Research Methodology, 7: 7.
38. Cherkin DC et al (2009) A randomized trial comparing acupuncture, simulated acupuncture, and usual care for chronic low back pain. Archives of Internal Medicine, 169(9): 858–66.

39. Guo R. Canter PH. Ernst E. (2007) A systematic review of randomised clinical trials of individualised herbal medicine in any indication. Postgraduate Medical Journal, 83: 633–7.

40. White A et al (2003) Individualised homeopathy as an adjunct in the treatment of childhood asthma: a randomised placebo controlled trial. Thorax, 58(4): 317–21.

41. Verhoef MJ et al (2004) Whole systems research: moving forward. Focus on Alternative Complementary Therapies, 9(2): 87–90.

42. Fleming K. (2007) The knowledge base for evidence-based nursing: a role for mixed methods research? Advances in Nursing Science, 30(1): 41–51.

43. Closs S. Cheater F. (1999) Evidence for nursing practice: a clarification of the issues. Journal of Advanced Nursing, 30(1): 10–17.

44. Fulbrook P. Harrison L. (2006) Linking evidence-based practice to clinical outcomes. Connect: The World of Critical Care Nursing, 5(1): 1.

45. Sackett D. Rosenberg W. (1995) The need for evidence-based medicine. Journal of the Royal Society of Medicine, 88(11): 620–4.

# 7
# Application – Integrative healthcare

## Chapter overview

Integrative healthcare is a comprehensive and holistic approach to healthcare in which all health professionals work together to safely and effectively meet the needs of the patient and the community. While such an approach is likely to increase healthcare choice, improve treatment outcomes and allow patients to more effectively navigate through the range of available treatment options, due consideration needs to be given to concerns about clinical evidence, practitioner competence and healthcare philosophy. These arguments for and against integrative healthcare will be discussed throughout this chapter. Examples will also be provided of existing models of integrative healthcare, and a framework for a new service delivery model will be proposed.

## Learning objectives

The content of this chapter will assist the reader to:
- explain the meaning of integrative healthcare
- discuss the merits and pitfalls of the conventional healthcare system
- recognise the forces driving the push towards integrative healthcare
- identify the factors opposing the assimilation of CAM into conventional healthcare
- recognise the merits of integrative healthcare
- describe existing models of integrative healthcare
- describe the integrative healthcare centre model.

## Chapter outline

- Introduction
- Defining integrative care
- Conventional system of healthcare
- Movement towards integration
- Problems with integration
- Merits of integration
- Models of integration
- Summary

## Introduction

In recent years, there has been a move towards the integration of CAM into mainstream healthcare. The emergence of new societies, academic chairs, forums, publications, referral networks, integrative clinics and centres of integrative healthcare are testament to this claim. Yet despite the level of progress in this area, few have questioned whether such a shift is appropriate or acceptable, and even fewer have explored how or why this approach should be implemented. This chapter will address these concerns by examining the merits and limitations of integrative healthcare and, further to this, highlight how these strengths may help to improve some of the shortfalls of a conventional system of care; it will also address the drawbacks of independent practice. But before addressing these issues, the term 'integrative' needs to be understood.

## Defining integrative care

Over the past few decades there has been a shift in the way healthcare has been delivered, from the traditional consultative, paternalistic and independent practice model, to the multidisciplinary approach and, more recently, to the integrative healthcare model. As one moves to the right of this consultative–integrative healthcare spectrum (see Figure 7.1), it is clear that these approaches become more holistic, complex and patient-centred as practitioner autonomy, hierarchy and reliance on the biomedical model decrease.[1] What this spectrum fails to differentiate, though, is integrative medicine from integrative healthcare, which are distinctly different, non-interchangeable approaches to care.

Integrative medicine is defined by Rees and Weil,[2] for instance, as 'practising medicine in a way that selectively incorporates elements of complementary and alternative medicine into comprehensive treatment plans alongside solidly orthodox methods of diagnosis and treatment'. What this definition implies is that integrative medicine is professionally exclusive because it applies only to the uptake of CAM by biomedical practitioners. By failing to consider other aspects of assimilation, such as the inclusion of CAM practitioners within mainstream settings, such a term holds little relevance to CAM practice. A more appropriate and inclusive term is 'integrative healthcare'.

Integrative healthcare is defined as a multidisciplinary, collaborative and patient-centred approach to healthcare in which the assessment, diagnostic and treatment processes of alternative and conventional medicine are equally considered.[3] This

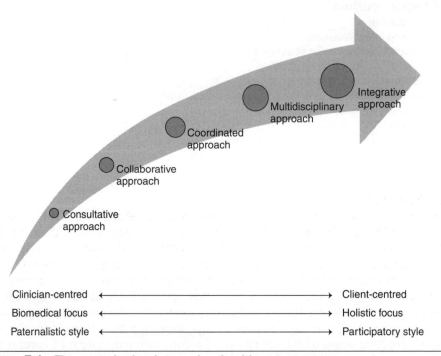

**Figure 7.1:** The consultative–integrative healthcare spectrum Modified from Boon et al 2004[1]

clinical approach also 'combines the strengths of conventional and alternative medicine with a bias towards options that are considered safe, and which, upon review of the available evidence, offer a reasonable expectation of benefit to the patient'.[4] Put simply, integrative healthcare is a comprehensive and holistic approach to healthcare in which all health professionals, including biomedical and CAM professions, work collaboratively in an equal and respectful manner, to safely and effectively meet the needs of the patient and the community.

## Conventional system of healthcare

Existing systems of healthcare are diverse and complex but are generally based on a similar purpose, that is, the treatment of disease and infirmity.[5] A more effective system of healthcare also needs to focus on preventing disease and promoting well-being,[5] as well as providing care that is individualised, holistic and patient-centred. Given the reductionist, fragmented, standardised and disempowering treatment often provided in conventional systems of healthcare at present,[6] particularly in secondary care settings, it is necessary that these systems be carefully evaluated and subsequently improved.

These systems of healthcare can be evaluated in terms of acceptability, efficiency and equity.[7] Acceptability for instance, refers to patient, community and provider acceptance of the system. System inefficiencies, quality of care, personal experience, beliefs and preferences are all likely to impact on this outcome.

The service, administrative and economic efficiencies of the healthcare system, or performance of the system, is influenced by a number of factors, such as skill mix, funding, resource allocation, infrastructure, system priorities, adaptability to change and outcomes of care.[7] Even though many healthcare systems have attempted to improve system efficiency through the introduction of casemix funding (an outcome-based funding model),[8] there are still ongoing issues relating to continuity of care, unavoidable costs, evaluation of service outcomes, adaptability to system level changes and the balance between medical and non-medical services.[7,8]

The final component of system evaluation is equity, which is concerned with indiscriminate access and outcomes of healthcare services.[7] Even though universal and equitable access to healthcare may be improved through the provision of national subsidy schemes, such as the Australian Medicare system, in most cases these public programs only subsidise the delivery of medical, hospital and laboratory services.[5,9] One exception to this is the Australian Medicare-funded enhanced primary care program, which allows eligible persons to gain access to a limited number of allied health services, albeit via referral from a general practitioner. The subsidisation of pharmaceutical agents through the pharmaceutical benefits scheme (PBS) is another long-standing national subsidy program,[9] although, once again, it only applies to specific medical treatments.

These examples illustrate that in Australia at least, the mainstream system of healthcare has been designed to perpetuate the interests of certain key stakeholders, such as medical practitioners and pharmaceutical companies.[5] The exclusion of other pertinent health services (such as naturopathy and massage therapy) and products (including most herbal medicines and nutritional supplements) from these subsidisation schemes indicates that this system is, by definition, unequitable. The following paragraph exemplifies this point further.

In Australia, health consumers have access to a wide range of CAM services, yet only a proportion of these services can be financially reimbursed through private insurance companies and none of the products prescribed by CAM practitioners are eligible for reimbursement. For consumers with chronic or complex care needs, there is limited access (i.e. maximum of five allied health services per year) to publicly funded CAM services, specifically, chiropractic and osteopathy. Thus, for the many individuals who wish to access CAM services but are uninsured, have an acute complaint or have long-term care needs, they will have to pay for these services out of pocket. According to a recent Australian survey of CAM consumers, these out-of-pocket expenses can range from AUD$1 to AUD$650 per month (mean = AUD$21.23) per user. This translates to AUD$1.3 billion per annum at the national level.[10]

The escalating cost of maintaining the current system is unlikely to be efficient, cost-effective or sustainable in the long term.[5] Measures that improve the efficiency, acceptability and equity of existing systems of healthcare need to be implemented so that the needs of all individuals can be better met.[5] These strategies also need to offer a significant cost–benefit to the system. One strategy that may fulfil these requirements is the development of an integrative system of healthcare.

## Movement towards integration

Over the last decade, there has been rising interest and increasing use of natural medicines and complementary practitioner services. This trend not only applies to consumers, but also to practitioner groups: orthodox clinicians now use and endorse a wide range of complementary therapies.[11,12] The scientific community is also pushing healthcare towards a more integrative approach,[13] with a number of integrative clinics, hospitals and academic centres now available across the globe, and pharmacies and pharmaceutical companies now selling a range of conventional and complementary medicines. Evidence also suggests that CAM practitioners are being accepted as legitimate health service providers.[14] One could argue that the legitimisation of CAM services, together with the integration of these services into mainstream care, may be influenced by the increasing biomedical content and evolving curricula of undergraduate CAM courses, the closer alignment of these courses with the scientific paradigm and subsequent improvements in biomedical language proficiency among CAM practitioners, but the impetus for these changes in practice remains unclear, although many factors have been proposed.

The shift towards CAM could be explained in part by mainstream medicine's inability to adequately address a number of patient needs,[15–17] including the need for respect, holism, choice, autonomy and time. The erosion of client–practitioner relationships, the dependence on invasive technologies and the primary focus on disease might also contribute to the move away from orthodox practice.[17] So, a change in patient needs and beliefs may be a factor driving the increasing use of CAM.[16,18]

Individuals with chronic and life-threatening conditions may also turn to CAM in order to find a solution to their problem. One reason why these patients may try CAM is that conventional practice, and the system it is situated in, does not allow for high-quality prevention or treatment of chronic disease.[19–23] Key stakeholders may need to consider an integrative model of practice in order to address the shortfalls of both the current system of healthcare and the medical model.[17]

Medical pluralism, or the utilisation of more than one form of healthcare, can increase the number of interventions made available to patients and, in turn, provide the client with a number of different treatment perspectives. As opposed to the paternalistic and universalistic model of healthcare that currently exists, the more pluralistic and individualised system of integrative care may foster collaboration between CAM services and mainstream practitioners, improve client outcomes and more effectively meet the needs of patients.[21] At present, however, the existing system of healthcare is the antithesis of pluralistic.[15]

The right to be informed about a range of therapeutic options from a variety of disciplines is a right of every individual. Yet, since most conventional clinicians are not sufficiently knowledgeable about CAM and preventative healthcare[11,20,24–26] and many CAM practitioners might not be familiar with the myriad orthodox treatment approaches,[27] a number of clinicians may not be equipped to inform patients about an appropriate range of therapies. Practitioner bias or lack of knowledge about other modalities could also deprive patients of suitable treatment options and, in effect, compromise the patient's ability to make an informed decision about their care.[24] Since practitioners have an obligation to inform patients about treatments that are well supported by evidence,[28] strategies that facilitate this process are in the best interests of the client. The inclusion of CAM content within medical degrees and the increasing biomedical content within CAM courses is a critical step towards addressing this problem.

## Problems with integration

In spite of the push towards an integrative system of healthcare, many issues need to be considered before accepting this approach (see Table 7.1). The first of these relates to the different paradigms of CAM and orthodox medicine. Since integrative healthcare is not just about adding therapies to a discipline, but is also about accepting a different mindset,[15] this is of some concern, as many practitioners who are well trained and experienced in their respective therapies may be unwilling to accept new healthcare philosophies or new challenges to convention.[29] In fact, conventional clinicians who simply choose a few isolated therapies to incorporate into their practice may be seen 'as orthodox biomedical cherry picking from the complementary field, [in order] to supplement conventional treatment'.[30] The same principle also applies to CAM practitioners who choose to adopt complementary therapies for which they have no formal training, for example, a chiropractor choosing to dabble in herbal medicine or a naturopath dabbling in acupressure. In either case, ignoring the philosophical foundations of a treatment may deem the approach as simply another tool and not an independent therapy in its own right.

| **Table 7.1:** Challenges facing the integrative healthcare movement |
|---|
| **Interprofessional issues** |
| • Conflicting philosophies or principles of care<br>• Disparate approaches to diagnosis and treatment<br>• Actual and/or perceived hierarchies of professions and treatments<br>• Differential access to diagnostic and specialist services<br>• Treatment interactions |
| **System issues** |
| • Disparate funding, reimbursement or subsidisation arrangements<br>• Diverse approaches to integrative healthcare<br>• Uncertainty about the cost-effectiveness and efficiency of integrative healthcare |

Clinicians choosing to incorporate CAM modalities into clinical practice need to be mindful of the level of competence required to deliver these therapies, as some practitioners may be adopting new modalities that they are not well equipped to use.[31] This is particularly important, as adequate training in CAM is critical to the safe and effective delivery of CAM.[15] The rate of adverse events per year of full-time traditional Chinese medicine (TCM) practice by 1278 non-medical practitioners (NMP) and 458 medical practitioners (MP) who practised TCM, for example, was 1/1009 consultations and 1/368 consultations respectively ($p<0.001$).[32] The authors attributed these differences to the inadequate training of MPs, with the average length of TCM training among MPs approximating 8 months, compared with 43.6 months among NMPs.[33] This disparity in MP and NMP training has also been identified elsewhere.[33] There is related concern that the therapies being integrated into clinical practice may not be supported by clinical evidence. Opponents of integrative care, for instance, argue that complementary therapies do not belong in orthodox medical settings because of scientific divide between the two settings.[34]

However, given that many conventional medical practices (including various surgical techniques (e.g. circumcision, tonsillectomy) and diagnostic methods (e.g. X-rays, screening tests)) have not been tested to the level expected of CAM,[35,36] that is, under double blind randomised placebo-controlled conditions, these arguments about the efficacy of treatments are not well founded. Instead, these concerns about the evidence-base of CAM may just be a smokescreen for other political or philosophical issues.[37]

Other factors impeding the assimilation of CAM into conventional healthcare settings relate to cost-effectiveness, funding, safety, financial reimbursement, infrastructure, and practitioner credentialling.[38,39] Unless these constraints are addressed, access to appropriate treatment options could be delayed. Furthermore, by failing to accept integrative care, clinicians may deny patients safe and effective treatments,[14] and, in effect, provide care that may not best meet the needs of the client. The continuation of sole practitioner practice models (where practitioners work independently of one another), for instance, may only serve to perpetuate this problem and further sustain the marginalisation of CAM practitioners.

## Merits of integration

The integration of credentialled CAM services into healthcare settings traditionally dominated by orthodox medicine (such as hospitals, rehabilitation centres and super-clinics) holds many benefits for consumers and practitioners (see Table 7.2). One of these merits is the capacity to 'bring together the strengths and to balance the weaknesses inherent in [the] different systems of healthcare',[27] and, in effect, provide a more favourable and complete system of care. CAM may also provide alternatives to treatment when conventional practice can no longer offer a solution[37,40] or when medical treatment is ineffective or harmful,[17] in, for example, the management of chronic pain, psoriasis, irritable bowel syndrome and menstrual complaints. In essence, integrative practices may increase healthcare choices, improve treatment outcomes and enable patients to more effectively navigate through the range of available treatment options.[41]

The fragmented and incomplete care provided by some professions may drive a number of practitioners to use CAM modalities or products in order to address the shortfalls of their discipline.[42] Integrating CAM philosophy into orthodox

| Table 7.2: Merits of integrative healthcare |
| --- |
| • Fosters client-centredness |
| • Addresses a range of client needs |
| • Approaches clinical assessment and care holistically |
| • Provides a wide scope of healthcare choices |
| • Has a non-hierarchical, participatory structure |
| • Increases access to services |
| • Fosters interdisciplinary collaboration and teamwork |
| • Improves treatment outcomes |
| • Reduces overlap or duplication of services |
| • Facilitates a smoother transition between services |

practice (including the principles of holism, client-centredness, illness prevention and wellness optimisation) may also provide practitioners with the means to deliver individualised healthcare[31] that is more holistic and less fragmented.[43]

Although the delivery of CAM services can be time and labour intensive, it is in many ways more cost-effective than the delivery of conventional care,[37,44] which leads to the argument that the inclusion of CAM practitioners within mainstream healthcare settings could generate substantial cost savings to the health service. This could be attributed in part to a reduction in the duplication of services or the use of less costly equipotent interventions. While earlier reports have found CAM to be no more cost-effective than conventional care, more recent evidence suggests otherwise.[45,46] As well as saving costs, an integrative approach to healthcare may also increase patient satisfaction.[47,48] One possible explanation for these improved outcomes may lie in the focus of care, with integrative healthcare being more client-centred than conventional care,[29,49] and, as a result, more likely to address patient needs.[48]

## Models of integration

In terms of complexity and skill mix, existing frameworks for the delivery of integrative medicine and/or integrative healthcare vary significantly. The level of integration reported in these models is also diverse, ranging from the basic uptake of selected CAM interventions by orthodox practitioners, to non-collaborative multidisciplinary clinics or networks, to the more complex integration of professional CAM services within a large collaborative interdisciplinary team. An integrative system of healthcare that would be of most benefit to patients is one that provides consumers with greater access to a full range of qualified practitioners and does not surrender practitioner or patient autonomy. A suitable model of healthcare should also inform patients about all appropriate treatment options, offer options in a prioritised manner and be focused on prevention, healing and health creation.[15,18] The model should also be holistic, promote evidence-based practice and be mindful of all individuals in a client's milieu.[15]

Leckridge[50] reports on four possible models of integrative healthcare: the market, regulated, assimilated and patient-centred models. The market model enables patients to access any healthcare product or service they desire. While such a model promotes freedom of choice, it is often chaotic, costly and unintegrated. A similar framework is the regulated model, although in this system, all products and services are regulated by government. The assimilated model builds on the regulated system by allowing biomedical practitioners to integrate CAM products and services into their care. However, not only does this model perpetuate the divide between CAM and orthodox clinicians, but it also disregards the comprehensive training required to safely and effectively implement CAM.

The patient-centred model turns the focus of healthcare towards the patient and away from the practitioner. Client's wishes become a pivotal part of any consultation and practitioners work closely together to more effectively meet patient needs. The benefit of this approach is that the divide between alternative and orthodox is narrowed and the true purpose of healthcare – the improvement of patient health and wellbeing – is accentuated.[50] By minimising practitioner ownership over health, the model also facilitates a more interdisciplinary approach to client care.[14]

There is now evidence to suggest that patient-centred models of integrative healthcare are being applied in clinical practice. In an Israeli study,[51] for instance, CAM practitioners were contracted to work within orthodox outpatient clinics or hospitals on a part-time basis; inside the hospitals, CAM practitioners worked within specific medical departments. Interviews with 10 alternative practitioners and nine biomedical clinicians across the four Jewish community hospitals found the integration of CAM practitioners into the hospital setting improved teamwork and collaborative attitudes, complemented other health services and addressed concerns relating to patient quality of life, although the extent of these benefits was not fully explored. The marginalisation of CAM practitioners was still evident, particularly with regards to employment status, office location, remuneration and participation in clinical rounds. Many CAM practitioners believed the holistic nature of their work was constrained by placement in specialised departments. The provision of complementary therapists at the hospital level rather than departmental level could address some of these concerns.

A number of integrative models have also been developed for the primary care setting. In one Israeli family practice,[52] the medical practitioner administered the role of gate keeper. In this capacity, the physician was required to review and diagnose all presenting cases, and then refer the cases onto the most suitable healthcare professional for clinical management. This gatekeeping primary care model is not dissimilar to that recently developed by a group of conventional and CAM practitioners in Sweden.[53] There is concern, however, that such a model could perpetuate medical dominance and control over patients and other healthcare professionals. Additionally, this model may be easily tainted by practitioner bias, therapy preference and level of knowledge. There are also philosophical and diagnostic differences between professions that need to be considered when triaging cases with a single practitioner.

Another integrative approach that may be used in the primary care setting is that recently administered by Get Well UK.[54] The CAM pilot project, which was conducted in 2007–08, involved 35 general practitioners (GPs) across two health centres in Northern Ireland, 713 patients with a variety of musculoskeletal and mental health problems, and 16 CAM practitioners from seven different CAM fields. The project encouraged GPs from participating health centres to refer eligible patients to pertinent CAM practitioners via the Get Well UK customer service team, which facilitated the selection of practitioners, the booking of appointments, the coordination of care and the reporting of outcomes. Appropriate assessment and care were provided by single or multiple CAM practitioners and, upon patient discharge, was summarised and reported back to the GP. Even though the outcomes of the pilot study strongly support an integrative healthcare approach, including improvements in patient symptoms, wellbeing, medication use and work absenteeism, it is not clear how the effectiveness of this approach compares to conventional care alone or to a single-centre integrative healthcare model, and whether this system offers similar benefits to patients with other illnesses.

A more collaborative model of integration, which addresses prior concerns about power, autonomy, respect and decision making, is that reported by Chung et al.[55] In this Hong Kong-based integrative health clinic (the first of its kind in Hong Kong), patients received initial screening and physical assessment by a registered nurse. The patient's case was then reviewed by a team of nurses, conventional physicians, TCM physicians and CAM practitioners working within the clinic. Although the majority of consumers using the clinic reported a high level of satisfaction with practitioner performance and various aspects of service delivery, there was concern that the case conferencing of every patient (including new and continuing cases) may be cost-prohibitive and time inefficient for regions demonstrating high service demand. The economic and clinical implications of this model warrant further investigation.

As well as the more traditional clinical settings, integrative healthcare may also be delivered through integrative wellness and health promotion programs in the work-place. These programs, which are often embraced by medium to large companies, can incorporate services from a range of health professionals, including naturopaths, chiropractors, medical practitioners, fitness trainers, ergonomists, massage therapists and/or registered nurses. Evidence to date indicates that the implementation of these programs reduces staff absenteeism and healthcare costs at the same time as improving work performance, job satisfaction and employee quality of life.[56] In addition to these positive outcomes, integrative wellness programs also demonstrate generous returns on program investment.[57] What remains unclear is how the skill mix affects these employee outcomes and whether the inclusion of CAM practitioners within these programs can contribute to significant improvements in work performance.

Despite the level or model of integration selected, physician support will be fundamental to the success of the service, as will practitioner competency (i.e. credentialling) and effective administration.[58] Other issues that need to be addressed in order to improve program success are equitable access, funding, practitioner hierarchy,[14] triage of cases, communication between clinicians and the selection of appropriate providers and therapies.[52]

A model of integrative healthcare that takes these concerns into consideration, at the same time as addressing the limitations of the systems previously discussed, is the integrative healthcare centre model (IHCCM). This interdisciplinary, publicly funded, non-hierarchical, client-centred model follows a four-stage process. The first stage of the model is patient registration. At this point, patients are required to register their details at centre reception, after which they will be directed either to the clinical waiting area (for follow-up visits) or to the triage officer (for newly presented cases). The triage officer, who may be a nurse practitioner, physician or other adequately qualified health professional, assesses the client and in conjunction with advanced diagnostic reasoning software (i.e. a modified clinical decision support system), determines which health professional will be the most appropriate to manage the presenting complaint. This person is referred to as the patient's 'primary practitioner'. As well as controlling for gatekeeping and practitioner bias, the decision support software alerts the triage officer of other team members who may need to be involved in the client's care. The primary and other practitioners who are identified by the software are collectively referred to as the 'core management team'. Once a team is identified, the patient is directed to the recommended primary practitioner for assessment, diagnosis and planning of care. Contingent on client choice, practitioner availability and workload, and the discretion of the primary practitioner, the client may be then referred to other members of the core management team so they can contribute to the patient's plan of care.

Stringent quality assurance systems monitor client progress during their episode of care to ensure that patient management is cost-effective and expected health outcomes are achieved in a timely and efficient manner. Overseeing these systems, as well as practitioner competency, performance, recruitment and clinic administration, is the centre operations manager. Regular team conferences are held in order to facilitate the management of complex patient cases and to foster collegiality, interprofessional understanding and respect, and professional development. These meetings, together with the utilisation of shared files, standardised documentation and shared clinical outcomes, also facilitate interprofessional communication. The use of non-hierarchical consensus voting during these review meetings also ensures that necessary changes to care are evaluated, endorsed and implemented by the team. While this equitable and accessible model of care is still in the conceptual phase of development, plans are currently in place to refine and test this model for future application in clinical practice. A visual representation of the IHCCM developed by the author is presented in Figure 7.2.

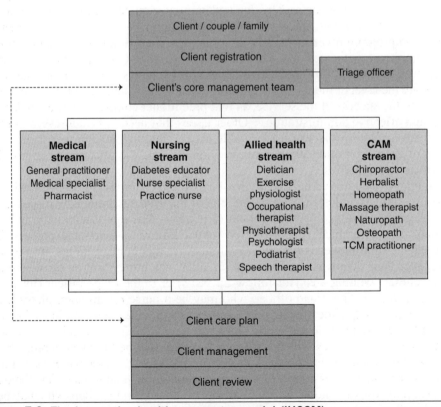

**Figure 7.2: The integrative healthcare centre model (IHCCM)** Note: TCM = traditional Chinese medicine

## Summary

The development of an integrative healthcare system will necessitate a major change in the current system of healthcare. These changes may require CAM and orthodox practitioners to redefine the parameters of their practice[31] and key stakeholders to redefine the hierarchical positions of these clinicians, as well as encourage amendments to legislation that will enable the provision of adequate funding of complementary medicines and services. Several models of integrative healthcare have been presented in this chapter, of which some are expected to address the many shortfalls of conventional healthcare. Despite the argument for an integrative system of care, there remains a paucity of evidence to demonstrate IHC is any more effective than conventional care at improving client health outcomes and quality of life. Because of the increasing shift towards integrative healthcare, research is urgently needed to justify the more rapid facilitation of this movement.

### Learning activities

1 From the perspective of your own profession, what is your interpretation of integrative healthcare?
2 Discuss how integrative healthcare may address some of the shortfalls of the conventional healthcare system.
3 Compared to independent practice, how might the inclusion of your profession into a client-centred integrative healthcare team change the role, scope of practice and professional development of your discipline?
4 How does the integrative healthcare centre model (IHCCM) address the limitations of existing integrative healthcare models?
5 Considering the information presented in this chapter and your responses to questions 2 and 4 above, develop an integrative healthcare model that you believe best serves the needs of the health consumer, medical and allied healthcare team, and the CAM profession.

## References

1. Boon H et al (2004) From parallel practice to integrative healthcare: a conceptual framework. BMC Health Services Research, 4: 15
2. Rees L. Weil A. (2001) Integrated medicine. British Medical Journal, 322: 119–20.
3. Hsiao AF et al (2006) Variations in provider conceptions of integrative medicine. Social Science and Medicine, 62(12): 2973–87.
4. Berndtson K. (1998) Integrative medicine: business risks and opportunities. Physician Executive, 24(6): 22–26.
5. van de Mortel T. (2002) Health for all Australians. Contemporary Nurse, 12(2): 169–75.
6. Russello A. (2007) Severe mental illness in primary care. Abingdon: Radcliffe Publishing.
7. Duckett S. (1999) Policy challenges for the Australian healthcare system. Australian Health Review, 22(2): 130–47.
8. Oliveira MD. Bevan G. (2008) Modelling hospital costs to produce evidence for policies that promote equity and efficiency. European Journal of Operational Research, 185(3): 933–47.
9. Gallagher C. Bailey-Flitter N. (2007) What can the NHS learn from healthcare provision in other countries? Pharmaceutical Journal, 279: 210–13.
10. MacLennan AH. Myers SP. Taylor AW. (2006) The continuing use of complementary and alternative medicine in South Australia: costs and beliefs in 2004. Medical Journal of Australia, 184(1): 27–31.
11. Leach MJ. (2004) Public, nurse and medical practitioner attitude and practice of natural medicine. Complementary Therapies in Nursing and Midwifery, 10(1): 13–21.
12. Sewitch MJ et al (2008) A literature review of healthcare professional attitudes toward complementary and alternative medicine. Complementary Health Practice Review, 13(3): 139–54.
13. Dalen J. (1999) Is integrative medicine the medicine of the future? Archives of Internal Medicine, 159(18): 2122–6.
14. Cohen M. (2004) CAM practitioners and 'regular' doctors: is integration possible? Medical Journal of Australia, 180: 645–6.

15. Myers S. (2003) Conclusion – challenges facing integrated medicine. In: An introduction to complementary medicine. Robson T, editor. Sydney: Allen & Unwin.
16. Sirois FM. (2008) Motivations for consulting complementary and alternative medicine practitioners: a comparison of consumers from 1997–8 and 2005. BMC Complementary and Alternative Medicine, 8: 16–26.
17. Snyderman R. Weil A. (2002) Integrative medicine: bringing medicine back to its roots. Archives of Internal Medicine, 162(4): 395–7.
18. Peters D. (2000) From holism to integration: is there a future for complementary therapies in the NHS? Complementary Therapies in Nursing and Midwifery, 6: 59–60.
19. Giordano J et al (2003) Complementary and alternative medicine in mainstream public health: a role for research in fostering integration. Journal of Alternative and Complementary Medicine, 9(3): 441–5.
20. Jones DS. Quinn S. (2006) Why functional medicine? importance of improving management of complex, chronic disease. In: Textbook of functional medicine. Jones DS, Quinn S, editors. Institute for Functional Medicine, Washington: Gig Harbor.
21. Mann D. Gaylord S. Norton S. (2004) Moving toward integrative care: rationales, models, and steps for conventional-care providers. Complementary Health Practice Review, 9: 155–72.
22. White A. (2003) Is integrated medicine respectable? Complementary Therapies in Medicine, 11(3): 140–1.
23. Wolff JL. Boult C. (2005) Moving beyond round pegs and square holes: restructuring Medicare to improve chronic care. Annals of Internal Medicine, 143(6): 439–45.
24. Adams K et al (2002) Ethical considerations of complementary and alternative medical therapies in conventional medical settings. Annals of Internal Medicine, 137(8): 660–4.
25. Giannelli M et al (2007) General practitioners' knowledge and practice of complementary/alternative medicine and its relationship with life-styles: a population-based survey in Italy. BMC Family Practice, 8: 30–8.
26. Kwan D. Hirschkorn K. Boon H. (2006) US and Canadian pharmacists' attitudes, knowledge, and professional practice behaviors toward dietary supplements: a systematic review. BMC Complementary and Alternative Medicine, 6: 31–41.
27. Owen D. Lewith G. Stephens C. (2001) Can doctors respond to patients' increasing interest in complementary and alternative medicine? British Medical Journal, 322: 154–7.
28. Verhoef MJ. Boon HS. Page SA. (2008) Talking to cancer patients about complementary therapies: is it the physician's responsibility? Current Oncology, 15(Suppl 2): S88–93.
29. Richardson J. (2001) Integrating complementary therapies into healthcare education: a cautious approach. Journal of Clinical Nursing, 10: 793–8.
30. St George D. (2001) Integrated medicine means doctors will be in charge. British Medical Journal, 322(7300): 1484.
31. Giordano J et al (2002) Blending the boundaries: steps toward an integration of complementary and alternative medicine into mainstream practice. Journal of Alternative and Complementary Medicine, 8(6): 897–906.
32. Bensoussan A. Myers S. Carlton A. (2000) Risks associated with the practice of traditional Chinese medicine. Archives of Family Medicine, 9(10): 1071–8.
33. Hughes E. (2001) Integrating complementary and alternative medicine into clinical practice. Clinical Obstetrics and Gynecology, 44(4): 902–6.
34. Robotin MC. Penman AG. (2006) Integrating complementary therapies into mainstream cancer care: which way forward? Medical Journal of Australia, 185: 377–9.
35. Clarke-Grill M. (2007) Questionable gate-keeping: scientific evidence for complementary and alternative medicines (CAM): response to Malcolm Parker. Journal of Bioethical Inquiry, 4(1): 21–8.
36. Parker M. (2007) Rejoinder. Journal of Bioethical Inquiry, 4(1): 29–31.
37. Stone J. (2002) Integrating complementary and alternative medicine: fresh challenges for RECs. Bulletin of Medical Ethics, (180): 13–16.
38. Barrett B. (2003) Alternative, complementary, and conventional medicine: is integration upon us? Journal of Alternative and Complementary Medicine, 9(3): 417–27.
39. Cohen M. (2005) Challenges and future directions for integrative medicine in clinical practice: 'Integrative', 'complementary' and 'alternative' medicine. Evidence-Based Integrative Medicine, 2(3): 117–22.
40. Paterson C. (2000) Primary healthcare transformed: complementary and orthodox medicine complementing each other. Complementary Therapies in Medicine, 8: 47–9.
41. Rakel D. (2005) Perspectives on integrative practice. In: Complementary medicine in clinical practice: integrative practice in American healthcare. Rakel D, Faass N, editors. Sudbury: Jones & Bartlett Publishers.
42. Michaeli D. (2000) Integrative medicine: who needs it and why? Archives of Internal Medicine, 160(8): 1205.
43. Davies P. (1999) Making sense of integrated care in New Zealand. Australian Health Review, 22(4): 25–47.
44. Herman PM. Craig BM. Caspi O. (2005) Is complementary and alternative medicine (CAM) cost-effective? a systematic review. BMC Complementary and Alternative Medicine, 5: 11–26.
45. Leach MJ. Pincombe J. Foster G. (2006) Using horsechestnut seed extract in the treatment of venous leg ulceration: a cost-benefit analysis. Ostomy/Wound Management, 52(4): 68–78.
46. Sarnat RL. Winterstein J. Cambron JA. (2007) Clinical utilization and cost outcomes from an integrative medicine independent physician Association: an additional 3-year update. Journal of Manipulative and Physiological Therapeutics, 30(4): 263–9.
47. Esch BM et al (2008) Patient satisfaction with primary care: an observational study comparing anthroposophic and conventional care. Health and Quality of Life Outcomes, 6: 74–89.
48. Myklebust M. Pradhan EK. Gorenflo D. (2008) An integrative medicine patient care model and evaluation of its outcomes: University of Michigan Experience. Journal of Alternative and Complementary Medicine, 14(7): 821–6.
49. Willms L. (2008) Blending in: Is integrative medicine the future of family medicine? Canadian Family Physician, 54(8): 1085–7.
50. Leckridge B. (2004) The future of complementary and alternative medicine – models of integration. Journal of Alternative and Complementary Medicine, 10(2): 413–16.
51. Shuval J. Mizrachi N. Smetannikov E. (2002) Entering the well-guarded fortress: alternative practitioners in hospital settings. Social Science and Medicine, 55(10): 1745–55.

52. Frenkel M. Borkan J. (2003) An approach for integrating complementary-alternative medicine into primary care. Family Practice, 20(3): 324–32.

53. Sundberg T et al (2007) Towards a model for integrative medicine in Swedish primary care. BMC Health Services Research, 7: 107–16.

54. McDade D. (2009) Evaluation of a CAM pilot project in Northern Ireland. Belfast: Social and Market Research.

55. Chung JWY et al (2008) Evaluation of services of the integrative health clinic in Hong Kong. Journal of Clinical Nursing, 17(19): 2550–7.

56. Mitchell SG. Goetzel RZ. Ozminkowski RJ. (2008) The value of worksite health promotion. ACSM's Health and Fitness Journal, 12(2): 23–7.

57. Young JM. (2006) Promoting health at the workplace: challenges of prevention, productivity, and program implementation. North Carolina Medical Journal, 67(6): 417–24.

58. Ananth S. Newman D. (2002) Risks and rewards. Hospitals and Health Networks, 60.

# 8
# Review

## Chapter overview

The final stage of DeFCAM is review – a continual and critical process aimed at improving client outcomes, quality of care and the professional advancement of CAM. Central to this process is the need to recognise and manage a range of elements that can affect these clinical outcomes. Consideration of these factors, together with comprehensive and holistic assessment, clinical expertise, reflective thinking and valid and reliable instrumentation will enable practitioners to better evaluate clinical care and, in effect, optimise client health, wellbeing and wellness.

## Learning objectives

The content of this chapter will assist the reader to:
* explain the meaning of clinical review
* recognise the merits of review
* identify data sources useful to the review process
* recognise the factors that influence the attainment of planned goals and expected outcomes
* outline the role of reflective practice in the review process.

## Chapter outline

* Introduction
* Defining review
* The importance of review
* Strategies for reviewing practice
* Reflective practice
* The review process
* Summary

## Introduction

The evaluation of client care is an ongoing process aimed at improving clinical outcomes, as well as advancing clinical practice, yet there is a dearth of literature to guide clinicians through this process. In order to improve individual health and wellbeing, and to improve the process and outcomes of care, CAM practitioners must be informed of the importance of client review and the range of methods capable of appraising clinical practice. Before presenting these approaches, however, the concept of review needs to be defined.

## Defining review

Review, or evaluation, is defined as 'attributing value to an intervention by gathering reliable and valid information about it in a systematic way, and by making comparisons, for the purposes of making more informed decisions or understanding causal mechanisms or general principles'.[1] The term is also described as 'a deliberate, systematic process in which a judgement is made about the *quality, value or worth* of something by comparing it to *previously identified criteria or standards*' (emphasis in the original).[2] In other words, review is a systematic process that uses valid and reliable instrumentation to quantify changes in a parameter in order to facilitate decision making. In clinical terms, review determines whether a client's presenting condition or state of imbalance improved after the delivery of care, which factors attributed to the client's outcome, whether the client moved towards expected outcomes or goals, whether the interventions were safe and effective, and whether the underlying cause of the complaint had been resolved.[3–5] Review can thus be likened to the evidence-based practice process in that the best available information on the client is gathered and appraised in order to inform practice. Research is another useful analogy, with the planning phase of care being akin to the generation of a hypothesis or expected outcome, and the review phase involving the testing of that expected endpoint.[6]

## The importance of review

Increasing demand for quality healthcare and evidence-based practice[7,8] suggests that CAM providers can no longer discount the evaluation of client care. As well as the increase in public pressure, the review of practice is also being driven by a need to quantify client outcomes, CAM practitioner performance and healthcare efficiency. This review of healthcare interventions and client outcomes not only provides useful feedback to improve the quality of care,[9,10] but by measuring the efficacy, cost-effectiveness and timeliness of healthcare,[3] can also provide essential data to improve the delivery of CAM services and to benchmark against best practice. The purposeful ongoing appraisal of client outcomes before, during and/or after each client appointment, for example, may promptly identify delays in the achievement of expected outcomes (by comparing actual progress against expected progress) and thus more effectively determine if a treatment needs to be modified or altered to better meet client needs and to deliver best practice care. The review of practice may also reduce treatment costs and client suffering by highlighting interventions that are neither safe nor useful[11] and, in some cases, determine if referral to another healthcare professional, either within or outside the integrative healthcare team, is needed. Put simply, the appraisal of CAM practice may improve the quality of client care by determining whether clinical outcomes have been achieved in the most beneficial, efficient and cost-effective manner.[7,10]

Practitioners who use review techniques may over time contribute significantly to the professional advancement of CAM. The evaluation of practice, for instance, encourages new ways of thinking and practising,[12] which, in turn, filters useful knowledge back into the profession.[9] This knowledge could help to improve personal and professional standards,[10] create new benchmarks for best practice care, and through subsequent improvements in client outcomes and client satisfaction, generate a more widely accepted, client-centred and ethically sound profession.

From the perspective of the clinician, practice review ensures that CAM practitioners maintain a sense of accountability for care given.[3] In other words, by self-appraising performance, competence, knowledge, experience and decision-making ability, a practitioner can identify areas for personal and professional development and thereby improve client care.[5,12,13] Given that CAM practitioners have a duty to deliver high-quality best practice care to all individuals, the importance of self-appraisal cannot be overemphasised.

From an ethical point of view, the critical appraisal of client outcomes provides some assurance that clinicians practise in a beneficent and non-maleficent manner. Nevertheless, for individual benefits to be seen, CAM practitioners need to not only measure the outcomes of care, but also to change practice when indicated.[10] Thus, review requires not only critical thinking and client interaction, but also action.

Practice review can also create mutual benefits for clinician and client. Fundamentally, evaluation provides useful information that facilitates shared decision making[9,14] and ameliorates client–practitioner communication.[7] These outcomes could lead to improvements in client rapport, which may further improve client health and wellbeing, and the efficiency of CAM services.[15]

## Strategies for reviewing practice

The review of clinical practice often requires a number of tools or outcome measures to effectively answer the clinical questions posed.[7] The use of multiple assessment methods is particularly important, including approaches that generate quantitative and qualitative data, to ensure that observer bias is minimised and practitioner confidence in findings can be increased.[16] Yet there is a limited number of freely available evaluation tools, with demonstrated validity and reliability, that can effectively review client outcomes in a clear, concise and quantifiable manner. Where suitable instruments are available, client outcomes should be evaluated using the same tools that were used during assessment[3] in order to improve the validity of inferences made about the efficacy of treatment[17] (see chapter 3).

Even though these evaluation instruments are useful in the review process, they are not the only source of information that can be drawn upon. CAM practitioners can, for instance, monitor the effectiveness of treatment through client interviews, physical assessment,[18] medical imaging and/or functional, pathology, invasive and miscellaneous tests. Client self-reporting through questionnaires and diaries is also adequate for monitoring and evaluating client outcomes and clinical progress.[7,19] As such, data for client review can be derived from a number of sources, including the client, family, caregivers, pertinent documentation, questionnaires, literature, other healthcare professionals, observations and objective measures such as blood pressure monitoring and pathology testing. Hence, depending on the type of data required and the timing of expected outcomes, information may be collected for review before, during and/or after client consultation. Other instruments that can be used to monitor individual progress are listed in Table 8.1.

While the sourcing of accurate and reliable data is important to the review process, it is only one of many considerations that need to be taken into account. An effective clinical review also requires CAM practitioners to be mindful of the factors that facilitate and impede the attainment of client outcomes (see Table 8.2). The achievement of these outcomes can, for example, be affected by the choice of intervention, the client–practitioner relationship and the treatment philosophy adopted by the clinician.[9,15] Social factors, such as environment,[18] family, culture, religion, language and education, can also influence the rate of progress towards defined clinical endpoints. A person with poor English proficiency or health literacy, for instance, may have difficulty understanding what is communicated by their clinician, including pertinent information about the disease process, complications of the condition and the management of their complaint. These difficulties could result in lower levels of knowledge and, consequently, poorer outcomes of care. The positive relationship between English fluency and diabetes knowledge scores reported in the Fremantle diabetes survey lends support to this claim.[20]

Equally important are the client-derived factors, including age, gender, functional ability, cognitive capacity, motivation, perceived health status, preference for

| **Table 8.1:** Examples of clinical review instruments |
| --- |
| • Acne severity index (ASI)<br>• Arthritis impact measurement scales (AIMS2)<br>• Asthma control scoring system (ACSS)<br>• Bristol stool scale (BSS)<br>• Claudication scale (CLAU-S)<br>• Diabetes quality of life measure (DQOL)<br>• Fibromyalgia impact questionnaire (FIQ)<br>• Hamilton anxiety scale (HAS-A)<br>• Hamilton rating scale for depression (HRSD)<br>• HIV quality of life questionnaire (HIV-QOL)<br>• Irritable bowel syndrome – quality of life questionnaire (IBS-QOL)<br>• International index of erectile dysfunction (IIED)<br>• International prostate symptom score (IPSS)<br>• MacNew heart disease health-related quality of life questionnaire (MacNew)<br>• McGill pain questionnaire (MPQ)<br>• Menopause rating scale (MRS)<br>• Osteoporosis assessment questionnaire (OPAQ)<br>• Polycystic ovary syndrome questionnaire (PCOSQ)<br>• Psoriasis disability index (PDI)<br>• Urinary incontinence-specific quality of life questionnaire (I-QOL)<br>• Wisconsin upper respiratory symptom survey (WURSS) |

| **Table 8.2:** Factors affecting the attainment of client outcomes or client adherence to treatment | | |
| --- | --- | --- |
| Age | Attitude to illness, treatment or practitioner | Availability/access to services and treatments |
| Chronicity/severity of presenting complaint | Chronicity, duration and number of comorbidities | Client–practitioner rapport |
| Client preference, expectations and faith in treatment | Client satisfaction with treatment | Complexity and safety of treatment |
| Culture and ethnicity | Educational attainment | Family influence and commitments |
| Financial constraints | Functional ability | Gender |
| Health literacy | Information about treatment | Level of follow-up or client review |
| Memory retention and recall | Motivation | Perceived health status |
| Physical and/or intellectual disability | Practitioner communication skills | Proficiency of local language |
| Psychiatric illness | Readiness to change | Religion |
| Support structure | Work commitments | |

treatment, readiness to change and treatment expectation. A person who has poor memory retention and recall, Alzheimer's disease for instance, may have difficulty adhering to a treatment plan and, as a result, may not receive optimal care. This may also be the case for clients suffering from depression, anxiety, or a physical or intellectual disability.

The review of practice also needs to appreciate the impact structural factors, such as the environment, resources and administrative and collegial support, have on client progress.[21] Product recalls, delivery delays, equipment failure and the absence of local health services or resources are just some examples of the many structural factors that can interfere with clinical progress.

Judicious consideration of process factors such as the coordination of services, collaboration, professionalism, interpersonal skills, clinician sensitivity, treatment compliance, waiting time, evidence-based practice and client education is also needed.[21] Indeed, any factor influencing treatment compliance is likely to affect client outcomes. Thus, changing an intervention when a client fails to meet a defined clinical endpoint may be premature if other factors influencing client outcomes have not been considered first. The questions listed in Table 8.3 take a number of these factors into account when evaluating client outcomes.

Another element that can hamper client progress is misdiagnosis. Two factors that might contribute to an incorrect diagnosis are inadequate diagnostic reasoning and/or insufficient clinical assessment, but by reassessing the client and revisiting the CAM diagnoses, aetiological factors, goals, expected outcomes and treatments, a practitioner can utilise the review process to identify and resolve misdiagnosis early.[3,5,18] An accurate diagnosis and the timely achievement of expected treatment outcomes (i.e. reaching the outcome by the predetermined date) can also be influenced by

---

**Table 8.3: Questions for reviewing clinical practice**

- Was the assessment accurate, holistic, complete and appropriate?
- Were the assessment data interpreted correctly?
- Was the assessment method valid, reliable and sensitive enough to detect changes in client outcomes?
- Did the assessment identify the underlying cause of the presenting complaint?
- Were the diagnosis or clinical problem accurate and appropriate?
- Was the treatment outcome positive or negative?
- What contributed to the treatment outcome?
- Did the client benefit in any way?
- Was the client harmed in any way? If yes, was this harm foreseeable or preventable?
- Was homeostasis or balance restored in the client?
- Was client suffering alleviated?
- What factors could have facilitated or impeded the client's progress?
- How does the client's actual outcome compare with the predicted treatment outcome?
- Were the treatment goals and expected outcomes realistic and measurable?
- Was sufficient time provided to achieve the client outcome?
- Was the treatment effective in clinical and financial terms?
- Were the treatment choices appropriate?
- Was the treatment tailored to the individual needs of the client?
- Were the treatments competently and effectively implemented?
- Was an important aspect of treatment omitted?
- How do the client outcomes compare to best practice benchmarks or other standards?
- Was the client compliant and satisfied with the treatment?
- Did the treatment optimise client health, wellbeing and/or wellness?
- Was there an improvement in the client's quality of life?
- Was good client rapport established in the first visit?
- What evidence is there to support the treatment approach used?
- What might other practitioners do in the same situation?
- What strategies, or changes in treatment, need to be implemented to achieve the expected best outcome of care?
- Should the client be referred to, or managed by, another member of the healthcare team?

Brownie;[12] Crisp & Taylor;[3] Leach;[22] Long;[17] Murray & Atkinson[23]

practitioner attitude, knowledge and skill.[4] The effect these attributes have on client outcomes can be identified and managed using reflective practice.

## Reflective practice

Rolfe, Freshwater and Jasper[24] define reflective practice as a rational and conscious process of systematically and rigorously reflecting on one's practice to challenge existing approaches and to learn from one's actions. Reflective practice is an effective lifelong learning tool that brings theory and practice closer together,[6,25] which, in accordance with the principles of evidence-based practice,[26] promotes safe, knowledgeable and informed care.[27] Reflective thinking also fosters an individualised, ethical, holistic and flexible approach to client care.[28] As well as meeting client needs more effectively, reflection also improves the quality of care[7] by identifying overlooked aspects of assessment, planning and treatment,[29] and by modifying practitioner decision making and performance.[30]

Reflection is an insightful strategy for which practitioners can view and approach situations from alternative perspectives to determine if the same approach would be repeated or changed if done again.[13,31,32] Without this insight, it is uncertain whether healthcare practices and client outcomes would improve.[30] Hence, reflection provides a means to evaluate performance, improve clinical competence and credibility, extend the scope of practice and aid the ongoing development of the CAM profession.[13,25,29,33]

A number of earlier studies have suggested that reflective strategies might improve clinical practice[34] and professional development.[13] Even so, there is still a paucity of evidence linking reflective thinking to positive clinical outcomes.[35,36] Sound clinical research is needed to investigate not only the potential benefits of reflective practice, but also the validity, reliability and sensitivity of useful review instruments.

Despite concerns regarding the subjectivity of reflective thinking, reflection does challenge 'the constraints of habituated thoughts and practices',[37] and furthermore, provides insight into the beliefs, values, assumptions, culture, history, theories, knowledge and practices that shape those decisions.[12,29,33] Questions that can facilitate reflective practice or introspective enquiry are listed in Table 8.4.

## The review process

As alluded to thus far, there are a number of important considerations when reviewing client care. Reflective and critical thinking, best available evidence, systematic clinical assessment and clinical expertise are just some of these core elements. These attributes are no different than those required at every other stage of DeFCAM. This is because review spans across all stages of the decision-making process and is not

| Table 8.4: Questions to facilitate reflective practice |
| --- |
| • Did my consultation style facilitate the development of client trust and rapport? |
| • Did my attitude towards the client foster an open and honest dialogue? |
| • Do I need to develop my skills to better identify the condition and/or the underlying causes of the complaint in future? |
| • Did I overlook any pertinent information during the clinical assessment of the client? |
| • Did I diagnose the client correctly? |
| • Do I need to further my knowledge base about the client's condition or treatment? |
| • Could I have provided a more effective treatment for the client? |
| • If given another chance, how would I treat the client? |

Adapted from Murray & Atkinson.[23]

restricted to the last and final stage of DeFCAM. Therefore, even though review plays a fundamental role in follow-up care, particularly in determining the safety and efficacy of prescribed treatment, and the degree to which a client has progressed towards planned goals and time-limited expected outcomes, it also informs clinical assessment, diagnostic reasoning, planning and the course of treatment. This relationship between review and other stages of DeFCAM is further illustrated in Figure 8.1.

Figure 8.1 also shows how a CAM practitioner can actively participate in the review process and how they should respond when a client is or is not making reasonable progress towards expected outcomes. If, for example, a client originally presenting with arthralgia (secondary to osteoarthritis) demonstrated a twenty-five

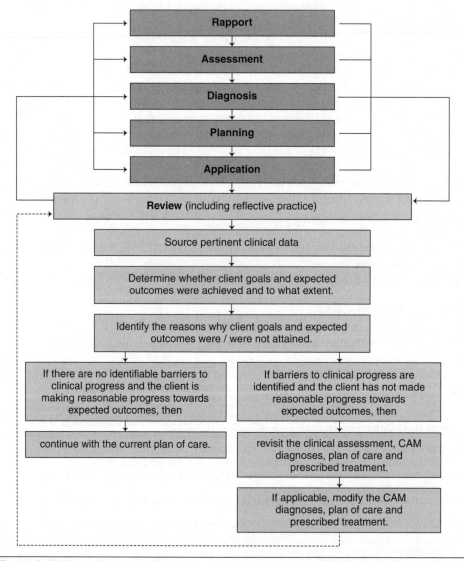

**Figure 8.1:** The review process

per cent improvement in bilateral knee pain after 2 weeks and the short-term expected outcome was a fifty per cent reduction in the severity of bilateral knee pain within 4 weeks, then the client would have made adequate clinical progress and the current plan of care should continue. If the client made no progress or knee pain worsened, then the practitioner should reassess the client to ascertain whether any pertinent data were overlooked during clinical assessment (e.g. joint laxity was not assessed), if the CAM diagnosis was accurate (the diagnosis ignored the impact of diet on osteoarthritis), whether the goals, expected outcomes and treatment were appropriate (e.g. the management plan did not incorporate local pain relief) and if there were any factors that may have affected client adherence to treatment or achievement of outcomes (e.g. recent cold weather exacerbated the arthralgia). If any of these issues are identified, the practitioner should employ measures to resolve the problem, where appropriate modify the treatment plan, and then review client progress again at the next follow-up visit.

## Summary

The evaluation of clinical practice is pivotal to delivering quality client care; it also provides assurance that client needs have been effectively met. Reviewing practice may therefore contribute to improvements in client, family and community health, as well as advances in CAM practice. A number of influential elements need to be taken into account when evaluating clinical practice, however, including social, client, structural and process factors. Consideration of these factors, together with comprehensive and holistic assessment, clinical expertise, reflective thinking, and valid and reliable instrumentation, will enable CAM practitioners to better evaluate clinical care and, in effect, improve client outcomes.

### Learning activities

1  What is your understanding of the term 'clinical review'?
2  How might the review process benefit the client, the practitioner and the wider CAM community?
3  Identify 10 different sources of information that may be used by your discipline to review client outcomes.
4  What structural, client-derived, process and social factors might influence the attainment of client goals and expected outcomes in CAM practice?
5  For each of the following scenarios, list five pertinent reflective practice questions that you would ask yourself in order to learn from the experience and improve your practice:
   a.  a 5-year-old boy with asthma demonstrates a twenty-five per cent decline in peak expiratory flow rate and a twenty per cent reduction in asthma quality of life 3 weeks after your initial consultation
   b.  a 36-year-old woman with depression reports a major adverse reaction to your prescribed treatment
   c.  a 13-year-old girl (and her mother) present to your clinic in need of treatment for premenstrual syndrome. The client does not engage in conversation, shares little information and does not respond to the advice given.

# References

1. Ovretveit J. (1998) Evaluating health interventions. Buckingham: Open University Press.
2. Wilkinson JM. (1992) Nursing process in action: a critical thinking approach. Redwood City: Addison-Wesley Nursing.
3. Crisp J. Taylor C. (2008) Potter and Perry's fundamentals of nursing. 3rd ed. Sydney: Elsevier Australia.
4. Harkreader H. Hogan MA. Thobaben M. (2007) Fundamentals of nursing: caring and clinical judgement. 3rd ed. Philadelphia: Elsevier Saunders.
5. Kulkarni K et al (2005) American dietetic association: standards of practice and standards of professional performance for registered dieticians (generalist, specialty, and advanced) in diabetes care. Journal of the American Dietetic Association, 105(5): 819–24.
6. Wilkinson JM. (2007) Nursing process and critical thinking. 4th ed. Upper Saddle River: Prentice Hall.
7. Marshall S. Haywood K. Fitzpatrick R. (2006) Impact of patient-reported outcome measures on routine practice: a structured review. Journal of Evaluation in Clinical Practice, 12(5): 559–68.
8. Shortell SM. Rundall TG. Hsu J. (2007) Improving patient care by linking evidence-based medicine and evidence-based management. Journal of the American Medical Association, 298(6): 673–6.
9. Long A. (2002) Outcome measurement in complementary and alternative medicine: unpicking the effects. Journal of Alternative and Complementary Medicine, 8(6): 777–86.
10. Lynn J et al (2007) The ethics of using quality improvement methods in healthcare. Annals of Internal Medicine, 146(9): 666–73.
11. Green J. South J. (2006) Evaluation. New York: McGraw-Hill International.
12. Brownie S. (2003) The role of reflective practice in case management. Journal of the Australian Traditional-Medicine Society, 9(3): 133–5.
13. Gustafsson C. Fagerberg I. (2004) Reflection, the way to professional development? Journal of Clinical Nursing, 13(3): 271–80.
14. Smith NL. (2007) Fundamental issues in evaluation. In: Fundamental issues in evaluation. Smith NL, Brandon PR, editors. New York: Guilford Press.
15. Leach MJ. (2005) Rapport: a key to treatment success. Complementary Therapies in Clinical Practice, 11(4): 262–5.
16. Joint Committee on Standards for Educational Evaluation. (2008) The personnel evaluation standards: how to assess systems for evaluating educators. 2nd ed. Thousand Oaks: Corwin Press.
17. Long A. Mercer G. Hughes K. (2000) Developing a tool to measure holistic practice: a missing dimension in outcomes measurement within complementary therapies. Complementary Therapies in Medicine, 8: 26–31.
18. Craven RF. Hirnle CJ. (2008) Fundamentals of nursing: human health and function. 6th ed. Philadelphia: Lippincott, Williams & Wilkins.
19. Eastwood CA et al (2007) Weight and symptom diary for self-monitoring in heart failure clinic patients. Journal of Cardiovascular Nursing, 22(5): 382–9.
20. Bruce DG et al (2003) Diabetes education and knowledge with type 2 diabetes from the community: the Fremantle diabetes study. Journal of Diabetes and Complications, 17: 82–9.
21. Byers JF. Brunell ML. (1998) Demonstrating the value of the advanced practice nurse: an evaluation model. AACN Clinical Issues, 9(2): 296–305.
22. Leach MJ. (2007) Revisiting the evaluation of clinical practice. International Journal of Nursing Practice 13(2): 70–4.
23. Murray ME. Atkinson LD. (2000) Understanding the nursing process in a changing care environment. 6th ed. New York: McGraw-Hill.
24. Rolfe G. Freshwater G. Jasper D. (2001) Critical reflection for nursing and the helping professions: a user's guide. Basingstoke: Palgrave.
25. Lachman N. Pawlina W. (2006) Integrating professionalism in early medical education: the theory and application of reflective practice in the anatomy curriculum. Clinical Anatomy, 19(5): 456–60.
26. Roberts AEK. (2002) Advancing practice through continuing professional education: the case for reflection. British Journal of Occupational Therapy, 65(5): 237–41.
27. Williams G. Lowes L. (2001) Reflection: possible strategies to improve its use by qualified staff. British Journal of Nursing, 10(22): 1482–8.
28. Gustafsson C. Asp M. Fagerberg I. (2007) Reflective practice in nursing care: embedded assumptions in qualitative studies. International Journal of Nursing Practice, 13(3): 151–60.
29. Donaghy M. Morss K. (2007) An evaluation of a framework for facilitating and assessing physiotherapy students' reflection on practice. Physiotherapy Theory and Practice, 23(2): 83–94.
30. Price A. (2004) Encouraging reflection and critical thinking in practice. Nursing Standard, 18(47): 46–52.
31. Clarke KA. (2004) Maslow: hierarchy of needs – or reflective framework? Nurse 2 Nurse Magazine, 4(2): 27–8.
32. O'Connor A. (2006) Clinical instruction and evaluation: a teaching resource. 2nd ed. Sudbury: Jones & Bartlett.
33. Murphy L. (2002) Enriching practice through reflection: an exemplar. Vision, 8(14): 16–19.
34. Page S. Meerabeau L. (2000) Achieving change through reflective practice: closing the loop. Nurse Education Today, 20: 365–72.
35. Duffy A. (2007) A concept analysis of reflective practice: determining its value to nurses. British Journal of Nursing, 16(22): 1400–7.
36. Schutz S. (2007) Reflection and reflective practice. Community Practitioner, 80(9): 26–9.
37. Wilkinson J. (1999) Implementing reflective practice. Nursing Standard, 13(21): 36–40.

# PART 2

# Practical application

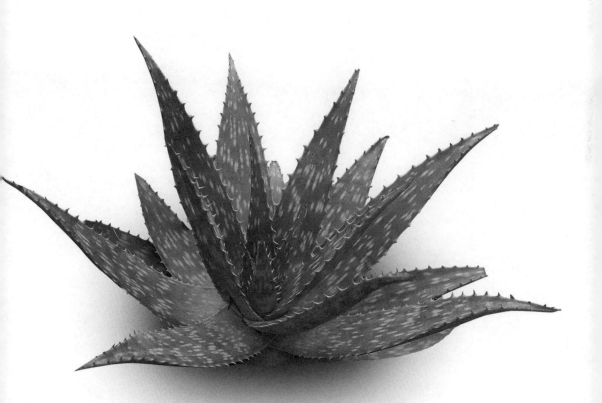

# 9
# Application of DeFCAM

## Chapter overview

The first part of this book discussed the theoretical foundations of the decision-making framework for complementary and alternative medicine (DeFCAM). In this final chapter, the reader will be guided through a number of hypothetical cases to better understand how each stage of DeFCAM can be applied in clinical practice and how evidence-based practice can be integrated into CAM care.

## Learning objectives

The content of this chapter will assist the reader to:

- recognise how DeFCAM can be applied to CAM practice
- know how each stage of DeFCAM is interrelated and how each phase is dependent on the outcomes of previous stages
- explain how evidence-based practice can be integrated into CAM practice
- recognise the level and quality of evidence for specific CAM interventions in particular health disorders.

## Chapter outline

- Introduction
- Methodology
- Case 1: Acne vulgaris/rosacea
- Case 2: Anxiety
- Case 3: Asthma
- Case 4: Chronic venous insufficiency
- Case 5: Dysmenorrhoea
- Case 6: Dermatitis/eczema
- Case 7: Irritable bowel syndrome
- Case 8: Migraine
- Case 9: Osteoarthritis
- Case 10: Psoriasis

## Introduction

The conditions described in this chapter are disorders that often present in CAM practice. The format for each of these conditions is the same – it begins with a general description of the disorder, which is followed by a representative case of that condition. Each case is structured around the six stages of DeFCAM, including rapport, clinical assessment, CAM diagnosis, planning, application and review. Most of these stages are self-explanatory, except for the application stage. In keeping with the need for rigour and transparency in evidence-based practice, the methodology of the application section is described below.

## Methodology

The application section in each of the 10 cases in this chapter identifies a wide range of dietary, lifestyle, nutritional, herbal and other modalities or interventions pertinent to CAM practice. To ensure that the content of this section was applicable to – or at least reflected – that used in CAM practice, several sources of information had to be reviewed. The first stage of the review consisted of a systematic search of the general CAM literature, specifically, a search of traditional and evidence-based texts on CAM, herbal medicine, nutrition, naturopathy, traditional Chinese medicine, chiropractic, osteopathy, homeopathy, mind–body medicine, aromatherapy, massage and reflexology. CAM texts were reviewed for content relevant to each of the 10 conditions presented. A systematic search of several online bibliographic databases (e.g. the Cochrane Library, CAM on PubMED, MEDLINE) was also performed to identify additional interventions. To locate the required information the search terms consisted of different combinations of conditions and CAM modalities. All interventions listed more than once in the general texts and/or bibliographic databases were considered potential treatments for the relevant condition.

A systematic search of the bibliographic databases was then performed to find the best available evidence of effectiveness for each potential intervention. The search strategy included all common and scientific names for the intervention and all alternative names for the condition. Treatments for which clinical evidence was available (i.e. level I to level IV evidence), were included in the application section. The evidence for these interventions was also appraised for quality.

To assess the quality of evidence, every eligible intervention was graded according to the hierarchy of evidence (Table 9.1), strength of evidence (Table 9.2) and direction of evidence (Table 9.3). A summary of each of these quality measures was provided for each intervention for which clinical evidence was available.

Interventions that demonstrated good to excellent evidence of effectiveness for the pertinent disorder (such as levels I, II or III-1, strength A or B and direction +), and were most compatible with the particular needs of the presenting case, that is, they targeted the planned goals, expected outcomes and CAM diagnoses, were listed as primary treatments in the CAM prescription. Interventions that addressed unmet needs of the presenting case but demonstrated lower levels of evidence (including levels III-2 or III-3 and strength C) were listed as secondary treatments.

| Table 9.1: The hierarchy of evidence | |
| --- | --- |
| **Level I** | Systematic reviews |
| **Level II** | Well-designed randomised controlled trials |
| **Level III-1** | Pseudorandomised controlled trials |
| **Level III-2** | Comparative studies with concurrent controls, such as cohort studies, case-control studies or interrupted time series studies |
| **Level III-3** | Comparative studies without concurrent controls, such as a historical control study, two or more single-arm studies or interrupted time series without a parallel control group |
| **Level IV** | Case series with post-test or pre-test/post-test outcomes; uncontrolled open label study |
| **Level V** | Expert opinion or panel consensus |
| **Level VI** | Traditional evidence |

Adapted from National Health and Medical Research Council (NHMRC 1999) and the Centre for Evidence-Based Medicine 2001[1,2]

**Table 9.2: Strength of evidence**

| Grade | Strength of evidence | Definition |
|---|---|---|
| A | Excellent | **Evidence:** multiple level I or II studies with low risk of bias<br>**Consistency:** all studies are consistent<br>**Clinical impact:** very large<br>**Generalisability:** the client matches the population studied<br>**Applicability:** findings are directly applicable to the CAM practice setting |
| B | Good | **Evidence:** one or two level II studies with low risk of bias, or multiple level III studies with low risk of bias<br>**Consistency:** most studies are consistent<br>**Clinical impact:** considerable<br>**Generalisability:** the client is similar to the population studied<br>**Applicability:** findings are applicable to the CAM practice setting with few caveats |
| C | Satisfactory | **Evidence:** level I or II studies with moderate risk of bias, or level III studies with low risk of bias<br>**Consistency:** there is some inconsistency<br>**Clinical impact:** modest<br>**Generalisability:** the client is different from the population studied, but the relationship between the two is clinically sensible<br>**Applicability:** findings are probably applicable to the CAM practice setting with several caveats |
| D | Poor | **Evidence:** level IV studies, level V or VI evidence, or level I to III studies with high risk of bias<br>**Consistency:** evidence is inconsistent<br>**Clinical impact:** small<br>**Generalisability:** the client is different from the population studied, and the relationship between the two is not clinically sensible<br>**Applicability:** findings are not applicable to the CAM practice setting |

Adapted from NHMRC 2009[3]

**Table 9.3: Direction of evidence**

| | |
|---|---|
| + | Positive evidence - intervention is more effective than the placebo or comparative agent |
| o | Neutral evidence – intervention is as effective or no different than the placebo or comparative agent |
| – | Negative evidence - intervention is less effective than the placebo or comparative agent |

# References

1. National Health and Medical Research Council (NHMRC). (1999) A guide to the development, implementation and evaluation of clinical practice guidelines. Canberra: NHMRC.
2. Centre for Evidence-Based Medicine (2001). Oxford Centre for Evidence-based Medicine Levels of Evidence. Oxford: Centre for Evidence-Based Medicine.
3. National Health and Medical Research Council (NHMRC). (2009) NHMRC additional levels of evidence and grades for recommendations for developers of guidelines – Stage 2 consultation. Canberra: NHMRC.

# Case 1
# Acne vulgaris/rosacea

## Description of acne vulgaris/rosacea

Definition
Acne is an integumentary disorder that affects the pilosebaceous units (acne vulgaris) and/or the underlying blood vessels (rosacea) of the skin. Some of the variants of the disease include acne vulgaris, acne conglobata, acne fulminans, acne excorié, mature onset, pyoderma faciale, rosacea, neonatal and infantile acne.

Epidemiology
Males and females of all ages can be affected by acne;[1] however, the type of acne can vary between sexes. The vulgaris, conglobata and fulminant variants of acne, for example, are most prevalent among adolescent males, while acne excorié, rosacea, mature onset and pyoderma faciale are more likely to manifest in women.[1]

Aetiology and pathophysiology
Many factors can be implicated in the pathogenesis of acne, including genetic, hormonal, infectious, dietary and environmental elements. In terms of hormonal influence, it is believed that elevated androgen levels increase sebum production and abnormal follicular keratinisation and desquamation, which leads to the blockage of pilosebaceous units and the formation of comedones.[1] The peak elevation in androgen, sebum and growth hormone levels during the adolescent period provides some explanation for the increased prevalence of this condition during adolescence.[2] Findings from a case study of 34 men and women with acne adds further support to the relationship between androgen levels and acne lesion count.[2]

The bacterium *Propionibacterium acnes* is another contributing factor in acne development. This is because the bacterium promotes inflammation by releasing chemotactic factors and proteases while hydrolysing sebum into proinflammatory free fatty acids.[1,3] In rosacea, an underlying vascular defect may be responsible,[3] although the actual aetiology of this disorder remains unclear. What is apparent is that rosacea can be triggered by a range of exogenous and endogenous stimuli, including cold or hot weather, wind, sun exposure, exercise, hot baths, emotional stress, alcohol, spicy foods, cosmetics and hot drinks.[4]

Other environmental factors that may be implicated in the pathogenesis of acne include medications (e.g. steroids, anticonvulsants), occlusive objects (e.g. shirt collars, helmets), topical agents (e.g. cosmetics, lotions, creams) and perspiration.[4,5]

The chronic consumption of foods with a high glycaemic index or glycaemic load also contributes to acne development by promoting hyperinsulinaemia and insulin resistance. This can be followed by elevated free levels of insulin growth factor and androgens, and a subsequent rise in keratinocyte proliferation, sebum production and acne formation.[6]

Clinical manifestations
Acne can range in severity from mild to severe. In mild cases, acneiform lesions might be limited to open (blackheads) and closed (whiteheads) comedones, and papules. In more severe cases, inflamed papules, pustules, nodules and cysts may develop, which can lead to scarring.[1,3] The presence of these lesions, as well as scarring, can impact negatively on the psychological wellbeing of the client and their family. Systemic manifestations of the disease can also present in certain variants, such as acne fulminans, with symptoms that include pyrexia, malaise, arthralgia and weight loss.[3] In most cases, acneiform lesions are confined to the face, upper back and chest where pilosebaceous units are most abundant. In rosacea, lesions are generally localised to the face and are often accompanied by facial erythema, oedema and telangiectasia.[5]

# Clinical case
*16-year-old male with acne vulgaris to the face and upper back*

## Rapport

Adopt the practitioner strategies and behaviours highlighted in Table 2.1 (chapter 2) to improve client trust, communication and rapport, as well as the accuracy and comprehensiveness of the clinical assessment.

## Assessment

Once measures have been put into place to build client–practitioner rapport, the clinician can begin the clinical assessment.

Health history

### History of presenting condition

A 16-year-old adolescent presents with concerns about long-standing *acne* to the face, as well as to the forehead, nose and cheeks, and to the upper back. The lesions began to emerge at the age of 13 and have since gradually increased in number and severity. When applied twice daily, five per cent benzoyl peroxide reduces the intensity of the inflammation, but chocolate and stress seem to aggravate the condition. A recent course of broad-spectrum antibiotics, prescribed by the client's general practitioner, produced a modest improvement in lesion severity, although this medicine had to be discontinued due to antibiotic-associated diarrhoea. The client is embarrassed by the condition and feels the acne is dampening his self-image and self-esteem.

### Medical history

**Family history**

Father had severe facial acne and scarring, paternal grandmother has type 2 diabetes mellitus, maternal grandfather has ischaemic heart disease.

**Allergies**

Bee venom.

**Medications**

Five per cent benzoyl peroxide ointment twice daily.

**Medical conditions**

Lactose intolerance.

**Surgical or investigational procedures**

Tonsillectomy and adenoidectomy (1999).

### Lifestyle history

**Tobacco use**

Nil.

**Alcohol consumption**

Nil.

**Illicit drug use**

Nil.

| Diet and fluid intake | |
| --- | --- |
| Breakfast | Large glass of full-cream milk. |
| Morning tea | Apple, muesli bar. |
| Lunch | Two sandwiches, made with white bread and spread with peanut butter or Vegemite®. |
| Afternoon tea | Sweet biscuits, toasted white bread spread with Vegemite®. |

| Diet and fluid intake | |
|---|---|
| Dinner | Spaghetti bolognaise, fettuccine carbonara, lasagne, supreme pizza. |
| Fluid intake | 1 cup of cordial daily, 1 cup of juice daily, 2 cups of water daily, 1 cup of milk daily. |
| **Food frequency** | |
| Fruit | 1–2 serves daily |
| Vegetables | 1–2 serves daily |
| Dairy | 2 serves daily |
| Cereals | 7 serves daily |
| Red meat | 6 serves a week |
| Chicken | 1 serve a week |
| Fish | 0 serves a week |
| Takeaway/fast food | 2–3 times a week |

**Quality and duration of sleep**
Continuous sleep; average duration is 6–7 hours.

**Frequency and duration of exercise**
Is not engaged in any sporting activities, is transported to and from school by car, engages in active play or exercise less than 1 hour a day, and sedentary activities (out of school) more than 5 hours a day.

**Socioeconomic background**
The client is Australian-born with an Australian-born mother and Italian-born father, who are married. He lives with his parents. His father works full time; his mother is a stay-at-home parent. He is studying Year 11 at a private school (which the client considers to be moderately stressful), is Roman Catholic and has three younger siblings, aged 9, 12 and 14. The client states he lives in a happy and supportive household.

Physical examination

**Inspection**
Multiple acneiform lesions are present on the forehead (18 lesions – papules and pustules), nose (6 lesions – open comedones), left cheek (3 lesions – papules), right cheek (4 lesions – closed comedones and papules) and upper back (17 lesions – closed comedones and papules). There is no bleeding, scarring, oedema, nodules, excoriation or ulceration. Finger and toenails are strong and intact, with no notable markings.

**Olfaction**
There is no abnormal odour to the lesions or patient.

**Palpation**
Skin to the face and upper back is oily. Papules and pustules are warm. The surrounding skin demonstrates good turgor, moisture and mobility.

**Percussion**
Not applicable.

**Auscultation**
Subcutaneous crepitus is not detectable.

**Additional signs**
Client is afebrile (36.4°C per oral) and overweight (body mass index (BMI) is 27 kg/m$^2$).

**Clinical assessment tools**

Using the Bikowski acne severity index (BASI), facial acne was graded as follows: forehead (moderate grade III acne), nose (mild grade II acne) and left and right cheeks (mild grade II acne).

## Diagnostics

CAM practitioners may request, perform and/or interpret findings from a range of diagnostic tests in order to add valuable data to the pool of clinical information. While several investigations are pertinent to this case (as described below), the decision to use these tests should be considered alongside factors such as cost, convenience, comfort, turnaround time, access, practitioner competence and scope of practice, and history of previous investigations.

**Pathology tests**

The use of culture and sensitivity tests to detect the presence of *P. acnes* is not a reliable diagnostic for acne as this bacterium is a normal resident of human skin. Testing serum androgen levels is also unreliable as most patients with acne demonstrate normal androgen levels.[1]

Low plasma concentrations of vitamin A are reported in people with acne.[7] Assessing hair or serum vitamin A levels may help to determine whether vitamin A deficiency is implicated in this condition.

**Radiology tests**

Not applicable.

**Functional tests**

Not applicable.

**Invasive tests**

Not applicable.

**Miscellaneous tests**

Not applicable.

## Diagnosis

Clusters of data extracted from the health history, clinical examination and pertinent diagnostic test results point towards the following differential CAM diagnosis.

Acne (actual), *related to* genetic predisposition (*client has a family history of acne*), hormonal imbalance (*androgen and growth hormone levels are typically elevated during adolescence*), high glycaemic load diet (*client's diet largely consists of highly refined carbohydrates; acne is exacerbated by chocolate consumption*), *P. acnes* colonisation (*the severity of acneiform lesions improved following antibiotic treatment*) and emotional stress (*acne is aggravated by stress*).

## Planning

The goals and expected outcomes that best serve the client's needs and that are most relevant to the presenting case (as determined by the clinical assessment and CAM diagnoses) are as follows.

Goal
1 Client will be free from acneiform lesions (client's primary concern is the long-standing acne).

Expected outcomes
Based on the degree of improvement reported in clinical studies that have used CAM interventions for the management of acne,[8–11] the following are anticipated.
1 Client will demonstrate a forty-five per cent decrease in the baseline number of acneiform lesions on the forehead, nose, cheeks and/or upper back in 9 weeks or by dd/mm/yyyy (measured by the severity component of the BASI).

2 Client will exhibit a forty-five per cent reduction in the baseline severity of acne-iform lesions in 9 weeks, or by dd/mm/yyyy (measured by the grade component of the BASI).

3 Client will report a twenty-five per cent improvement in baseline self-esteem in 9 weeks or by dd/mm/yyyy (measured by a 0–10 visual analogue scale).

## Application

The range of interventions reported in the CAM literature that can be used in the treatment of acne are appraised below.

### Diet

**Low glycaemic-load diet (Level II, Strength A, Direction +)**

The consumption of foods with a high glycaemic index or glycaemic load may, as discussed earlier, contribute to the pathogenesis of acne. Hence, the substitution of high glycaemic-load foods such as sweetened, refined and highly processed products with foods that have a low glycaemic-load, such as wholegrains and fruits with edible skins or are high in protein, including eggs and lean meat, may be of benefit to those suffering from acne. Indeed, two controlled clinical trials have shown young males who follow a 12-week low glycaemic-load diet demonstrate a significant reduction in insulin resistance, fasting insulin, free androgen levels, BMI, total acneiform lesion counts and inflammatory lesion counts when compared to those consuming a high glycaemic-load diet.[9,10]

### Lifestyle

**Relaxation therapy (Level II, Strength B, Direction +)**

Psychological stress is positively correlated with the severity of acne.[12,13] It is therefore reasonable to assume that successful attempts at reducing stress could lead to clinical improvements in acne. This assumption was tested in a small randomised controlled trial (RCT) of thirty dermatology patients with acne vulgaris, and found 6 weeks of biofeedback-assisted relaxation and cognitive imagery was significantly more effective than attention-comparison and medical control at reducing acne severity.[14] Further research is now needed to determine whether similar effects can be observed using other stress reduction techniques, including meditation, yoga and tai chi.

### Nutritional supplementation

**Ascorbic acid (Level II, Strength C, Direction +)**

Vitamin C has the potential to attenuate the pathogenesis of acne by reducing cutaneous lipid peroxidation, *P. acnes* replication[15] and serum C-reactive protein (CRP) levels (a marker of acute inflammation).[16] Findings from an open comparative study add some support to this theory, with topically applied five per cent sodium ascorbyl phosphate (SAP) (a vitamin C derivative) twice daily for 12 weeks shown to be more effective than five per cent benzoyl peroxide in reducing the number of inflammatory and non-inflammatory acneiform lesions in 49 subjects.[15] A small double-blind RCT (n = 30) also found five per cent SAP lotion (applied twice daily for 8 weeks) to reduce inflammatory lesion count in adults with acne vulgaris, although the difference between the SAP and 0.2 per cent retinol groups was not statistically significant.[17] Given that studies have used different active controls, no firm conclusions can yet be made about the efficacy of topical SAP in acne.

**Nicotinamide (Level II, Strength B, Direction +)**

Vitamin $B_3$ reduces inflammatory mediator release[18] and, as such, may play a role in the treatment of inflammatory skin disorders. Several controlled clinical trials have confirmed this, with topically administered nicotinamide gel (four per cent) found to be as effective as antibiotic gel in reducing the number and severity of inflamed acneiform lesions.[11,19] Whether this affect can be demonstrated with orally administered vitamin $B_3$ is not yet clear.

**Vitamin A (Level II, Strength B, Direction +)**
Collagen synthesis, phagocytosis, antibody production and epithelial cell differentiation are key functions of vitamin A.[20] Given these actions and the significantly lower plasma concentration of vitamin A reported in people with acne,[7] it is not surprising that many studies (albeit methodologically limited studies) have found synthetic vitamin A derivatives to be effective at reducing the severity of acne vulgaris when administered as oral or topical preparations.[21–26] Whether these effects translate to betacarotene and/or natural vitamin A is not yet certain.

**Zinc (Level II, Strength C, Direction o)**
Zinc modulates inflammatory and immune activity[27] and demonstrates antimicrobial activity against *Propionibacterium* strains.[28] While low serum and epidermal zinc concentrations have been reported in people with acne vulgaris,[29,30] the evidence is not conclusive. Likewise, evidence from trials investigating the clinical efficacy of zinc in acne has not been consistent.[31–35]

***Lactobacillus* spp., omega 3 fatty acids, selenium and vitamin E**
These supplements exhibit myriad effects that are desirable in the management of acne, including anti-inflammatory and immunomodulatory activity; however, there is insufficient clinical evidence to justify the administration of these agents in individuals with acne.

## Herbal medicine

***Commiphora molmol* (Level II, Strength C, Direction o)**
Myrrh has long been used as an anti-inflammatory, vulnerary and antimicrobial herb. These effects appear to be of some benefit to patients with nodulocystic acne, with a small RCT of 20 patients finding oral Gugulipid extract (equivalent to 25 mg guggulsterone), administered twice daily for 3 months, to be as effective as oral tetracycline at reducing the number of inflamed acneiform lesions.[36] No firm conclusions can be made about the efficacy of myrrh until further evidence from larger studies becomes available.

***Vitex agnus-castus* (Level III-1, Strength D, Direction +)**
Chaste tree may exert a mild antiandrogenic effect by reducing serum prolactin levels[37] and thus may attenuate the sequence of events leading to the manifestation of acne. This action may explain why an earlier controlled trial of 161 subjects found chaste tree treatment to be significantly superior to placebo at improving the signs of acne at 12 weeks.[38] In view of the paucity of corroborating data and the insufficient details of the study, these results should be interpreted with caution.

**Other herbs**
*Arctium lappa* (burdock), *Galium aparine* (cleavers), *Trifolium pratense* (red clover), *Rumex crispus* (yellow dock) *and Scrophularia nodosa* (figwort) have long been used as treatments for skin complaints because of their depurative action. Experimental data suggest that *Glycyrrhiza glabra* (licorice) and *Echinacea* spp. (echinacea) may also be indicated for the treatment of acne because of their anti-inflammatory, immunomodulatory and antimicrobial activity against *P. acnes*.[39,40] Despite the availability of traditional and/or experimental evidence in this area, there is insufficient clinical evidence to support or refute the effectiveness of these herbs in acne.

## Other

**Acupuncture (Level II, Strength D, Direction +)**
Many case reports have been published on the effectiveness of acupuncture in acne;[41–43] however, given the methodological limitations of these reports, no firm conclusions can be drawn. A more recent RCT of 52 patients with acne conglobata adds much-needed rigour to this body of evidence. Four weeks of treatment, daily encircling acupuncture, together with twice weekly venesection and cupping, was found to be as effective as orally administered isotretinoin (10 mg three times a day)

at reducing the signs of acne, and superior to isotretinoin at lowering serum inter-leukin-6 levels.[44] The risk of placebo bias in this trial and the unknown confounding effect of venesection and cupping makes the translation of these findings into clinical practice difficult.

### *Melaleuca alternifolia* (aromatherapy) (Level II, Strength B, Direction +)
Indigenous Australians traditionally used tea tree for its anti-inflammatory, antimicro-bial and antiseptic properties. These effects, as well as the sensitivity of *P. acnes* to tea tree oil,[45] indicate that tea tree may be effective as a treatment for acne. Find-ings from a systematic review of one RCT (n = 124) support this proposition,[46] with the topical application of five per cent tea tree oil gel found to be as effective as five per cent benzoyl peroxide at reducing the number and severity of acneiform lesions, albeit with a relatively slower onset of action.[47] Similar outcomes were observed in a more recent RCT (n = 60) that compared five per cent tea tree oil gel to placebo in 60 adolescents and young adults.[8]

### Chiropractic, homeopathy, massage, osteopathy and reflexology
There is insufficient clinical evidence to support the use of these therapies in the management of acne.

## CAM prescription
The CAM interventions that are most appropriate for the management of the pre-senting case – that is, they target the planned goals, expected outcomes and CAM diagnoses, they are supported by the best available evidence, they are pertinent to the client's needs and they are most relevant to CAM practice – are outlined below.

### Primary treatments
- Commence low-glycaemic-load (GL) diet (e.g. substitute high-GL foods, such as sweetened, refined and highly processed products, including chocolate, with foods that have a low-GL, including wholegrains and fruits with edible skins) (*client consumes a high-GL diet; the consumption of a low-GL diet is shown to be effective in reducing the number and severity of acneiform lesions*).
- Commence relaxation therapy (e.g. progressive muscle relaxation and guided imagery), at least 30 minutes twice a week (*stress aggravates the client's acne; relaxation therapy induces the relaxation response and may be helpful in de-creasing the severity of acne*).

Consider one of the following biological interventions:
1. Four per cent nicotinamide gel, applied to lesions twice a day (*nicotinamide gel is effective in reducing the number and severity of inflamed acneiform lesions*).
2. Five per cent tea tree oil gel, applied to lesions daily (*tea tree oil gel is effective in reducing the number and severity of acneiform lesions*).

### Secondary treatments
Consider oral gugulipid extract, equivalent to 25 mg guggelsterone, twice a day (*P. acnes colonisation may be contributing to the client's acne; C. molmol is an antimi-crobial and anti-inflammatory herb, and may help to reduce the number of inflamed acneiform lesions*).

### Referral
- Refer the client to a general practitioner, family physician, endocrinologist or dermatologist if the condition deteriorates, if serious pathology is suspected (such as Cushing's syndrome or diabetes mellitus) or if a serious complication arises (such as an abscess or skin ulceration).
- Refer the client to another CAM practitioner if acne vulgaris, or the treatment of acne vulgaris, is outside the clinician's area of expertise.
- Liaise with the general practitioner about the client's overall management plan.

## Review

To determine whether pertinent client goals and expected outcomes have been achieved at follow-up, and if any aspects of the client's care need to be improved, consider the factors listed in Table 8.2 (chapter 8) and the questions listed below.

- Was there a reduction in the severity component of the BASI for the four facial regions and upper back?
- Was there a reduction in the grade component of the BASI for the four facial regions and upper back?
- Was there an improvement in client self-esteem?
- Has there been a general reduction in the glycaemic index or glycaemic load of foods consumed since the initial consultation?
- Has the need for benzoyl peroxide decreased?

# References

1. Cargnello JA. (2005) Acne: what's new? In: Marks R, editor. Dermatology. 2nd ed. Sydney: Australasian Medical Publishing Company.

2. Cappel M. Mauger D. Thiboutot D. (2005) Correlation between serum levels of insulin-like growth factor 1, dehydroepiandrosterone sulfate, and dihydrotestosterone and acne lesion counts in adult women. Archives of Dermatology, 141: 333–8.

3. Buchanan P. Courtenay M. (2006) Prescribing in dermatology. Cambridge: Cambridge University Press.

4. Porter R et al, editors. (2008). The Merck manual. Whitehouse Station: Merck Research Laboratories.

5. Feldman S et al (2004) Diagnosis and treatment of acne. American Family Physician, 69: 2123–30.

6. Cordain L. (2005) Implications for the role of diet in acne. Seminars in Cutaneous Medicine and Surgery, 24(2): 84–91.

7. El-Akawi Z. Abdel-Latif N. Abdul-Razzak K. (2006) Does the plasma level of vitamins A and E affect acne condition? Clinical and Experimental Dermatology, 31(3): 430–4.

8. Enshaieh S et al (2007) The efficacy of 5% topical tea tree oil gel in mild to moderate acne vulgaris: a randomized, double-blind placebo-controlled study. Indian Journal of Dermatology, Venereology and Leprology, 73(1): 22–5.

9. Smith RN et al (2007) A low-glycemic-load diet improves symptoms in acne vulgaris patients: a randomized controlled trial. American Journal of Clinical Nutrition, 86(1): 107–15.

10. Smith R et al (2008) A pilot study to determine the short-term effects of a low glycemic load diet on hormonal markers of acne: a nonrandomized, parallel, controlled feeding trial. Molecular Nutrition and Food Research, 52(6): 718–26.

11. Weltert Y et al (2004) Double-blind clinical assessment of the efficacy of a 4% nicotinamide gel (Exfoliac NC Gel) versus a 4% erythromycin gel in the treatment of moderate acne with a predominant inflammatory component. Nouvelles Dermatologiques, 23(7): 385–94.

12. Schulpis K et al (1999) Psychological and sympathoadrenal status in patients with cystic acne. Journal of the European Academy of Dermatology and Venereology, 13(1): 24–7.

13. Yosipovitch G et al (2007) Study of psychological stress, sebum production and acne vulgaris in adolescents. Acta Dermato-Venereologica, 87(2): 135–9.

14. Hughes H et al (1983) Treatment of acne vulgaris by biofeedback relaxation and cognitive imagery. Journal of Psychosomatic Research, 27(3): 185–91.

15. Klock J et al (2005) Sodium ascorbyl phosphate shows in vitro and in vitro efficacy in the prevention and treatment of acne vulgaris. International Journal of Cosmetic Science, 27(3): 171–6.

16. Wannamethee SG et al (2006) Associations of vitamin C status, fruit and vegetable intakes, and markers of inflammation and hemostasis. American Journal of Clinical Nutrition, 83(3): 567–74.

17. Ruamrak C. Lourith N. Natakankitkul S. (2009) Comparison of clinical efficacies of sodium ascorbyl phosphate, retinol and their combination in acne treatment. International Journal of Cosmetic Science, 31(1): 41–6.

18. Namazi MR. (2003) Nicotinamide: a potential addition to the anti-psoriatic weaponry. FASEB Journal, 17: 1377–9.

19. Shalita AR et al (1995) Topical nicotinamide compared with clindamycin gel in the treatment of inflammatory acne vulgaris. International Journal of Dermatology, 34(6): 434–7.

20. Leach MJ. (2004) A critical review of natural therapies in wound management. Ostomy/Wound Management, 50(2): 36–51.

21. Fatum B. Hansen HHV. Mortensen E. (1980) Topical treatment of acne vulgaris with the vitamin A acid derivate motretinide (Tasmaderm®), tretinoin (Airol®) and a placebo cream. Ugeskrift for laeger, 142(51): 3364–6.

22. Gandola M et al (1976) Topical vitamin A acid in the treatment of acne vulgaris (a controlled multicenter trial). Archives for Dermatological Research, 255(2): 129–38.

23. Lucky AW et al (1998) Comparative efficacy and safety of two 0.025% tretinoin gels: results from a multicenter double-blind, parallel study. Journal of the American Academy of Dermatology, 38(4): S17–23.

24. Peck GL et al (1982) Isotretinoin versus placebo in the treatment of cystic acne. A randomized double–blind study. Journal of the American Academy of Dermatology, 6(4 Suppl 2): 735–45.

25. Schumacher A. Stuttgen G. (1971) Vitamin A acid in hyperkeratoses, epithelial tumors and acne. Deutsche Medizinische Wochenschrift, 96: 1547–51.

26. Shalita AR et al (1999) Tazarotene gel is safe and effective in the treatment of acne vulgaris: a multicenter, double-blind, vehicle-controlled study. Cutis, 63(6): 349–54.

27. Kahmann L et al (2008) Zinc supplementation in the elderly reduces spontaneous inflammatory cytokine release and restores T cell functions. Rejuvenation Research, 11(1): 227–37.
28. Fluhr JW et al (1999) In-vitro and in-vivo efficacy of zinc acetate against propionibacteria alone and in combination with erythromycin. Zentralblatt fur Bakteriologie, 289(4): 445–56.
29. Amer M et al (1982) Serum zinc in acne vulgaris. International Journal of Dermatology, 21(8): 481–4.
30. Michaelsson G. Ljunghall K. (1990) Patients with dermatitis herpetiformis, acne, psoriasis and Darier's disease have low epidermal zinc concentrations. Acta Dermato-Venereologica, 70(4): 304–8.
31. Agrawal P et al (1985) Oral zinc in acne vulgaris (a double blind evaluation). Indian Journal of Dermatology, Venereology and Leprology, 51(1): 38–9.
32. Dreno B et al (1989) Low doses of zinc gluconate for inflammatory acne. Acta Dermato-Venereologica, 69(6): 541–3.
33. Goransson K. Liden S. Odsell L. (1978) Oral zinc in acne vulgaris: a clinical and methodological study. Acta Dermato-Venereologica, 58(5): 443–8.
34. Orris L et al (1978) Oral zinc therapy of acne. Absorption and clinical effect. Archives of Dermatology, 114(7): 1018–20.
35. Verma KC. Saini AS. Dhamija SK. (1980) Oral zinc sulphate therapy in acne vulgaris: a double-blind trial. Acta Dermato-Venereologica, 60(4): 337–40.
36. Thappa DM. Dogra J. (1994) Nodulocystic acne: oral gugulipid versus tetracycline. Journal of Dermatology, 21(10): 729–31.
37. Bone K. (2003) A clinical guide to blending liquid herbs. St Louis: Churchill Livingstone.
38. Amann W. (1967) Improvement of acne vulgaris following therapy with Agnus castus (Agnolyt). Therapie der Gegenwart, 106(1): 124–6.
39. Nam C et al (2003) Anti-acne effects of Oriental herb extracts: a novel screening method to select anti-acne agents. Skin Pharmacology and Applied Skin Physiology, 16(2): 84–90.
40. Sharma M et al (2008) Echinacea extracts contain significant and selective activities against human pathogenic bacteria. Pharmaceutical Biology, 46(1–2): 111–16.
41. Ding LN. (1985) 50 cases of acne treated by puncturing acupoint dazhui in combination with cupping. Journal of Traditional Chinese Medicine, 5(2): 128.
42. Hou H. Wu T. (2002) Fifty-six cases of acne treated by auricular needle-embedding. Journal of Traditional Chinese Medicine, 22(2): 115–16.
43. Xu YH. (1989) Treatment of acne with ear acupuncture – a clinical observation of 80 cases. Journal of Traditional Chinese Medicine, 9(4): 238–9.
44. Liu CZ. Lei B. Zheng JF. (2008) Randomized control study on the treatment of 26 cases of acne conglobata with encircling acupuncture combined with venesection and cupping. Zhen Ci Yan Jiu, 33(6): 406–8.
45. Raman A. Weir U. Bloomfield SF. (1995) Antimicrobial effects of tea-tree oil and its major components on Staphylococcus aureus, Staph. epidermidis and Propionibacterium acnes. Letters in Applied Microbiology, 21(4): 242–5.
46. Ernst E. Huntley A. (2000) Tea tree oil: a systematic review of randomized clinical trials. Forschende Komplementarmedizin und Klassische Naturheilkunde, 7(1): 17–20.
47. Bassett IB. Pannowitz DL. Barnetson RS. (1990) A comparative study of tea-tree oil versus benzoylperoxide in the treatment of acne. Medical Journal of Australia, 153(8): 455–8.

# Case 2
# Anxiety

## Description of anxiety

### Definition

Anxiety is an unpleasant and often distressing sense of uneasiness, apprehension and/or nervousness. Anxiety is considered to be a standalone, non-pathological symptom (i.e. a normal response to an environmental stessor such as workplace or examination stress), as well as a central feature of 'anxiety disorder', a term that is inclusive of generalised anxiety disorder (GAD), phobias, panic disorder, obsessive–compulsive disorder (OCD) and post-traumatic stress disorder (PTSD).[1]

### Epidemiology

The lifetime prevalence rate of GAD ranges from 10.6 per cent to 16.6 per cent. This disorder is most prevalent in women, and appears to increase with advancing age. For the more specific anxiety disorders, the lifetime prevalence rates range from 0.5–1.3 per cent for OCD, 1.0–1.2 per cent for panic disorder, 1.2–2.1 per cent for PTSD, 3.6–5.3 per cent for phobias and 2.6–6.2 per cent for GAD.[2]

### Aetiology and pathophysiology

Anxiety disorders are complex conditions that appear to originate from a number of causes. Genetic predisposition and/or familial history, for instance, have been associated with panic disorder, GAD, phobias and OCD.[3] Physiological factors, including group A beta-hemolytic *Streptococcus* infection and trauma or postpartum events are, respectively, also implicated in OCD and panic disorder. But most attention has focused on the neurochemical aetiology of these disorders. Elevated central nervous system catecholamine levels (e.g. panic disorder), impaired gamma-amino butyric acid metabolism (e.g. panic disorder), carbon dioxide sensitivity (e.g. panic disorder), abnormal serotoninergic and noradrenergic activity (e.g. GAD and PTSD), reduced dopamine (D2) receptor and transporter binding (e.g. phobias), abnormal number and/or function of serotinergic receptors (e.g. OCD), neurological disease (e.g. OCD), increased limbic system activity (e.g. PTSD), impaired lactate metabolism (e.g. panic disorder), and basal ganglia dysfunction and prefrontal hyperactivity (e.g. OCD) are just some of the many neurochemical causes of these disorders.[4]

The pathogenesis of anxiety disorders is only partly explained by these physiological elements. The development of these conditions is also influenced by socioenvironmental factors such as stress, illicit drug use (e.g. marijuana and lysergic acid diethylamide, or LSD), diet (e.g. caffeine), poor social support (e.g. PTSD) and the demise of close relationships (e.g. panic disorder). Behavioural elements also may be implicated in the pathogenesis of anxiety disorder, including the development of abnormal or irrational conditioned responses to fearful situations (e.g. panic disorder), life events (e.g. GAD) or stressful situations (e.g. OCD).[4,5]

### Clinical manifestations

Anxiety is an elusive symptom that can manifest in any person, at any time, in any given situation and to any degree. Anxiety can manifest in any health condition and the physiological features of anxiety can mimic other disorders. As a result, distinguishing anxiety from other medical conditions may be a challenge for some clinicians. A critical first step to identifying anxiety disorder is to understand that anxiety is only one symptom of this condition. Other symptoms that commonly manifest in this group of disorders are irritability, poor concentration, insomnia, restlessness, muscle tension, avoidance behaviour, preoccupation with an event or situation, easy fatigability, tachycardia, palpitations, shortness of breath and an exaggerated startle response.[1,3,4]

The duration of anxiety is also important. Panic disorder, for instance, is an acute condition that manifests rapidly and peaks within 10 minutes. PTSD can be acute (i.e. occurring soon after an event) and chronic (i.e. occurring more than 3 months after an event). Conditions such as GAD, OCD and phobias are chronic and can exist for many months, years or decades. While the intensity of symptoms is often most severe in acute panic disorder, the severity of symptoms in other anxiety disorders varies greatly.[1,3,4]

---

## Clinical case
*33-year-old woman with generalised anxiety disorder*

### Rapport

Adopt the practitioner strategies and behaviours highlighted in Table 2.1 (chapter 2) to improve client trust, communication and rapport, and to assure the accuracy and comprehensiveness of the clinical assessment.

### Assessment

Once measures have been established to build client–practitioner rapport, the clinician can begin the clinical assessment.

Health history

**History of presenting condition**
A 33-year-old woman presents to the clinic complaining of *anxiety*. The anxiety (defined by the patient as tremulousness and uneasiness) began 12 months ago when she decided to move to Australia to further her career and get married. The anxiety has continued to increase since then, and it was only one month before her consultation with the CAM practitioner that the client decided to speak to her general practitioner (GP). The GP prescribed temazepam for the insomnia and alprazolam for the anxiety. The GP advised the client that she may have generalised anxiety disorder (GAD), and that if the condition did not improve within 3 months, she would refer the client to a psychiatrist. The GP recommended that the client also take up daily meditation and commence an exercise program to assist with coping.

While the temazepam has helped increase the duration of sleep and the alprazolam has reduced the severity of the anxiety, the client is reluctant to continue with the anxiolytic in the long term. The client also has not commenced meditation or exercise. This is because up until now she was not sure who to approach for this advice. The client has found the anxiety, including concomitant sighing, shortness of breath, muscle tension, restlessness, poor concentration and insomnia, worsens when her husband is away or when she steps up as acting manager at work. These symptoms often improve during the weekends, and even more so during recreational leave.

**Medical history**
**Family history**
Mother has depression, father has type 2 diabetes mellitus, paternal grandmother has agoraphobia.
**Allergies**
Nil.
**Medications**
Temazepam 10 mg nocte, alprazolam 0.5 mg daily, salbutamol inhaler as needed.
**Medical conditions**
Mild asthma, insomnia, GAD.
**Surgical or investigational procedures**
Tonsillectomy (1978).

## Lifestyle history

**Tobacco use**
Nil.

**Alcohol consumption**
Nil.

**Illicit drug use**
Nil.

| Diet and fluid intake | |
|---|---|
| Breakfast | Cornflakes® cereal with skim milk, coffee. |
| Morning tea | Coffee. |
| Lunch | Wholemeal sandwich with tomato, low fat cheese, lettuce and/or ham. |
| Afternoon tea | Coffee, sweet biscuits. |
| Dinner | Lamb and vegetable curry, fish in coconut cream, baked cod with tomato and onion, beef meatballs with sweet potato bake. |
| Fluid intake | 4–5 cups of percolated coffee a day, 1–2 cups of water a day. |
| **Food frequency** | |
| Fruit | 1 serve daily |
| Vegetables | 2–3 serves daily |
| Dairy | 2 serves daily |
| Cereals | 5 serves daily |
| Red meat | 1 serve a week |
| Chicken | 1 serve a week |
| Fish | 3 serves a week |
| Takeaway/fast food | 1 time a week |

**Quality and duration of sleep**
Broken sleep, has difficulty falling asleep; average duration is 5 hours.

**Frequency and duration of exercise**
Dislikes gyms. Drives to work. Engages in incidental exercise (e.g. work-related walking, gardening, cleaning) less than 3 hours a day and sedentary activities more than 5 hours a day.

## Socioeconomic background

The client is Fijian-born with Fijian-born parents. She moved to Australia 12 months ago, leaving behind her parents and all her family members. The client has an English-born husband but no children. She works full time as an optician in an optical store, which she finds stressful at times. The client is buying her own home and is responsible for all household activities and finances as her husband is away every second week for mining-related work. The client finds these periods of absence from her husband distressing, although she does find some peace in her Christian practice.

## Physical examination

### Inspection

The client is cooperative, well groomed, appropriately dressed and maintains good attention and eye contact. Gait and posture are normal. Skin is dark brown in colour with no abnormal pigmentary signs. Nails are strong and intact. There is no evidence of goitre, proptosis, tremors or virilisation.

### Olfaction
There is no abnormal odour to the patient, and the patient does not perceive there to be any abnormal odours.

### Palpation
The skin is warm, with good skin turgor and moisture. There is no palpable goitre, thyroid tenderness or thyroid thrill.

### Percussion
All deep tendon reflexes are normal.

### Auscultation
The patient voices concerns about the anxiety in a clear, well-paced and articulate manner. There is no evidence of delusions, obsessions, compulsions, paranoid thoughts or impaired memory recall and retention. There is also no evidence of a thyroid bruit.

### Additional signs
Client is afebrile (36.4°C, per oral), hypertensive (140/85) and of normal weight (BMI is 24.2 kg/m$^2$). Heart rate (89 beats per minute) and respiratory rate (26 breaths per minute) are slightly elevated.

### Clinical assessment tools
The state trait anxiety inventory (STAI) provided a total score of 42/120, which is within the 'mild anxiety' range. As for the client's other concerns, using the Hamilton anxiety rating scale (HAM-A) subscales the client rated 2/4 each for anxious mood, tension, insomnia and difficulty concentrating.

## Diagnostics
CAM practitioners can request, perform and/or interpret findings from a range of diagnostic tests in order to add valuable data to the pool of clinical information. While several investigations are pertinent to this case (as described below), the decision to use these tests should be considered alongside factors such as cost, convenience, comfort, turnaround time, access, practitioner competence and scope of practice, and history of previous investigations.

### Pathology tests
There are no specific diagnostic tests for anxiety. Clinical examination suggests that other causes of anxiety are also unlikely, including perimenopause, hyperthyroidism, phaeochromocytoma and depression. If there was uncertainty about the cause of anxiety, it would be appropriate to test thyroid function, serum follicle-stimulating hormone levels and/or catecholamine levels.

### Radiology tests
Not applicable.

### Functional tests
Not applicable.

### Invasive tests
Not applicable.

### Miscellaneous tests
Not applicable.

## Diagnosis

Clusters of data extracted from the health history, clinical examination and pertinent diagnostic test results point towards the following differential CAM diagnoses.

Anxiety (actual), *related to* emotional stress (*anxiety symptoms heighten when husband is away and when work responsibilities increase; anxiety is alleviated when client is not at work*), life-changing event (*anxiety symptoms emerged around the time the client moved to Australia*), poor social support (*client's family is overseas, and husband is frequently away for work – limited access to these social supports may predispose the client to anxiety*), and/or excess caffeine intake (*high caffeine intake may cause anxiety symptoms in susceptible individuals – the client consumes 4–5 cups of percolated coffee a day, which is equivalent to approximately 360–450 mg of caffeine daily*).

## Planning

The goals and expected outcomes that best serve the client's needs, and which are most relevant to the presenting case (as determined by the clinical assessment and CAM diagnoses), are as follows.

### Goal
Client will be free from GAD (*client's principal concern is the anxiety*).

### Expected outcomes
Based on the degree of improvement reported in clinical studies that have used CAM interventions for the management of anxiety,[6–8] the following are anticipated.

1 Client will demonstrate a fifty-five per cent reduction in baseline STAI total score in 4 weeks, or by dd/mm/yyyy.
2 Client will demonstrate a fifty-five per cent decrease in baseline severity of anxiety in 4 weeks or by dd/mm/yyyy (according to HAM-A anxious mood subscore).
3 Client will demonstrate a fifty-five per cent improvement in baseline severity of nervous tension in 4 weeks or by dd/mm/yyyy (according to HAM-A tension subscore).
4 Client will demonstrate a fifty-five per cent reduction in baseline severity of insomnia in 4 weeks or by dd/mm/yyyy (according to HAM-A insomnia subscore).
5 Client will demonstrate a fifty-five per cent improvement in baseline mental concentration in 4 weeks, or by dd/mm/yyyy (according to HAM-A concentration subscore).

## Application

The range of interventions reported in the CAM literature that can be used in the treatment of anxiety are appraised below.

### Diet
**Low-fat, Mediterranean and/or low-sodium diets (Level II, Strength C, Direction o)**
Several studies have examined the effect of diet on psychological function, but there is no convincing evidence that diet, including low-fat, Mediterranean and low-sodium diets, are any more effective than controls or standard diet at improving anxiety or psychological wellbeing.[9–11] Thus, rather than prescribe a particular type of diet for this client, it may be more pertinent to increase dietary consumption of foods and nutrients that demonstrate anxiolytic activity (see 'Nutritional supplementation' below for specific examples).

### Lifestyle
**Physical exercise (Level I, Strength A, Direction +)**
Increasing levels of physical activity are associated with improvements in physiological and psychological health and wellbeing.[12] According to findings from a meta-analysis of 49 RCTs, exercise therapy also demonstrates moderate reductions in anxiety when compared to no-exercise controls or other anxiolytic treatment.[13] The anxiolytic effect of exercise appears to be less significant in children and adolescents.[14]

**Relaxation therapy (Level I, Strength A, Direction +)**
Relaxation therapy describes a range of mind–body techniques that induce the relaxation response and attenuate sympathetic nervous system activity. Many studies have explored the effectiveness of relaxation therapy in anxiety, including 19 RCTs. A meta-analysis of these RCTs found relaxation therapy to be effective at reducing anxiety, particularly state and trait anxiety, with meditation found to be superior to

progressive relaxation, autogenic training and multimethod approaches.[6] These findings were consistent across studies, although the significant heterogeneity of these trials, including the various types of anxiety and the range of treatment approaches used, suggests results should be interpreted with caution.

### Tai chi (Level II, Strength C, Direction +)
Tai chi is an ancient Chinese therapy often used as a meditative technique, soft martial art or form of physical exercise. It is not surprising, then, that the physical and psychological benefits of tai chi are similar to exercise.[15,16] In terms of psychological effects, evidence from a number of RCTs suggests that tai chi is superior to sedentary controls in reducing anxiety,[15–17] but given that studies are small and methodologically different, further research is needed before any firm conclusions can be made.

### Yoga (Level I, Strength C, Direction +)
Yoga is an ancient Indian practice that integrates stretching, exercise, posture and breathing with meditation. Given that these techniques are likely to induce a relaxation response, yoga may be helpful in alleviating emotional stress and anxiety. Findings from a systematic review of eight controlled clinical trials (including six RCTs)[18] and results from four recent trials[19–22] show that yoga brings about positive improvements in various types of anxiety, including OCD, phobia, anxiety neurosis, psychoneurosis and examination anxiety. Given the high risk of bias attributed to inadequate randomisation, high rates of attrition and uncertainty about allocation concealment or blinding, these findings should be interpreted with caution.

## Nutritional supplementation

### 5-hydroxytryptophan (5-HTP) (Level II, Strength C, Direction +)
The amino acid 5-HTP is a metabolite of tryptophan and a precursor of the neurotransmitter serotonin. Because serotonin plays a key role in the pathogenesis of anxiety, it is postulated that 5-HTP supplementation may increase brain serotonin production and release, and subsequently elevate mood. Few high-level studies have explored this hypothesis, however. In one RCT, 5-HTP supplementation (200 mg single dose) was found to be significantly more effective than placebo at reducing anxiety levels (i.e. panic symptom list score, visual analogue scale of anxiety, number of panic attacks) in 24 patients with agoraphobia ($p = 0.012$), but not in 24 healthy volunteers.[23] Another RCT, which looked at the effect of 5-HTP supplementation (variable dose for 8 weeks) in 45 participants with anxiety disorder, found 5-HTP to be as effective as clomipramine and more effective than placebo at reducing state trait anxiety, yet less effective than clomipramine and as effective as placebo at reducing HAM-A scores.[24] Even though 5-HTP shows promise as an anxiolytic agent, the small size of these studies limits the generalisability of these results.

### Inositol (Level II, Strength B, Direction + (for panic disorder only))
Inositol is a B-complex vitamin that serves as a second-messenger precursor. Given that the phosphatidyl-inositol second messenger system is linked to serotonin and noradrenalin receptor subtypes,[25] inositol may be useful in the treatment of anxiety disorder. As a treatment for panic disorder, two RCTs found inositol 12–18 g daily for 4 weeks to be superior to fluvoxamine ($p = 0.049$)[26] and statistically significantly superior to placebo ($p = 0.03$)[25] in reducing the number of panic attacks. As a treatment for OCD, inositol (18 g daily for 6 weeks) was found to be no more effective than placebo at reducing anxiety or OCD severity under RCT conditions. It is probable that this small study (n = 10) did not have sufficient power to detect a significant difference between groups, which suggests that evidence from larger studies is needed.

### Melatonin (Level II, Strength B, Direction +)
Melatonin is a hormone secreted by the pineal gland. The hormone is responsible for regulating the body's sleep–wake cycle and, as such, may play a part in promoting

sedation, as well as reducing anxiety. Many studies have explored the effectiveness of melatonin in short-term anxiety, specifically, preoperative anxiety. While most of these studies show melatonin to be superior to placebo, and as effective as conventional anxiolytics in reducing preoperative anxiety,[27–32] little is known about the effectiveness of melatonin in chronic anxiety disorder.

**Multivitamins (Level II, Strength C, Direction o)**
Nutrient deficiencies can lead to a number of psychological manifestations. It seems logical, therefore, that these symptoms might improve with micronutrient supplementation. According to one double-blind RCT of 80 healthy male volunteers, this appears to be the case. The trial found multivitamin and/or mineral supplementation for 28 days significantly reduced anxiety levels and perceived stress when compared to placebo.[33] In an RCT of 59 older people, micronutrient supplementation was found to be inferior to placebo at 8 weeks.[34] These conflicting results suggest further research is needed in this area.

**Omega 3 fatty acids (Level II, Strength B, Direction +)**
The essential fatty acids, eicosapentaenoic acid (EPA) and docosahexaenoic acid (DHA), are purported to produce psychotropic effects.[35] A small double-blind RCT adds support to this claim: the administration of omega 3 polyunsaturated fatty acids (3 g) for 12 weeks in 21 substance abusers significantly reduced anger and anxiety scores when compared to soybean oil control.[36] This is consistent with findings from an earlier controlled trial of healthy subjects with test anxiety.[37] The effectiveness of omega 3 fatty acid supplementation in GAD is not yet known.

**Selenium (Level II, Strength B, Direction o)**
Selenium, an essential trace element, is responsible for a number of structural and enzymatic functions within the body. Not surprisingly, a deficiency in selenium may lead to a wide range of adverse effects, including hostility, confusion, depression and anxiety.[38] This has led many researchers to investigate the effect of supplemental selenium on mood. In one double-blind crossover RCT (n = 50), participants treated with 100 µg selenium daily for 5 weeks demonstrated, using the profile of moods states (POMS) tool, a significant reduction in anxiety when compared to patients receiving placebo.[39] In another RCT, HIV+ drug users (n = 63) administered 200 µg selenium daily for 12 months demonstrated a marginally significant reduction in state anxiety and a statistically significant reduction in trait anxiety when compared to placebo-treated individuals.[40] A more recent and much larger RCT (n = 448) found no statistically significant difference in POMS-bipolar form scores between placebo and selenium (100, 200 and 300 µg) groups after 6 months.[41] Evidence of the effectiveness of selenium in anxiety is therefore inconclusive.

**Glycine**
This amino acid has been found to exhibit anxiolytic activity in experimental studies; however, there is a paucity of clinical data to support its use in clinical practice.

Herbal medicine
***Bacopa monnieri* (Level II, Strength B, Direction +)**
Brahmi is an Ayurvedic herb traditionally used in the treatment of nervous disorders, including anxiety. While the anxiolytic effects of *Bacopa monnieri* might be attributed to serotonin, gamma-amino butyric acid (GABA) and/or brain stress hormone modulation,[42] the mechanisms of action are still uncertain. Even though data from mechanistic studies are lacking, there is emerging clinical evidence to suggest that brahmi may be useful as a treatment for anxiety. In two similarly designed double-blind RCTs, treatment with brahmi extract (300 mg) significantly reduced state anxiety scores at 12 weeks in healthy adults (n = 46)[43] and healthy elderly subjects (n = 48)[42] when compared to placebo.

### *Centella asiatica* (Level II, Strength C, Direction +)

Gotu kola is used in Ayurvedic and traditional Chinese medicine as an adaptogenic, nervine tonic and anxiolytic.[44] The latter action may be attributed to glutamic acid decarboxylase modulation and subsequent elevations in brain GABA levels.[45] With the exception of one double-blind RCT, few studies have explored the efficacy of gotu kola in anxiety. This small trial of 40 healthy volunteers found that, when compared to placebo, the administration of a single 12 g oral dose of gotu kola significantly attenuated the acoustic startle response at 30 and 60 minutes after treatment, but it had no significant effect on self-rated anxiety.[46] Further investigation now needs to determine whether these anxiolytic effects are any different following long-term gotu kola administration.

### *Cymbopogon citratus* (Level II, Strength C, Direction o)

This lemongrass variety is native to India. Aside from its role in cooking, the herb is traditionally used as a nervine tonic. Even so, the best available evidence for this herb has not been favourable. In a small double-blind RCT of 18 patients with high trait anxiety scores, a single-dose of lemongrass tea was found to be no more effective than placebo at reducing cognitive test-induced anxiety 30 minutes after administration.[47] There is some doubt whether the single-dose administration of the herb, the method of extraction and the short-term outcome measure were appropriate for evaluating the efficacy of lemongrass.

### *Hypericum perforatum* (Level II, Strength C, Direction + (for somatisation complaints only))

St John's wort is a well-recognised antidepressive agent. Given the serotonergic, domaminergic and GABAminergic activity of the herb,[48] it is probable that *Hypericum* may also be useful as a treatment for anxiety disorder. However, evidence from a number of clinical trials has been inconsistent. An RCT of 151 outpatients suffering from somatisation complaints, for example, found St John's wort to be statistically significantly superior to placebo in reducing HAM-A total scores, as well as psychic and somatic subscores.[49] Yet, in people with social phobia[48] and OCD[50], *Hypericum* was found to be no more effective than placebo at improving clinical outcomes. Given the heterogenous patient populations and differences in study duration and size, it is difficult to draw any conclusions from these findings.

### *Passiflora incarnata* (Level I, Strength A, Direction +)

Passionflower is traditionally indicated in nervous system disorders due to its sedative, anxiolytic and hypnotic effects. While the mechanism of action of passionflower is not yet clear, the anxiolytic effect of the constituent chrysin has been linked to the activation of GABA-A receptors.[51] Emerging clinical evidence adds further support to this anxiolytic effect. Three RCTs, involving 258 patients, found *P. incarnata* to be significantly more effective than placebo at reducing preoperative anxiety scores (when administered as a single 500 mg dose),[52] and as effective as benzodiazepines at reducing GAD anxiety scores (when administered at a dose of 45 drops per day or 90 mg per day for 4 weeks).[53] Since these studies demonstrate low risk of bias, these findings are promising.

### *Piper methysticum* (Level I, Strength B, Direction o)

Kava kava, a native to the Pacific Islands, has long been used as an anxiolytic, sedative and hypnotic agent. Although the modulation of GABA receptors and/or the downregulation of beta-adrenergic activity may contribute to the anxiolytic effect of the herb, these effects have yet to be confirmed.[54] Despite the paucity of mechanistic data, there is a wealth of clinical data on the effectiveness of kava kava in anxiety. In a Cochrane review of 12 double-blind RCTs, of which seven were eligible for meta-analysis, a small but marginally significant reduction in HAM-A total scores was demonstrated in patients receiving *P. methysticum* when compared to patients receiving placebo.[55] Studies postdating this review have yielded inconsistent results.[56–59] An updated meta-analysis of the effectiveness of kava kava in anxiety is therefore warranted.

### *Scutellaria laterifolia* (Level III-1, Strength C, Direction +)

Baicalin and baicalein are two constituents of skullcap that have been shown to activate the benzodiazepine binding site of GABA-A receptors,[60] which may be responsible for the sedative and anxiolytic effects of the plant. To date, only one published RCT has investigated the anxiolytic effect of skullcap monopreparation. The double-blind, placebo controlled crossover trial compared the effects of three different single doses of skullcap (350 mg vs 200 mg vs 100 mg) to a single-dose placebo in 19 healthy volunteers. The two higher doses of skullcap were found to be most effective at reducing anxiety 60 minutes after administration.[61] Given the descriptive nature of the analysis it is uncertain whether the difference between groups was statistically significant.

### *Valeriana officinalis* (Level II, Strength B, Direction o)

Valerian has a long history of use as a sedative, hypnotic and anxiolytic. The anxiolytic effect of *Valeriana*, in particular, may be credited to glutamic acid decarboxylase stimulation and subsequent elevations in brain GABA levels.[45] According to a systematic review of the literature, only one controlled clinical trial has investigated the efficacy of valerian monopreparation in anxiety.[53] The 4-week RCT involving 36 patients with GAD found no significant difference between the valerian (50–150 mg daily) and diazepam (2.5–7.5 mg daily) groups, and the valerian and placebo groups in HAM-A total scores.[62] Larger studies may help to determine whether valerian is effective in the treatment of anxiety disorder.

### Other herbs

*Chamomilla recutita* (chamomile), *Eschscholzia californica* (Californian poppy), *Humulus lupulus* (hops), *Leonurus cardiaca* (motherwort), *Paullinia cupana* (guarana), *Piscidia erythrina* (Jamaican dogwood), *Tilia* spp. (lime flower) and *Withania somnifera* (ashwaganda) are traditionally used as nervine, anxiolytic and/or sedative agents. There is insufficient clinical evidence to support or refute the efficacy of these herbs as monopreparations in humans with anxiety.

### Other

### Acupuncture (Level I, Strength C, Direction +)

Many studies have examined the effectiveness of acupuncture in anxiety, including GAD, anxiety neurosis, procedure-related anxiety, and substance abuse and withdrawal anxiety, though few of these studies were rigorously designed. A systematic review of 10 RCTs provides the best available evidence for this treatment. The review reports positive findings for the use of acupuncture in the treatment of GAD or anxiety neurosis, and limited evidence in favour of auricular acupuncture in perioperative anxiety.[63] The lack of methodological detail and the range of comparative interventions and outcome measures used meant the data were not amenable to meta-analysis and suggests that larger and more rigorously designed studies are needed.

### Aromatherapy (Level I, Strength C, Direction o)

The therapeutic application of essential oils can induce a range of psychological effects, including the alleviation of stress and anxiety. These effects are partly supported by a systematic review of six RCTs.[64] While the review found a weak positive association between massage aromatherapy (with lavender, orange and/ or chamomile essential oil) and anxiety, the effect was transient and the methodological quality of the studies poor. Methodological rigour continues to be a limitation of recent studies, but perhaps the biggest concern with controlled studies on aromatherapy inhalation or massage and anxiety is the paucity of positive findings.[65–67] These inconsistent results do little to assist clinicians in making effective clinical decisions about the use of aromatherapy in anxiety disorder.

### Chiropractic (Level II, Strength C, Direction o)

Chiropractic manipulation is often used to treat nervous and musculoskeletal disorders. While chiropractic manipulation is not a primary treatment of anxiety, it is not outside the scope of chiropractic care. In fact, a pilot study examining the effect of chiropractic manipulation on salivary cortisol levels suggested chiropractic could cause short-term reductions in client stress and anxiety, with healthy adult male students demonstrating a progressive and statistically significant decrease in cortisol levels from 15 minutes post treatment to 60 minutes post treatment ($p < 0.05$).[68] Findings from a RCT demonstrate no significant difference in state anxiety levels between active chiropractic, placebo chiropractic and no treatment control in 21 hypertensive patients.[69]

### Flower essences (Level I, Strength B, Direction o)

Flower essence therapy is an energetic form of medicine that uses the vital force of a flower to treat physiological and psychological complaints, including anxiety.[70] According to a systematic review of four placebo-controlled RCTs (n = 370), Bach flower essences were found to be no more effective than placebo at reducing anxiety disorder severity or examination anxiety scores.[71] The short duration of these studies (from 3 hours to 14 days), and the predominant use of Bach flower rescue remedy, suggests further investigation is needed to determine whether a longer duration of treatment or the use of other flower essences yields different results.

### Homeopathy (Level I, Strength C, Direction o)

Several uncontrolled and observational studies have reported positive changes in anxiety following homeopathic treatment, although the high risk of bias in these studies limits any conclusions that can be made.[72] The best available evidence comes from a systematic review of eight RCTs, which found the effectiveness of homeopathy in anxiety disorder, specifically, test anxiety, GAD and anxiety related to medical or physical conditions, was contradictory.[72] Meta-analysis of the data was also unsuitable given differences in homeopathic and control interventions, outcome measures and treatment duration.

### Massage therapy (Level I, Strength B, Direction +)

Massage is the systematic manipulation of soft tissues of the body. This manipulative therapy may help to reduce anxiety, depression and pain by stimulating parasympathetic nervous system activity, as well as elevating serotonin and endorphin release.[8] Many controlled studies have examined the effectiveness of massage therapy in anxiety, including a systematic review of 28 RCTs. This review found that massage therapy (ranging from 5 to 60 minutes per session) significantly improved state and trait anxiety by thirty-seven per cent and seventy-seven per cent, respectively ($p < 0.01$).[8] These effect sizes were found to be similar in magnitude to those provided by psychotherapy.[8] While these findings are promising, the effect of massage on anxiety in more recent RCTs has been inconsistent.[73-76]

### Reflexology (Level III-2, Strength D, Direction o)

Reflexology is a tactile therapy based on a premise that stimulating specific zones of the feet, hands and/or ears can generate neurophysiological reflexes or responses in distant organs, glands and tissues. Like most tactile therapies, reflexology can also be used to treat stress and anxiety, although evidence of this effect has been inconsistent. In short-term controlled studies, for example, single reflexology treatments in healthy individuals and patients with various types of cancer demonstrated significant anxiety-reducing effects when compared to controls.[77-80] In longer term studies, multiple reflexology treatments over a period of 5 days to 19 weeks were found to be no more effective than controls at improving anxiety in individuals experiencing menopause or in patients undergoing cardiac bypass surgery.[81,82] These findings highlight the need for much larger studies on the long-term effects of reflexology on anxiety.

CAM prescription
The CAM interventions that are most appropriate for the management of the presenting case – that is, they target the planned goals, expected outcomes and CAM
diagnoses, they are supported by the best available evidence, they are pertinent to
the client's needs and they are most relevant to CAM practice – are outlined below.

**Primary treatments**
- Instigate regular physical exercise program (such as walking or cycling to work,
  or swimming with colleagues), at least 20 minutes daily (*client does not engage
  in intentional physical exercise – regular physical exercise is shown to be effective in reducing anxiety*).
- Commence meditation (such as mindfulness meditation), at least 30 minutes
  daily (*meditation induces the relaxation response, and is effective in reducing
  state and trait anxiety*).
- Commence oral passionflower extract, 90 mg three times a day (*P. incarnata
  extract is effective in reducing GAD anxiety scores*).

**Secondary treatments**
- Consider full body massage, 30 minutes twice a week (*massage may be helpful
  in reducing emotional stress, as well as state and trait anxiety*).
- Reduce daily coffee intake, and/or substitute percolated coffee with instant
  coffee, decaffeinated coffee or coffee alternatives (*high caffeine intake may induce anxiety symptoms in the client; moderating the consumption of coffee may
  reduce total daily caffeine intake and, in doing so, may mitigate the symptoms of
  anxiety – this is based on theoretical evidentiary support only*).
- Encourage client to engage in social networking activities (such as web-
  based, church or workplace networks, or Fijian societies) (*the move to Australia, as well as the limited social supports available to the client, may have
  contributed to the development of her anxiety symptoms – social networking
  may help to mitigate the effects of these stressors on the client's psychological wellbeing*).[25,83,84]

Referral
- Refer client to general practitioner, family physician, psychologist or psychiatrist
  if the condition deteriorates, if serious pathology is suspected (such as hyperthyroidism or pheochromocytoma) or if a serious complication arises (such as
  substance abuse).
- Refer client to another CAM practitioner if GAD, or the treatment of GAD, is
  outside the clinician's area of expertise.
- Liaise with the general practitioner about the client's overall management plan.

**Review**

To determine whether pertinent client goals and expected outcomes have been
achieved at follow-up and if any aspects of the client's care need to be improved, consider the factors listed in Table 8.2 (chapter 8), as well as the questions listed below.
- Was there a reduction in the HAM-A total score?
- Were there improvements in the anxiety, tension, insomnia and/or concentration subscores of HAM-A?
- Has the frequency and/or intensity of concomitant sighing, shortness of breath
  and restlessness reduced?
- Has the need for temazepam decreased?
- Does the severity of GAD symptoms diminish each time the client is re-exposed
  to the triggers of anxiety?

# References

1. Thornhill JT. (2007) Anxiety disorders. In: Thornhill JT, editor. NMS Psychiatry. 5th ed. Baltimore: Lippincott Williams & Wilkins.
2. Somers JM et al (2006) Prevalence and incidence studies of anxiety disorders: a systematic review of the literature. Canadian Journal of Psychiatry, 51: 100–13.
3. Tomb DA. (2007) Psychiatry. 7th ed. Philadelphia: Lippincott Williams & Wilkins.
4. Andreasen NC. Black DW. (2006) Introductory textbook of psychiatry. 4th ed. Arlington: American Psychiatric Publishing.
5. Broderick P. Benjamin AB. (2004) Caffeine and psychiatric symptoms: a review. Journal of the Oklahoma State Medical Association, 97(12): 538–42.
6. Manzoni GM et al (2008) Relaxation training for anxiety: a ten-years systematic review with meta-analysis. BMC Psychiatry, 8: 41.
7. Miyasaka LS, Atallah ÁN, Soares B. (2007) Passiflora for anxiety disorder. Cochrane Database of Systematic Reviews, (1): CD004518.
8. Moyer CA. Rounds J. Hannum JW. (2004) A meta-analysis of massage therapy research. Psychological Bulletin, 130(1): 3–18.
9. Beerendonk C et al (1999) The influence of dietary sodium restriction on anxiety levels during an in vitro fertilization procedure. Journal of Psychosomatic Obstetrics and Gynaecology, 20(2): 97–103.
10. Wardle J et al (2000) Randomized trial of the effects of cholesterol-lowering dietary treatment on psychological function. American Journal of Medicine, 108(7): 547–53.
11. Wells AS et al (1998) Alterations in mood after changing to a low-fat diet. British Journal of Nutrition, 79(1): 23–30.
12. Ussher MH et al (2007) The relationship between physical activity, sedentary behaviour and psychological wellbeing among adolescents. Social Psychiatry and Psychiatric Epidemiology, 42(10): 851–6.
13. Wipfli BM. Rethorst CD. Landers DM. (2008) The anxiolytic effects of exercise: a meta-analysis of randomized trials and dose-response analysis. Journal of Sport and Exercise Psychology, 30(4): 392–410.
14. Larun L et al (2006) Exercise in prevention and treatment of anxiety and depression among children and young people. Cochrane Database of Systematic Reviews, (3): CD004691.
15. Frye B et al (2007) Tai chi and low impact exercise: effects on the physical functioning and psychological well-being of older people. Journal of Applied Gerontology, 26(5): 433–53.
16. Jin P. (1992) Efficacy of tai chi, brisk walking, meditation, and reading in reducing mental and emotional stress. Journal of Psychosomatic Research, 36(4): 361–70.
17. Tsai JC et al (2003) The beneficial effects of tai chi chuan on blood pressure and lipid profile and anxiety status in a randomized controlled trial. Journal of Alternative and Complementary Medicine, 9(5): 747–54.
18. Kirkwood G et al (2005) Yoga for anxiety: a systematic review of the research evidence. British Journal of Sports Medicine, 39(12): 884–91.
19. Kozasa EH et al (2008) Evaluation of Siddha Samadhi yoga for anxiety and depression symptoms: a preliminary study. Psychological Reports, 103(1): 271–4.
20. Michalsen A et al (2005) Rapid stress reduction and anxiolysis among distressed women as a consequence of a three-month intensive yoga program. Medical Science Monitor, 11(12): CR555–61.
21. Rao MR et al (2009) Anxiolytic effects of a yoga program in early breast cancer patients undergoing conventional treatment: a randomized controlled trial. Complementary Therapies in Medicine, 17(1): 1–8.
22. Smith C et al (2007) A randomised comparative trial of yoga and relaxation to reduce stress and anxiety. Complementary Therapies in Medicine, 15(2): 77–83.
23. Schruers K et al (2002) Acute L-5-hydroxytryptophan administration inhibits carbon dioxide-induced panic in panic disorder patients. Psychiatry Research, 113(3): 237–43.
24. Kahn RS et al (1987) Effect of a serotonin precursor and uptake inhibitor in anxiety disorders; a double-blind comparison of 5-hydroxytryptophan, clomipramine and placebo. International Clinical Psychopharmacology, 2(1): 33–45.
25. Benjamin J. Fux M. Belmaker R. (1996) Time course of inositol treatment of panic disorder. Ninth European College of Neuropsychopharmacology Congress. Amsterdam, Netherlands.
26. Palatnik A et al (2001) Double-blind, controlled, crossover trial of inositol versus fluvoxamine for the treatment of panic disorder. Journal of Clinical Psychopharmacology, 21(3): 335–9.
27. Acil M et al (2004) Perioperative effects of melatonin and midazolam premedication on sedation, orientation, anxiety scores and psychomotor performance. European Journal of Anaesthesiology, 21(7): 553–7.
28. Caumo W. Levandovski R. Hidalgo MP. (2009) Preoperative anxiolytic effect of melatonin and clonidine on postoperative pain and morphine consumption in patients undergoing abdominal hysterectomy: a double-blind, randomized, placebo-controlled study. Journal of Pain, 10(1): 100–8.
29. Caumo W et al (2007) The clinical impact of preoperative melatonin on postoperative outcomes in patients undergoing abdominal hysterectomy. Anesthesia and Analgesia, 105(5): 1263–71.
30. Naguib M. Samarkandi AH. (1999) Premedication with melatonin: a double-blind, placebo-controlled comparison with midazolam. British Journal of Anaesthesia, 82(6): 875–80.
31. Naguib M. Samarkandi AH. (2000) The comparative dose-response effects of melatonin and midazolam for premedication of adult patients: a double-blinded, placebo-controlled study. Anesthesia and Analgesia, 91(2): 473–9.
32. Samarkandi A et al (2005) Melatonin vs. midazolam premedication in children: a double-blind, placebo-controlled study. European Journal of Anaesthesiology, 22(3): 189–96.
33. Carroll D et al (2000) The effects of an oral multivitamin combination with calcium, magnesium, and zinc on psychological well-being in healthy young male volunteers: a double-blind placebo-controlled trial. Psychopharmacology, 150(2): 220–5.
34. Gosney MA et al (2008) Effect of micronutrient supplementation on mood in nursing home residents. Gerontology, 54(5): 292–9.

35. Young GS. Conquer J. (2005) Omega-3 fatty acids and neuropsychiatric disorders. Reproduction Nutrition Development, 45: 1–28.
36. Buydens-Branchey L. Branchey M. Hibbeln JR. (2007) Associations between increases in plasma n-3 polyunsaturated fatty acids following supplementation and decreases in anger and anxiety in substance abusers. Progress in Neuro-Psychopharmacology and Biological Psychiatry, 32(2): 568–75.
37. Fontani G et al (2005) Cognitive and physiological effects of omega-3 polyunsaturated fatty acid supplementation in healthy subjects. European Journal of Clinical Investigation, 35(11): 691–9.
38. Rayman M. (2000) The importance of selenium to human health. Lancet, 356: 233–41.
39. Benton D. Cook R. (1991) The impact of selenium supplementation on mood. Biological Psychiatry, 29(11): 1092–8.
40. Shor-Posner G et al (2003) Psychological burden in the era of HAART: impact of selenium therapy. International Journal of Psychiatry in Medicine, 33(1): 55–69.
41. Rayman M et al (2006) Impact of selenium on mood and quality of life: a randomized, controlled trial. Biological Psychiatry, 59(2): 147–54.
42. Calabrese C et al (2008) Effects of a standardized Bacopa monnieri extract on cognitive performance, anxiety, and depression in the elderly: a randomized, double-blind, placebo-controlled trial. Journal of Alternative and Complementary Medicine, 14(6): 707–13.
43. Stough C et al (2001) The chronic effects of an extract of Bacopa monniera (brahmi) on cognitive function in healthy human subjects. Psychopharmacology, 156(4): 481–4.
44. Bone K. (2003) A clinical guide to blending liquid herbs. Churchill Livingstone, Missouri, St Louis.
45. Awad R et al (2007) Effects of traditionally used anxiolytic botanicals on enzymes of the gamma-aminobutyric acid (GABA) system. Canadian Journal of Physiology and Pharmacology, 85(9): 933–42.
46. Bradwejn J et al (2000) A double-blind, placebo-controlled study on the effects of gotu kola (Centella asiatica) on acoustic startle response in healthy subjects. Journal of Clinical Psychopharmacology, 20(6): 680–6.
47. Leite JR et al (1986) Pharmacology of lemongrass (Cymbopogon citratus Stapf). III. Assessment of eventual toxic, hypnotic and anxiolytic effects on humans. Journal of Ethnopharmacology, 17(1): 75–83.
48. Kobak KA et al (2005) St. John's wort versus placebo in social phobia: results from a placebo-controlled pilot study. Journal of Clinical Psychopharmacology, 25(1): 51–8.
49. Volz HP et al (2002) St John's wort extract (LI 160) in somatoform disorders: results of a placebo-controlled trial. Psychopharmacology, 164(3): 294–300.
50. Kobak KA et al (2005) St John's wort versus placebo in obsessive-compulsive disorder: results from a double-blind study. International Clinical Psychopharmacology, 20(6): 299–304.
51. Zanoli P. Avallone R. Baraldi M. (2000) Behavioral characterisation of the flavonoids apigenin and chrysin. Fitoterapia, 71(1): S117–23.
52. Movafegh A et al (2008) Preoperative oral Passiflora incarnata reduces anxiety in ambulatory surgery patients: a double-blind, placebo-controlled study. Anesthesia and Analgesia, 106(6): 1728–32.
53. Miyasaka LS. Atallah ÁN. Soares B. (2006) Valerian for anxiety disorders. Cochrane Database of Systematic Reviews, (4): CD004515.
54. Sarris J. (2007) Herbal medicines in the treatment of psychiatric disorders: a systematic review. Phytotherapy Research, 21: 703–16.
55. Pittler MH. Ernst E. (2003) Kava extract versus placebo for treating anxiety. Cochrane Database of Systematic Reviews, (1): CD003383.
56. Connor KM. Payne V. Davidson JR. (2006) Kava in generalized anxiety disorder: three placebo-controlled trials. International Clinical Psychopharmacology, 21(5): 249–53.
57. Geier FP. Konstantinowicz T. (2004) Kava treatment in patients with anxiety. Phytotherapy Research, 18(4): 297–300.
58. Jacobs BP et al (2005) An internet-based randomized, placebo-controlled trial of kava and valerian for anxiety and insomnia. Medicine, 84(4): 197–207.
59. Lehrl S. (2004) Clinical efficacy of kava extract WS 1490 in sleep disturbances associated with anxiety disorders. Results of a multicenter, randomized, placebo-controlled, double-blind clinical trial. Journal of Affective Disorders, 78(2): 101–10.
60. Awad R et al (2003) Phytochemical and biological analysis of skullcap (Scutellaria lateriflora L.): a medicinal plant with anxiolytic properties. Phytomedicine, 10(8): 640–9.
61. Wolfson P. Hoffmann DL. (2003) An investigation into the efficacy of Scutellaria lateriflora in healthy volunteers. Alternative Therapies in Health and Medicine, 9(2): 74–8.
62. Andreatini R et al (2002) Effect of valepotriates (valerian extract) in generalised anxiety disorder: a randomised placebo-controlled pilot study. Phytotherapy Research, 16: 650–4.
63. Pilkington K et al (2007) Acupuncture for anxiety and anxiety disorders: a systematic literature review. Acupuncture in Medicine, 25(1–2): 1–10.
64. Cooke B. Ernst E. (2000) Aromatherapy: a systematic review. British Journal of General Practice, 50: 493–6.
65. Holm L. Fitzmaurice L. (2008) Emergency department waiting room stress: can music or aromatherapy improve anxiety scores? Pediatric Emergency Care, 24(12): 836–8.
66. Muzzarelli L. Force M. Sebold M. (2006) Aromatherapy and reducing preprocedural anxiety: a controlled prospective study. Gastroenterology Nursing, 29(6): 466–71.
67. Soden K et al (2004) A randomized controlled trial of aromatherapy massage in a hospice setting. Palliative Medicine, 18(2): 87–92.
68. Whelan TL et al (2002) The effect of chiropractic manipulation on salivary cortisol levels. Journal of Manipulative and Physiological Therapeutics, 25(3): 149–53.
69. Yates RG et al (1988) Effects of chiropractic treatment on blood pressure and anxiety: a randomized, controlled trial. Journal of Manipulative and Physiological Therapeutics, 11(6): 484–8.
70. Heneka N. White I. (2003). Flower essences: Bach flowers/Australian bush flower essences. In: An introduction to complementary medicine. Robson T, editor. Sydney: Allen & Unwin.
71. Thaler K et al (2009) Bach flower remedies for psychological problems and pain: a systematic review. BMC Complementary and Alternative Medicine, 9: 16.
72. Pilkington K et al (2006) Homeopathy for anxiety and anxiety disorders: a systematic review of the research. Homeopathy: the Journal of the Faculty of Homeopathy, 95(3): 151–62.

73. Billhult A et al (2008) The effect of massage on cellular immunity, endocrine and psychological factors in women with breast cancer: a randomized controlled clinical trial. Autonomic Neuroscience Basic and Clinical, 140(1–2): 88–95.

74. Bost N. Wallis M. (2006) The effectiveness of a 15 minute weekly massage in reducing physical and psychological stress in nurses. Australian Journal of Advanced Nursing, 23(4): 28–33.

75. Campeau MP et al (2007) Impact of massage therapy on anxiety levels in patients undergoing radiation therapy: randomized controlled trial. Journal of the Society for Integrative Oncology, 5(4): 133–8.

76. Fernandez-Perez AM et al (2008) Effects of myofascial induction techniques on physiologic and psychologic parameters: a randomized controlled trial. Journal of Alternative and Complementary Medicine, 14(7): 807–11.

77. McVicar AJ et al (2007) Evaluation of anxiety, salivary cortisol and melatonin secretion following reflexology treatment: a pilot study in healthy individuals. Complementary Therapies in Clinical Practice, 13(3): 137–45.

78. Quattrin R et al (2006) Use of reflexology foot massage to reduce anxiety in hospitalized cancer patients in chemotherapy treatment: methodology and outcomes. Journal of Nursing Management, 14(2): 96–105.

79. Stephenson NL et al (2007) Partner-delivered reflexology: effects on cancer pain and anxiety. Oncology Nursing Forum Online, 34(1): 127–32.

80. Stephenson NL. Weinrich SP. Tavakoli AS. (2000) The effects of foot reflexology on anxiety and pain in patients with breast and lung cancer. Oncology Nursing Forum, 27(1): 67–72.

81. Gunnarsdottir TJ. Jonsdottir H. (2007) Does the experimental design capture the effects of complementary therapy? A study using reflexology for patients undergoing coronary artery bypass graft surgery. Journal of Clinical Nursing, 16(4): 777–85.

82. Williamson J et al (2002) Randomised controlled trial of reflexology for menopausal symptoms. BJOG: an international journal of obstetrics and gynaecology, 109(9): 1050–5.

83. Kuo WH. Tsai YM. (1986) Social networking, hardiness and immigrant's mental health. Journal of Health and Social Behavior, 27(2): 133–49.

84. Tsai JH. (2006) Use of computer technology to enhance immigrant families' adaptation. Journal of Nursing Scholarship, 38(1): 87–93.

# Case 3
# Asthma

## Description of asthma

### Definition

Asthma is a chronic inflammatory disease of the airways, characterised by acute exacerbations of reversible airway obstruction. The condition was formerly divided into two main types – extrinsic and intrinsic asthma. These classifications have since changed. Asthma is now separated into more specific aetiological subtypes, including, for example, allergic, exercise-induced, nocturnal, aspirin-sensitive and occupational asthma.

### Epidemiology

This distressing, often disabling, and sometimes fatal disorder affects around ten per cent of the Australian population.[1] A slightly higher prevalence rate is evident among adult women (eleven per cent) and among the 15–24 and 75 years and over age groups (eleven per cent). Higher rates of asthma are also observed among socially disadvantaged, unemployed and Indigenous populations.[1]

### Aetiology and pathophysiology

The aetiology of asthma is multifactorial, with genetic and familial factors playing a major part in the pathogenesis of the disease. There is some suggestion that the growing prevalence of asthma is also due to a number of environmental contacts, such as vaccination, early introduction of foods, early exposure to antibiotics and food additives,[2,3] but there are insufficient data to support these theories. Emerging evidence does indicate that exposure to infectious agents may be a risk factor; one recent longitudinal study reported significantly higher odds of asthma and respiratory wheeze among 5-year-old children who reported severe respiratory infections during infancy, particularly those with atopy.[4] Other factors linked to the development of asthma are obesity, exposure to household allergens (e.g. dust mite, cockroaches, pets), omega 3 fatty acid intake and perinatal issues (e.g. lack of breastfeeding, poor maternal nutrition, young maternal age, prematurity, low birthweight).[3,5] Evidence linking nutrient deficiency (e.g. vitamin C, vitamin E) with asthma is not convincing.[6,7]

The acute onset of asthma in susceptible individuals can be initiated by a range of allergic and non-allergic triggers, including household allergens (e.g. dust mite, cockroaches, animal dander), respiratory irritants (e.g. air pollution, cigarette smoke, perfumes, cleaning agents, sulfur dioxide), grass and tree pollens, occupational irritants (e.g. latex, solder, flour), hormonal changes, exercise, emotions (e.g. anger, anxiety, excitement), respiratory infections, cold air, aspirin and gastro-oesophageal reflux disease.[3,8] It is not yet established how these factors trigger respiratory distress, although the prevailing theory suggests that heightened inflammatory activity could be a precipitating factor. The predominance of T-helper cell type 2 (Th2) activity observed in asthmatics and the subsequent increase in pro-inflammatory cytokine levels, airway eosinophilia and immunoglobulin (IgE) production, all appear to promote the development of smooth muscle hypertrophy and airway remodelling.[9] These changes lead to airway hyper-responsiveness, which, upon exposure to any one of the aforementioned triggers, causes airway inflammation, submucosal oedema, increased mucus production, bronchoconstriction, mucus plugging and respiratory distress.[3,9]

### Clinical manifestations

People with mild asthma are normally asymptomatic between exacerbations. In more severe cases of asthma, and during acute exacerbations of asthma, people typically present with dyspnoea, tachypnoea, chest tightness, cough, audible wheezing and anxiety. As airway obstruction progresses, and oxygen exchange diminishes, more serious manifestations begin to emerge, including hypoxia, cyanosis and altered consciousness, and at worst, respiratory failure and death.[3,8]

## Clinical case
*23-year-old woman with exercise-induced asthma*

### Rapport

Adopt the practitioner strategies and behaviours highlighted in Table 2.1 (chapter 2) to improve client trust, communication and rapport, and the accuracy and comprehensiveness of the clinical assessment.

### Assessment

Once measures have been put into place to build client–practitioner rapport, the clinician can begin the clinical assessment.

Health history

#### History of presenting condition

A 23-year-old woman presents to her CAM practitioner with concerns about relapsing *asthma*. The client developed mild asthma at the age of 5, that went into remission in mid-adolescence. In the past 12 months, the signs of asthma have returned, specifically, wheezing, coughing, *dyspnoea* and chest tightness. These symptoms, which manifest at least 2–3 times a week, are mild and short-lived, and are no more than 10–15 minutes in duration. The symptoms, relieved by salbutamol inhaler and rest, are infrequently aggravated by cold air and frequently *triggered by intense exercise*. The exercise-induced asthma is particularly problematic for the client as it is interfering with her ability to perform as a personal trainer. The client is deeply concerned that without adequate treatment, she may have to turn to another career.

#### Medical history

##### Family history
Mother has asthma, maternal grandmother has severe eczema, paternal grandfather has peripheral vascular disease, paternal grandmother had breast cancer.

##### Allergies
Penicillin (caused a generalised rash).

##### Medications
Salbutamol inhaler 2 puffs as needed, eformoterol 1 inhalation daily, 1 multivitamin tablet daily.

##### Medical conditions
Asthma, allergic rhinitis, recurrent sinusitis (for the past 5 years, often during spring).

##### Surgical or investigational procedures
Tonsillectomy and adenoidectomy (1989), right knee anterior cruciate ligament repair (2001).

#### Lifestyle history

##### Tobacco use
Nil (partner is also a non-smoker).

##### Alcohol consumption
Light social drinker. Consumes 1–2 × 375 mL premixed Vodka drinks per fortnight.

##### Illicit drug use
Nil.

| Diet and fluid intake | |
| --- | --- |
| Breakfast | Wholemeal toast with low-fat cream cheese, coffee. |
| Morning tea | Protein bar, banana, walnuts. |
| Lunch | Tossed salad or wholemeal sandwich with turkey or chicken, tomato, low-fat cheese and lettuce. |

| Diet and fluid intake | |
|---|---|
| Afternoon tea | 150 g vanilla yoghurt. |
| Dinner | Egg white omelette with tomato and cheese, grilled salmon or whiting with carrots and beans, stirfry with chicken breast, carrots, capsicum and onion. |
| Fluid intake | 1–2 cups of instant coffee a day, 7–8 cups of water a day. |
| **Food frequency** | |
| Fruit | 1–2 serves daily |
| Vegetables | 2–3 serves daily |
| Dairy | 2–3 serves daily |
| Cereals | 4–5 serves daily |
| Red meat | 1 serve a week |
| Chicken | 6 serves a week |
| Fish | 1 serve a week |
| Takeaway/fast food | 0–1 times a week |

**Quality and duration of sleep**
Continuous sleep, average duration is 6–7 hours. In winter, sleep is often broken due to cold-air induced exacerbations of asthma.

**Frequency and duration of exercise**
Client is very active. Drives to work, but participates in personal training activities (e.g. weights, circuit) more than 4 hours a day; recently had to cease aerobic training due to asthma. Engages in incidental exercise (e.g. cleaning, cooking, work-related walking) more than 3 hours a day and sedentary activities less than 2 hours a day.

## Socioeconomic background
The client is German-born with German-born parents. She completed tertiary education 18 months ago and has since been employed as a full-time personal trainer, which she enjoys. The client lives with her supportive partner in a new home in the outer suburbs, away from arterial roads and heavy industry. She has no children, nor any firm religious or cultural beliefs.

Physical examination

### Inspection
Client is able to maintain a normal conversation in a sitting and lying position without becoming short of breath. Respiratory rate (16 breaths per minute), rhythm (regular), depth and effort are unremarkable. There are no visible signs of respiratory distress (e.g. accessory muscle use), hypoxia (e.g. clubbing or cyanosis), oropharyngeal inflammation, chest deformities or scarring.

### Olfaction
Mild halitosis is evident. The client denies any sinus, chest or oral infections.

### Palpation
Paranasal sinuses, lymph nodes and chest wall are non-tender and unremarkable. Chest expansion is symmetrical and tactile fremitus is normal.

### Percussion
All lung fields are resonant; no abnormal percussive tones were detected.

### Auscultation
Vesicular breath sounds are heard equally over all lung fields. Mild late expiratory polyphonic wheeze is also evident across all lung fields. Bronchophony, aegophony and whispered pectoriloquy are absent.

### Additional signs

Client is afebrile (36.7°C, per oral) and of normal weight (BMI is 21.4 kg/m², waist circumference is 67 cm).

### Clinical assessment tools

The asthma control scoring system (ACSS) revealed a clinical subscore of twenty per cent (a measure of symptom frequency, physical limitation and rescue medication use), a physiological subscore of eighty per cent (a measure of peak expiratory flow rate), and an inflammatory subscore of eighty per cent (a measure of airway eosinophil count).[10] This provided a mean global asthma control score of 60 per cent, signifying modest asthma control and moderate asthma severity (a higher percentage score indicates better control and reduced severity).

## Diagnostics

CAM practitioners may request, perform and/or interpret findings from a range of diagnostic tests in order to add valuable data to the pool of clinical information. While several investigations are pertinent to this case (as described below), the decision to use these tests should be considered alongside factors such as cost, convenience, comfort, turnaround time, access, practitioner competence and scope of practice, and history of previous investigations.

### Pathology tests

#### Eosinophil count

This count is a useful marker of asthma activity because activated eosinophils release histamine, which triggers bronchial smooth muscle contraction and mucus production, all of which are implicated in the pathogenesis of asthma.[9]

#### Immunoglobulin E (IgE)

IgE is an antibody primarily involved in allergic reactions. When IgE is cross-linked with an antigen, it stimulates the release of vasoactive substances (e.g. histamine) from basophils and mast cells. This results in smooth muscle contraction, increased vascular permeability and inflammation,[11] and the subsequent manifestation of symptoms such as wheeze and dyspnoea. Elevated levels of serum IgE are positively associated with the severity of asthma.[12]

#### Plasma or red cell fatty acid analysis

This assesses the concentration of fatty acids within the plasma or erythrocyte, including omega 3, omega 6 and omega 9 polyunsaturated fatty acids, saturated fatty acids and trans fatty acids. Given that high dietary omega 3 fatty acid intake is associated with decreased odds of developing wheeze and asthma when compared with lower omega 3 fatty acid intake,[5] this test may help to determine whether poor omega 3 fatty acid consumption is a contributing factor in asthma.

#### Sputum culture and sensitivity testing

These tests may be warranted if infectious triggers of asthma are suspected, in particular, the presence of bacterial, viral or fungal infections of the respiratory tract.[11]

### Radiology tests

It is not routine practice to use medical imaging in the diagnosis of asthma. Chest X-ray and CT scans may be indicated, however, in complicated asthma, atypical presentations of asthma, and/or suspicions of more serious pathology.[7]

### Functional tests

#### Pulmonary function tests (PFTs)

PFTs are often used to evaluate the presence and severity of asthma. The PFT can incorporate any number of different measures of lung volume and capacity, including total lung capacity, tidal volume, maximal mid-expiratory flow (MMEF), maximal volume ventilation (MVV), peak inspiratory flow rate (PIFR), forced vital capacity (FVC), forced expiratory volume in 1 second ($FEV_1$), and peak expiratory flow rate (PEFR). Reductions in the latter three measures are often evident in obstructive airway diseases such as asthma.[11]

**Invasive tests**

Invasive procedures are not typically used in the diagnosis of asthma unless there are suspicions of serious underlying pathology.

**Miscellaneous tests**

Bronchial provocation tests use either direct (e.g. inhaled histamine or methacholine) or indirect (e.g. exercise, cold air hyperventilation) stimuli to trigger bronchial smooth muscle contraction in hyperresponsive airways. There is some debate as to whether the results of these tests are specific to a diagnosis of asthma.[13,14]

## Diagnosis

Clusters of data extracted from the health history, clinical examination and pertinent diagnostic test results point towards the following differential CAM diagnoses.
- Dyspnoea (actual), *secondary to* asthma, *related to* genetic predisposition (*client has a family history of asthma*), chronic inflammation (*if supported by an elevated serum IgE and eosinophil count*), exercise (*asthma symptoms are triggered by intense exercise*), cold air (*asthma symptoms are aggravated by cold air*), and/or low omega 3 fatty acid intake (*low omega 3 fatty acid intake is associated with increased odds of developing asthma; while the client reports the consumption of approximately one serve of fish a week, dietary recall bias cannot be excluded*).
- Exercise intolerance (actual), *secondary to* asthma, *related to* genetic predisposition, chronic inflammation, exercise, cold air and/or low omega 3 fatty acid intake.

## Planning

The goals and expected outcomes that best serve the client's needs and that are most relevant to the presenting case (as determined by the clinical assessment and CAM diagnoses) are as follows.

Goals
1 Client will report a reduction in acute asthmatic episodes (*client is concerned about the relapsing asthma*).
2 Client will experience an improvement in exercise tolerance (*client has expressed concern about the asthma interfering with personal training activities*).

Expected outcomes
Based on the degree of improvement reported in clinical studies that have used CAM interventions for the management of asthma,[15,16] the following are anticipated.
1 Client will demonstrate a forty per cent reduction in the baseline number of asthma attacks experienced per week in 6 weeks or by dd/mm/yyyy (measured by asthma diary and ACSS clinical assessment subscore).
2 Client will exhibit a forty per cent decrease in baseline asthma severity in 6 weeks or by dd/mm/yyyy (measured by mean global asthma control score).
3 Client will report a forty per cent increase in the baseline duration of exacerbation-free exercise per week in 3 weeks or by dd/mm/yyyy (measured by exercise diary).

## Application

The range of interventions reported in the CAM literature that may be used in the treatment of asthma are appraised below.

Diet
**Low-calorie diet (Level I, Strength C, Direction +)**
As previously stated, there are a number of factors that elevate a person's risk of developing asthma. A risk factor that is generally responsive to dietary change is obesity. There is, for instance, convincing evidence that high body weight at birth and/or during middle childhood increases the risk of developing asthma.[17] Whether weight-reduction strategies are able to reverse this risk or improve asthma outcomes requires evidence from intervention studies. According to a Cochrane review, only one RCT has explored this hypothesis. The trial found the consumption of a low-energy diet plus education for 14 weeks to be statistically significantly superior to normal diet plus education at improving $FEV_1$, FVC and rescue medication use in obese people with asthma.[18] Given that low-calorie diets also reduce serum levels of inflammatory markers[19] suggests that the low-energy diet could have improved respiratory function via an anti-inflammatory effect.

**Miscellaneous diets (Level I, Strength C, Direction o)**
Dietary modification is central to the overall management of asthma in many fields of CAM. While there is adequate theoretical justification to recommend many of these dietary interventions to people with asthma, such as a low-reactive or anti-inflammatory diet, there is a paucity of evidence to support these practices. A number of systematic reviews have also found insufficient or inconclusive evidence to link fish oil supplementation,[20,21] dietary salt reduction[22] and tartrazine avoidance[23] to improvements in asthma outcomes. A recent meta-analysis of 10 observational studies also failed to find a significant correlation between dietary intake of antioxidants (including vitamin C, vitamin E and beta-carotene) and risk of asthma.[6] By contrast, the consumption of whole foods (e.g. apples, pears, whole milk, butter) appears to offer some protection against asthma, according to a community-based, cross-sectional study of 1601 young adults.[24] Several controlled trials have also found the dietary consumption of sulfur dioxide to exacerbate asthma in adults[25] and to significantly reduce lung function in children with asthma.[26] Nonetheless, these studies were small and, despite being published more than 15 years ago, have yet to be replicated using larger samples and more rigorous methodology.

Lifestyle
**Buteyko breathing (Level II, Strength B, Direction + (for bronchodilatator use) and o (for respiratory function))**
The Buteyko breathing technique (BBT) is a set of breathing exercises that serve to control the rate and depth of respirations. In doing so, Buteyko is believed to benefit people suffering from conditions characterised by hyperventilation, such as asthma. Five small RCTs have tested this claim,[27–31] none of which found BBT to be effective at improving the physiological outcomes of asthma (e.g. $FEV_1$, PEFR). Changes in quality of life and asthma control were also inconsistent across studies. On the other hand, all studies consistently showed BBT to be statistically significantly superior to controls at reducing inhaled beta-2 agonist and corticosteroid medication use. This suggests that the inclusion of BBT within a client's asthma management plan may help to reduce the overall cost of asthma treatment.

**Relaxation therapy (Level I, Strength C, Direction + (for bronchodilatator use) and o (for respiratory function))**
The relaxation response can be induced by a number of behavioural therapies, such as progressive muscle relaxation, guided imagery and autogenic training. Many RCTs and systematic reviews have examined the effect of these therapies on asthma outcomes, although the results of these studies have been inconsistent. There are conflicting findings regarding, for instance, the effect of relaxation therapy (RT) on asthma symptoms and respiratory function (e.g. $FEV_1$ and PEFR) in asthmatic adults.[32–35] In asthmatic children, evidence suggests that RT may be effective at improving PEFR.[36] A meta-analysis of two small RCTs indicates that RT may also be effective at reducing bronchodilator

use,[35] but the small size and methodological limitations of these studies, as well as the short duration of the interventions, limits any conclusions that can be made.

### Yoga (Level II, Strength B, Direction o)
Yoga is an ancient Indian practice that integrates stretching, posture, exercise and breathing with meditation. Given that these techniques are likely to bring on a relaxation response, yoga has been thought to be helpful in improving asthma symptoms, but with the exception of one controlled trial,[37] many RCTs have found yoga to be no more effective than controls at improving asthma symptoms, physiological parameters or quality of life.[38–42] Still, studies using bronchial provocation tests have demonstrated significantly greater tolerance to airway provocation among people practising yoga than people receiving controls.[39,41] This suggests that yoga might be more effective in certain subtypes of asthma, although given the uncertain specificity of this test, further investigation is needed.

## Nutritional supplementation
### Ascorbic acid (Level 1, Strength C, Direction o)
When compared with normal subjects lower levels of vitamin C have been reported in asthmatic adults and children.[43,44] Low vitamin C levels are also associated with poor respiratory function.[45] A meta-analysis of seven studies (n = 13,653) found no significant association between dietary intake of vitamin C and risk of asthma.[6] Similarly, a Cochrane review of nine RCTs that involved 330 adults and children found no significant difference for the effect of orally administered vitamin C on lung function or symptoms.[46]

### Beta-carotene (Level III-1, Strength C, Direction +)
Beta-carotene demonstrates immunomodulatory and antioxidant activity in experimental and clinical studies.[47] While a meta-analysis of seven studies (n = 13,653) found no significant association between dietary intake of beta-carotene and risk of asthma,[6] this does not seem to apply to supplemental beta-carotene. In a small RCT, the acute effect of beta-carotene supplementation (64 mg daily for 1 week) was compared with placebo in 37 patients with exercise-induced asthma. Exercise-induced asthma was prevented in fifty-two per cent of people receiving the beta-carotene. All people in the placebo group demonstrated a decline in lung function.[16] Whether these effects can be replicated using lower doses of beta-carotene over a longer period of time is not yet certain.

### Magnesium (Level II, Strength B, Direction o)
Magnesium is involved in many enzymatic reactions and physiological processes throughout the body. Hence, a deficiency of this mineral can result in a number of adverse manifestations. Low serum magnesium levels, for example, have been shown to intensify neuromuscular cell excitability, resulting in increased smooth muscle contractility. High serum levels of magnesium cause smooth muscle relaxation.[48] In addition to this bronchodilating effect, magnesium also plays a role in modulating inflammation.[49] Although these properties have influenced the use of intravenous magnesium in the emergency management of asthma, for which there is sound evidence,[50] this approach to asthma is not congruent with CAM philosophy or compatible with the scope of CAM practice. Using orally administered magnesium to prevent asthma exacerbations would be a more suitable approach. Even though several RCTs have examined the effectiveness of orally administered magnesium in children and adults with asthma (with doses ranging from 200–450 mg/day of Mg chelate, to 18.3 g/day of Mg), results have been conflicting with regards to lung function, bronchial reactivity, asthma symptoms and bronchodilator use.[51–53]

### Omega 3 fatty acids (Level I, Strength B, Direction o)
High dietary omega 3 fatty acid intake is associated with decreased odds of developing wheeze and asthma when compared with lower omega 3 fatty acid intake.[5] It is likely that this protective effect may be attributed, among other reasons, to

the anti-inflammatory action of the fatty acids.[54] While findings from epidemiological studies are promising, a systematic review of 26 clinical studies (including 11 RCTs) found inadequate or inconclusive evidence to support the use of fish oil supplementation in the primary and secondary prevention of asthma.[20] Studies postdating this review[55–57] have also demonstrated conflicting results. There is some evidence to suggest that prenatal administration of fish oil may be effective in the primary prevention of asthma, allergic asthma[58] and asthma symptoms.[59]

**Pyridoxine (Level III-1, Strength C, Direction + (for medication use only))**
Vitamin $B_6$ is a water-soluble vitamin and an important coenzyme in carbohydrate, lipid and protein metabolism. Emerging data suggest pyridoxine also may be useful in the treatment of inflammatory disorders. Clinical data indicate that, for instance, pyridoxine supplementation (300 mg twice a day for 7 days) significantly reduces thromboxane $B_2$ and leukotriene $E_4$ excretion ($p<0.05$) in male subjects, although the effect in females is not certain.[60] Despite the results of this small mechanistic study, evidence from two double-blind controlled clinical trials is somewhat difficult to interpret because of the small size of the studies, the lack of randomisation, different control groups, the variable dosage and duration of $B_6$ treatment, and the different outcomes measured. In the first study, oral pyridoxine (200 mg daily for 20 weeks) significantly reduced bronchodilator and cortisone use when compared with lower dose pyridoxine (100 mg daily).[61] In the second study, oral pyridoxine (300 mg daily for 9 weeks) was found to be no more effective than placebo at improving asthma symptoms or lung function,[62] which highlights the need for further research in this area.

**Selenium (Level II, Strength B, Direction o)**
Selenium is a mineral involved in the regulation of inflammation and immunity, specifically, the inhibition of nuclear factor-kappaB activation,[63] the enhancement of T-cell function, and B-cell activation and proliferation.[64] Selenium has also been shown to lower oxidative stress in asthmatics with selenium deficiency.[65] Despite these favourable results, findings from controlled trials have yet to support the use of this mineral in people with asthma. Two controlled clinical trials have, for instance, failed to demonstrate a statistically significant difference between patients receiving selenium (100 μg daily for 14–24 weeks) and patients receiving placebo with regards to lung function, medication use, asthma symptoms and quality of life.[66,67] While selenium supplementation was significantly ($p = 0.04$) more effective than placebo at improving a composite score of these measures (excluding quality of life), the validity and reliability of this score is questionable. The effectiveness of higher doses of selenium in people with asthma is a matter for further research.

**Vitamin E (Level II, Strength C, Direction o)**
Tocopherols exhibit a number of actions that may target the mechanisms of asthma; for instance, the inhibition of proinflammatory cytokine release, and the reduction in monocyte adhesion to endothelial tissue.[68] Even so, observational studies have failed to find a significant correlation between dietary vitamin E intake and risk of asthma.[6] Likewise, a 6-week double-blind RCT involving 72 adults with asthma found vitamin E supplementation (500 mg daily) to be no more effective than placebo at improving bronchial hyperresponsiveness, lung function, asthma symptom scores and bronchodilator use.[69]

**Quercetin**
Quercetin exhibits myriad effects that are considered desirable in the management of asthma, including anti-inflammatory, immunomodulatory and antiallergic activity; however, there is insufficient clinical evidence regarding its efficacy to justify the administration of this nutrient in people with asthma.

Herbal medicine
**Boswellia serrata (Level II, Strength B, Direction +)**
Frankincense has long been used as an anti-inflammatory herb in Ayurvedic medicine. Data from experimental studies support this anti-inflammatory effect; the boswellic acids in

frankincense gum resin have been shown to inhibit 5-lipo-oxygenase and cyclo-oxygenase activity, and the subsequent release of proinflammatory mediators.[70] While frankincense was traditionally used as a treatment for arthritis, the action of the herb suggests it may also be useful in the management of asthma. Findings from one well-designed RCT (n = 80 adults with asthma) lend support to this claim. This trial found *B. serrata* extract (350 mg three times a day for 6 weeks) to be significantly more effective than placebo at improving lung function, particularly $FEV_1$ (p<0.0001). *B. serrata* was also effective at reducing asthma symptoms, number of asthma attacks, eosinophilic count and erythrocyte sedimentation rate.[15] Further research is now required to corroborate these findings.

### *Ginkgo biloba* (Level III-2, Strength C, Direction +)
Maidenhair tree has demonstrable anti-inflammatory and antioxidant effects.[71,72] Despite these useful properties, and the long history of its use in traditional Chinese medicine, only one published study has explored the clinical efficacy of ginkgo in people with asthma. This study, which compared the effectiveness of a concentrated ginkgo leaf liquor (15 g three times a day) to placebo in 61 adults and children with asthma, found ginkgo to be significantly more effective than placebo (p<0.05) at improving $FEV_1$ at 8 weeks.[72] While this outcome is promising, further research is needed to determine if standardised extracts of *G. biloba* exhibit similar activity to ginkgo liquor.

### *Picrorhiza kurroa* (Level II, Strength B, Direction o)
Katuka is traditionally used in Ayurvedic medicine for the treatment of respiratory disease, particularly asthma and bronchitis. The anti-inflammatory, antioxidant, smooth muscle relaxant and immunomodulatory effects of the herb, which have been demonstrated experimentally,[73,74] offer a pathophysiological rationale for the use of katuka in asthma. That said, the best available evidence fails to support this theory. In the only known RCT of katuka and asthma, *P. kurroa* root (300 mg three times a day for 14 weeks) was found to be no more effective than placebo at improving lung function (i.e. $FEV_1$) or asthma symptoms in 72 children and adults with asthma.[75]

### *Tylophora indica* (Level I, Strength B, Direction o)
Indian ipecac is an Ayurvedic herb traditionally prescribed for the treatment of asthma, bronchitis, allergy and respiratory complaints. The anti-inflammatory, antihistaminic and smooth muscle relaxant properties of *T. indica*, which are supported by a number of experimental studies,[76] are desirable for the effective management of asthma. At least five controlled clinical trials have explored the effectiveness of monopreparations of *T. indica* in adults and children with asthma.[77] Firm conclusions cannot be made about the effectiveness of this herb, as improvements in lung function and asthma symptoms have not been consistent across studies. This may be partly explained by differences in treatment duration (i.e. 1–12 weeks), as well as differences in the active and control preparations used. One study did find the alkaloid extract of Indian ipecac to be significantly more effective than control at reducing medication use at 12 weeks, though the relevance of this preparation to conventional CAM practice is not certain. Given that all five studies are more than 30 years old, and that the clinical efficacy of *T. indica* in people with asthma is still inconclusive, further research in this area is well justified.

### Other herbs
*Adhatoda zeylanica* (adhatoda), *Albizia lebbeck* (albizzia), *Aloe barbadensis* (aloe vera), *Althaea officinalis* (marshmallow), *Chamomilla recutita* (German chamomile), *Coleus forskohlii* (coleus), *Euphorbia hirta* (euphorbia), *Inula helenium* (elecampane), *Grindelia camporum* (grindelia), *Rehmannia glutinosa* (rehmannia), *Schisandra chinensis* (schisandra), *Scutellaria baicalensis* (baical skullcap), *Viburnum prunifolium* (black haw) and *Withania somnifera* (ashwaganda) have all been used traditionally and/or tested under experimental conditions for their antiallergic, antimicrobial, anti-inflammatory and/or immunostimulant activity,[78,79] but there is insufficient clinical data to support the use of these herbs in asthma.

## Other

### Acupuncture (Level I, Strength C, Direction o)

Acupuncture originated in China more than 4000 years ago.[80] Since then, the therapy has established a large traditional evidence base. In the case of asthma, the best available evidence indicates that acupuncture is not an effective treatment for this condition. According to a Cochrane review of 12 RCTs (n = 350), for instance, neither needle nor laser acupuncture were found to be effective at improving lung function or wellbeing in people with asthma, while changes in asthma symptoms were shown to be inconsistent across studies. Needle acupuncture did demonstrate statistically significant superiority to sham acupuncture in reducing medication usage.[81] Given the range of interventions or techniques used, the lack of consideration given to contextual effects, and the differences in study design and outcomes measures, no firm conclusions can be drawn.

### Chiropractic (Level II, Strength C, Direction o)

Chiropractic manipulation is generally indicated in the treatment of nervous and musculoskeletal disorders. While chiropractic is also used to treat a range of non-musculoskeletal complaints, such as asthma,[82,83] there is insufficient evidence to support the use of chiropractic manipulation in asthma. Findings from three small RCTs indicate that chiropractic spinal manipulation is no more effective than sham manipulation at reducing bronchodilator use or improving PEFR, $FEV_1$ or FVC in children and adults with asthma.[84-86] As for asthma severity and quality of life, results have not been consistent across studies.

### Homeopathy (Level I, Strength C, Direction o)

Homeopathy is a system of medicine that uses highly diluted and potentised remedies to influence the body's vital force and restore balance. The therapy can be used to treat a wide range of acute and chronic complaints, including asthma. A number of trials have investigated the effectiveness of homeopathy in asthma, the results of which have been synthesised in a Cochrane review.[87] The six randomised double-blind placebo-controlled trials included in the review examined the effect of individualised and formula homeopathy in adults and children with mild to severe asthma, for a period ranging from 1 day to 12 months. Changes in lung function (e.g. $FEV_1$, FVC, PEFR), asthma symptoms, quality of life, frequency, duration or intensity of asthma exacerbations and medication use were not consistent across studies; thus the effectiveness of homeopathy for asthma is still uncertain. There is some concern that the outcomes of these studies might have been influenced by the concurrent administration of allopathic medication, as well as the omission of important contextual effects of homeopathic treatment (i.e. client–practitioner interaction). A more appropriate way of investigating the effectiveness of homeopathic management in future may be through whole systems research.

### Massage therapy (Level II, Strength C, Direction + (for some measures of respiratory function))

Massage is the systematic manipulation of soft tissues of the body. This therapy may be helpful in reducing the symptoms of asthma, such as anxiety, wheezing and tachypnoea, by stimulating parasympathetic nervous system activity.[88] The best available evidence to date comes from two small RCTs, both of which investigated the effects of parent-administered massage (20 minutes every night for 30 days) in children. In the first study (n = 32), massage was found to be more effective than progressive muscle relaxation in reducing child anxiety,[89] although the level of significance was not clear. In the second trial (n = 44), massage was shown to be more effective than standard care in improving $FEV_1$ (p = 0.04) and FVC (p = 0.05), though the difference between groups was only marginally significant.[90] Reported changes in MMEF were inconsistent across studies. Whether massage is effective in adults with asthma or at reducing the frequency or severity of asthma attacks is yet to be investigated.

## Reflexology (Level II, Strength B, Direction o)

Reflexology is a tactile therapy based on a theory that stimulating specific zones of the feet, hands and/or ears can generate neurophysiological reflexes or responses in distant organs, glands and tissues. Some claim that this therapy may be of benefit to those with asthma. Findings from two RCTs have failed to support this claim. Both studies found foot reflexology (45–60 minutes per week for 10 weeks) to be no more effective than usual care[91] or simulated foot reflexology[92] at improving objective lung function, quality of life or reducing beta-2 agonist use in patients with asthma.

## Aromatherapy and osteopathy

There is insufficient clinical evidence supporting the use of aromatherapy and osteopathy in the management of asthma.

## CAM prescription

The CAM interventions that are most appropriate for the management of the presenting case – that is, they target the planned goals, expected outcomes and CAM diagnoses, they are supported by the best available evidence, they are pertinent to the client's needs and they are most relevant to CAM practice – are outlined below.

## Primary treatments

- Commence oral *Boswellia serrata* resin extract, 350 mg three times a day (*frankincense attenuates inflammatory activity, and may be of benefit in reducing asthma symptoms and the number of asthma attacks*).
- Consider training in BBT (*buteyko breathing is effective in reducing inhaled beta-2 agonist and corticosteroid use in people with asthma*).

## Secondary treatments

Consider one of the following treatments.
- Oral beta-carotene, 64 mg for 1 week, then titrate dose to minimum effective dose (*beta-carotene supplementation may help to reduce the incidence of exercise-induced asthma attacks*).
- Minimise exposure to cold air (*consider installing central heating in the home to control for cold air-induced asthma attacks; this is based on theoretical evidentiary support only*).
- Consume at least two serves of fruit a day that includes apples and/or pears (*client seldom consumes apples and pears; increased consumption of apples and pears may offer some protection against asthma progression*).

## Referral

- Refer client to general practitioner, family physician, respiratory physician or emergency department if the condition deteriorates, if a serious complication arises (such as respiratory failure) or if another pathology is suspected (such as a pulmonary tumour).
- Refer client to another CAM practitioner if asthma, or the treatment of asthma, is outside the clinician's area of expertise.
- Liaise with the general practitioner about the client's overall management plan.

## Review

To determine whether pertinent client goals and expected outcomes have been achieved at follow-up, and if any aspects of the client's care need to be improved, consider the factors listed in Table 8.2 (chapter 8), as well as the questions listed below.
- Was there a reduction in the total number of asthma attacks experienced per week?
- Did asthma severity improve?
- Was there an improvement in exercise tolerance (i.e. an increased duration of exacerbation-free exercise)?

- Has the need for salbutamol decreased?
- Does the severity of asthma symptoms lessen each time the client is re-exposed to cold air or intense exercise?
- Is the asthma still interfering with the client's ability to perform as a personal trainer?

# References

1. Australian Bureau of Statistics (ABS). (2009) 2007–08 National health survey: summary of results. Canberra: Australian Bureau of Statistics. Cat 4364.0.
2. Pizzorno JE. Murray MT. (2006) Textbook of natural medicine. 3rd ed. Philadelphia: Elsevier.
3. Porter R et al, editors. (2008). The Merck manual. Whitehouse Station: Merck Research Laboratories.
4. Kusel MMH et al (2007) Early-life respiratory viral infections, atopic sensitization, and risk of subsequent development of persistent asthma. Journal of Allergy and Clinical Immunology, 119(5): 1105–10.
5. Burns JS et al (2007) Low dietary nutrient intakes and respiratory health in adolescents. Chest, 132(1): 238–45.
6. Gao J et al (2008) Observational studies on the effect of dietary antioxidants on asthma: a meta-analysis. Respirology, 13(4): 528–36.
7. Woods AQ. Lynch DA. (2009) Asthma: an imaging update. Radiologic Clinics of North America, 47(2): 317–29.
8. Levy M. Weller T. Hilton S. (2006) Asthma. 4th ed. London: Class Publishing.
9. Barrios RJ et al (2006) Asthma: pathology and pathophysiology. Archives of Pathology and Laboratory Medicine, 130(4): 447–51.
10. Boulet LP. Boulet V Milot J. (2002) How should we quantify asthma control. Chest, 122(6): 2217–23.
11. Pagana KD. Pagana TJ. (2008) Mosby's diagnostic and laboratory test reference. 9th ed. St Louis: Elsevier Mosby.
12. Borish L et al (2005) Total serum IgE levels in a large cohort of patients with severe or difficult-to-treat asthma. Annals of Allergy, Asthma and Immunology, 95: 247–53.
13. Brannan JD. Koskela H. Anderson SD. (2007) Monitoring asthma therapy using indirect bronchial provocation tests. Clinical Respiratory Journal, 1(1): 3–15.
14. Freed R. Anderson SD. Wyndham J. (2002) The use of bronchial provocation tests for identifying asthma: a review of the problems for occupational assessment and a proposal for a new direction. ADF Health, 3: 77–85.
15. Gupta I et al (1998) Effects of Boswellia serrata gum resin in patients with bronchial asthma: results of a double-blind, placebo-controlled, 6-week clinical study. European Journal of Medical Research, 3(11): 511–14.
16. Neuman I. Nahum H. Ben-Amotz A. (1999) Prevention of exercise-induced asthma by a natural isomer mixture of beta-carotene. Annals of Allergy, Asthma and Immunology, 82(6): 549–53.
17. Flaherman V. Rutherford GW. (2006) A meta-analysis of the effect of high weight on asthma. Archives of Disease in Childhood, 91(4): 334–9.
18. Cheng J. Pan T. (2003) Calorie controlled diet for chronic asthma. Cochrane Database of Systematic Reviews, (2): CD004674.
19. Forsythe CE et al (2008) Comparison of low fat and low carbohydrate diets on circulating fatty acid composition and markers of inflammation. Lipids, 43(1): 65–77.
20. Agency for Healthcare Research and Quality. (2004) Health effects of omega-3 fatty acids on asthma. Rockville: Agency for Healthcare Research and Quality.
21. Thien FCK et al (2002) Dietary marine fatty acids (fish oil) for asthma in adults and children. Cochrane Database of Systematic Reviews, (2): CD001283.
22. Ardern K. (2004) Dietary salt reduction or exclusion for allergic asthma. Cochrane Database of Systematic Reviews, (2): CD000436.
23. Ardern K. (2001) Tartrazine exclusion for allergic asthma. Cochrane Database of Systematic Reviews, (4): CD000460.
24. Woods RK et al (2003) Food and nutrient intakes and asthma risk in young adults. American Journal of Clinical Nutrition, 78(3): 414–21.
25. Freedman BJ. (1977) Asthma induced by sulphur dioxide, benzoate and tartrazine contained in orange drinks. Clinical allergy, 7(5): 407–15.
26. Steinman HA. Le Roux M. Potter PC. (1993) Sulphur dioxide sensitivity in South African asthmatic children. South African Medical Journal, 83(6): 387–90.
27. Bowler SD. Green A. Mitchell CA. (1998) Buteyko breathing techniques in asthma: a blinded randomised controlled trial. Medical Journal of Australia, 169(11–12): 575–8.
28. Cooper S et al (2003) Effect of two breathing exercises (Buteyko and pranayama) in asthma: a randomised controlled trial. Thorax, 58(8): 674–9.
29. Cowie RL et al (2008) A randomised controlled trial of the Buteyko technique as an adjunct to conventional management of asthma. Respiratory Medicine, 102(5): 726–32.
30. McHugh P et al (2003) Buteyko breathing technique for asthma: an effective intervention. New Zealand Medical Journal, 116(1187): U710.
31. Opat AJ et al (2002) A clinical trial of the Buteyko breathing technique in asthma as taught by a video. Journal of Asthma, 37(7): 557–64.
32. Chiang LC et al (2009) Effect of relaxation-breathing training on anxiety and asthma signs/symptoms of children with moderate-to-severe asthma: a randomized controlled trial. International Journal of Nursing Studies, 46(8): 1061–70.
33. Huntley A. White AR. Ernst E. (2002) Relaxation therapies for asthma: a systematic review. Thorax, 57(2): 127–31.
34. Lahmann C et al (2009) Functional relaxation and guided imagery as complementary therapy in asthma: a randomized controlled clinical trial. Psychotherapy and Psychosomatics, 78(4): 233–9.
35. Yorke J. Fleming SL. Shuldham C. (2006) Psychological interventions for adults with asthma. Cochrane Database of Systematic Reviews, (1): CD002982.

36. Yorke J. Fleming SL. Shuldham C. (2005) Psychological interventions for children with asthma. Cochrane Database of Systematic Reviews, (4): CD003272.
37. Nagarathna R. Nagendra HR. (1985) Yoga for bronchial asthma: a controlled study. British Medical Journal, 291(6502): 1077–9.
38. Fluge T et al (1994) Long-term effects of breathing exercises and yoga in patients suffering from bronchial asthma. Pneumologie, 48(7): 484–90.
39. Manocha R et al (2002) Sahaja yoga in the management of moderate to severe asthma: a randomised controlled trial. Thorax, 57(2): 110–15.
40. Sabina AB et al (2005) Yoga intervention for adults with mild-to-moderate asthma: a pilot study. Annals of Allergy, Asthma and Immunology, 94(5): 543–8.
41. Singh V et al (1990) Effect of yoga breathing exercises (pranayama) on airway reactivity in subjects with asthma. Lancet, 335(8702): 1381–3.
42. Vedanthan PK et al (1998) Clinical study of yoga techniques in university students with asthma: a controlled study. Allergy and Asthma Proceedings, 19(1): 3–9.
43. Aderele WI et al (1985) Plasma vitamin C (ascorbic acid) levels in asthmatic children. African Journal of Medical Science, 14(3–4): 115–20.
44. Olusi SO et al (1979) Plasma and white blood cell ascorbic acid concentrations in patients with bronchial asthma. Clinica Chimica Acta, 92(2): 161–6.
45. Schwartz J. Weiss ST. (1994) Relationship between dietary vitamin C intake and pulmonary function in the first national health and nutrition examination survey (NHANES I). American Journal of Clinical Nutrition, 59(1): 110–14.
46. Kaur B. Rowe BH. Arnold E. (2009) Vitamin C supplementation for asthma. Cochrane Database of Systematic Reviews, (1): CD000993.
47. Hughes D. (1999) Effects of carotenoids on human immune function. Proceedings of the Nutrition Society, 58(3): 713–18.
48. Kowal A et al (2007) The use of magnesium in bronchial asthma: a new approach to an old problem. Archivum Immunologiae et Therapiae Experimentalis, 55(1): 35–9.
49. Cairns CB. Kraft M. (1996) Magnesium attenuates the neutrophil respiratory burst in adult asthmatic patients. Academic Emergency Medicine, 3: 1093–7.
50. Cheuk DK. Chau TC. Lee SL. (2005) A meta-analysis on intravenous magnesium sulphate for treating acute asthma. Archives of Disease in Childhood, 90(1): 74–7.
51. Bede O et al (2003) Urinary magnesium excretion in asthmatic children receiving magnesium supplementation: a randomized, placebo-controlled, double-blind study. Magnesium Research, 16(4): 262–70.
52. Fogarty A et al (2003) Oral magnesium and vitamin C supplements in asthma: a parallel group randomized placebo-controlled trial. Clinical and Experimental Allergy, 33(10): 1355–9.
53. Gontijo-Amaral C et al (2007) Oral magnesium supplementation in asthmatic children: a double-blind randomized placebo-controlled trial. European Journal of Clinical Nutrition, 61(1): 54–60.
54. Jho DH et al (2004) Role of omega-3 fatty acid supplementation in inflammation and malignancy. Integrative Cancer Therapies, 3(2): 98–111.
55. Marks GB et al (2006) Prevention of asthma during the first 5 years of life: a randomized controlled trial. Journal of Allergy and Clinical Immunology, 118(1): 53–61.
56. Mickleborough TD et al (2006) Protective effect of fish oil supplementation on exercise-induced bronchoconstriction in asthma. Chest, 129(1): 39–49.
57. Moreira A et al (2007) Pilot study of the effects of n-3 polyunsaturated fatty acids on exhaled nitric oxide in patients with stable asthma. Journal of Investigational Allergology and Clinical Immunology, 17(5): 309–13.
58. Olsen SF et al (2008) Fish oil intake compared with olive oil intake in late pregnancy and asthma in the offspring: 16 y of registry-based follow-up from a randomized controlled trial. American Journal of Clinical Nutrition, 88(1): 167–75.
59. Mihrshahi S et al (2004) Effect of omega-3 fatty acid concentrations in plasma on symptoms of asthma at 18 months of age. Pediatric Allergy and Immunology, 15(6): 517–22.
60. Saareks V et al (2002) Opposite effects of nicotinic acid and pyridoxine on systemic prostacyclin, thromboxane and leukotriene production in man. Pharmacology and Toxicology, 90(6): 338–42.
61. Collipp PJ et al (1975) Pyridoxine treatment of childhood bronchial asthma. Annals of Allergy, 35(2): 93–7.
62. Sur S et al (1993) Double-blind trial of pyridoxine (vitamin B6) in the treatment of steroid-dependent asthma. Annals of Allergy, 70(2): 147–52.
63. Vunta H et al (2007) The anti-inflammatory effects of selenium are mediated through 15-deoxy-Delta12,14-prostaglandin J2 in macrophages. Journal of Biological Chemistry, 282(25): 17964–73.
64. Hawkes WC et al (2001) The effects of dietary selenium on the immune system in healthy men. Biological Trace Element Research, 81(3): 189–213.
65. Voitsekhovskaia IuG et al (2007) Assessment of some oxidative stress parameters in bronchial asthma patients beyond add-on selenium supplementation. Biomeditsinskaia Khimiia, 53(3): 577–84.
66. Hasselmark L et al (1993) Selenium supplementation in intrinsic asthma. Allergy, 48(1): 30–6.
67. Shaheen SO et al (2007) Randomised, double blind, placebo-controlled trial of selenium supplementation in adult asthma. Thorax, 62(6): 483–90.
68. Singh U. Devaraj S. Jialal I. (2005) Vitamin E, oxidative stress, and inflammation. Annual Review of Nutrition, 25: 151–74.
69. Pearson PJ et al (2004) Vitamin E supplements in asthma: a parallel group randomised placebo controlled trial. Thorax, 59(8): 652–6.
70. Ammon HP. (2006) Boswellic acids in chronic inflammatory diseases. Planta Medica, 72(12): 1100–16.
71. Li GH et al (2008) Studies on the effect of Ginkgo biloba extracts on NF-kappaB pathway. Journal of Chinese Medicinal Materials, 31(9): 1357–60.
72. Li MH. Zhang HL. Yang BY. (1997) Effects of Ginkgo leaf concentrated oral liquor in treating asthma. Chinese Journal of Integrated Traditional and Western Medicine, 17(4): 216–18.
73. Govindarajan R et al (2003) Free radical scavenging potential of Picrorhiza kurrooa Royle ex Benth. Indian Journal of Experimental Biology, 41(8): 875–9.
74. Khare CP. (2004) Indian herbal remedies: rational Western therapy, Ayurvedic, and other traditional usage, botany. New York: Springer Verlag.
75. Doshi VB et al (1983) Picrorrhiza kuroa in bronchial asthma. Journal of Postgraduate Medicine, 29(2): 89–9
76. Patel NJ et al (2008) Anti-inflammatory and antinociceptive activities of leaf extracts of Tylophora indica. Pharmacognosy Magazine, 4(Suppl 15): S31–6.

77. Huntley A. Ernst E. (2000) Herbal medicines for asthma: a systematic review. Thorax, 55(11): 925–9.
78. Bone K. (2003) A clinical guide to blending liquid herbs. St Louis: Churchill Livingstone.
79. Yaniv Z, Bachrach U, editors. (2005) Handbook of medicinal plants. New York: Haworth Press.
80. O'Brien KA. Xue CC. (2003) Acupuncture. In: Robson T, editor. An introduction to complementary medicine. Sydney: Allen & Unwin.
81. McCarney RW et al (2003) Acupuncture for chronic asthma. Cochrane Database of Systematic Reviews, (3): CD000008.
82. Andrews L et al (1998) The use of alternative therapies by children with asthma: a brief report. Journal of Paediatrics and Child Health, 34: 131–4.
83. Sidora-Arcoleo K et al (2007) Complementary and alternative medicine use in children with asthma: prevalence and sociodemographic profile of users. Journal of Asthma, 44(3): 169–75.
84. Balon J et al (1998) A comparison of active and simulated chiropractic manipulation as adjunctive treatment for childhood asthma. New England Journal of Medicine, 339(15): 1013–20.
85. Bronfort G et al (2001) Chronic pediatric asthma and chiropractic spinal manipulation: a prospective clinical series and randomized clinical pilot study. Journal of Manipulative and Physiological Therapeutics, 24(6): 369–77.
86. Nielsen NH et al (1995) Chronic asthma and chiropractic spinal manipulation: a randomized clinical trial. Clinical and Experimental Allergy, 25(1): 80–8.
87. McCarney RW. Linde K. Lasserson TJ. (2004) Homeopathy for chronic asthma. Cochrane Database of Systematic Reviews, (1): CD000353.
88. Moyer CA. Rounds J. Hannum JW. (2004) A meta-analysis of massage therapy research. Psychological Bulletin, 130(1): 3–18.
89. Field T et al (1998) Children with asthma have improved pulmonary functions after massage therapy. Journal of Pediatrics, 132(5): 854–8.
90. Nekooee A et al (2008) Effect of massage therapy on children with asthma. Iranian Journal of Pediatrics, 18(2): 123–9.
91. Petersen LN et al. (1992) Foot zone therapy and bronchial asthma: a controlled clinical trial. Ugeskrift for Laeger, 154(30): 2065–2068.
92. Brygge T et al. (2001) Reflexology and bronchial asthma. Respiratory Medicine, 95(3): 173–9.

# Case 4
# Chronic venous insufficiency

## Description of chronic venous insufficiency

Definition
Chronic venous insufficiency (CVI) is a pathological condition of the venous system, characterised by impaired venous blood flow in the lower limbs. The disorder presents as pathological changes to the skin, subcutaneous tissue and vascular tissue, and is a precursor to varicose veins and venous leg ulceration.

Epidemiology
CVI affects between 0.1 per cent and seventeen per cent of men, and from 0.2 per cent to twenty per cent of women.[1] While evidence that links CVI occurrence to gender is inconsistent, being female is associated with an increased risk of CVI manifestations, including varicose veins[1] and venous leg ulceration.[2] CVI prevalence is also associated with increasing age, a relationship that may be attributed to the decline in blood vessel wall integrity and calf muscle strength over time.[1]

Aetiology and pathophysiology
A number of risk factors are connected with the development of CVI. Family history and increasing age, for instance, are both associated with an increased risk.[1] In terms of modifiable risk factors, several studies have observed a higher prevalence and severity of CVI and varicose veins among people in occupations that typically require prolonged periods of standing, such as nurses, flight attendants and factory workers.[1] The reduced calf-muscle pump activity associated with prolonged standing may contribute to the pathogenesis of CVI because of excessive lower limb venous congestion and pressure.

Another modifiable risk factor of CVI is macrovascular insult, the cause of which may be credited to lower limb trauma, surgery, deep vein thrombosis (DVT) and/or pregnancy. The injury to the venous system triggers a cascade of events that contribute to CVI, including valvular incompetence, venous reflux (or retrograde blood flow), ambulatory venous hypertension, venous wall dilatation and elevated capillary filtration. Over time, these pathological changes lead to the formation of interstitial oedema, localised hypoxia, malnutrition and tissue destruction. Two mechanisms are believed to be responsible for the progression from a state of elevated capillary filtration pressure to changes in tissue perfusion and local architecture, including the extravasation or leakage of fibrinogen into the subcutaneous tisues and the subsequent formation of pericapillary cuffs, the intraluminal trapping of leucocytes and subsequent release of toxic metabolites, proteolytic enzymes and tissue necrosis factor-alpha. The extravasation of fibrinogen and leucocyte products into pericapillary tissue may also mediate inflammation, which suggests that CVI may be a disease of chronic inflammation.[3]

Clinical manifestations
The early stages of CVI typically manifest as lower leg fatigue, heaviness, discomfort and pruritus. As the disease progresses, visible changes to the skin and subcutaneous tissue begin to emerge, such as lower leg oedema, ochre pigmentation, stasis dermatitis and lipodermatosclerosis. In the more advanced stages of CVI, a person may also present with superficial and deep varicose veins, as well as venous leg ulceration. The functional and cosmetic implications of these manifestations can significantly affect a person's quality of life.[4]

## Clinical case
*44-year-old woman with mild chronic venous insufficiency*

### Rapport

Adopt the practitioner strategies and behaviours highlighted in Table 2.1 (chapter 2) to improve client trust, communication and rapport, as well as the accuracy and comprehensiveness of the clinical assessment.

### Assessment

Once measures have been put into place to build client–practitioner rapport, the clinician can begin the clinical assessment.

Health history

**History of presenting condition**
A 44-year-old woman presents to the clinic with bilateral lower leg heaviness and discomfort. These symptoms began around 10 years ago and, until the last 6 months, have been short-lived, mild and tolerable. These symptoms are now persistent for most of the day, are frequently aggravated by prolonged standing and sitting, and relieved by leg elevation, lying in bed and with the use of support stockings. The lower limb heaviness and constant dull ache (pain score = 3/10) are accompanied by afternoon leg fatigue and intermittent pruritus to the bilateral, posterior lower legs. These symptoms are often problematic because as a flight attendant the client is required to stand for prolonged periods. Over the past month, the client has needed to rest her legs at least two to three times during long-haul flights, which is not only unusual but also disruptive to work. This disruption to work concerns the client, who has also expressed concern about developing a leg ulcer, as did her mother, if the condition goes untreated.

Medical history

**Family history**
Mother has hypertension and severe leg ulceration, father has hypertension, maternal grandmother had breast cancer.

**Allergies**
Latex (causes contact dermatitis), penicillin (causes a systemic cutaneous rash).

**Medications**
Vitamin B complex 1 daily, alpha-lipoic acid 100 mg daily.

**Medical conditions**
Varicose veins, mild endometriosis.

**Surgical or investigational procedures**
Diagnostic laparoscopy (1985), left anterior cruciate ligament repair (1987).

**Lifestyle history**

**Tobacco use**
Nil.

**Alcohol consumption**
Consumes 2–3 standard drinks (e.g. white wine, Irish cream) every 2–4 weeks.

**Illicit drug use**
Nil.

| Diet and fluid intake | |
| --- | --- |
| Breakfast | Coffee, porridge with skim milk. |
| Morning tea | Coffee, apple. |

| Lunch | Vegetable hotpot, sandwich with white bread, lettuce, tomato and carrot, chicken salad with tomato, cucumber, mixed greens and mushrooms. |
|---|---|
| Afternoon tea | Cheese and water crackers, apple juice, coffee. |
| Dinner | Beef and onion stew, chicken curry with white rice, grilled haddock with steamed carrot, cauliflower and broccoli. |
| Fluid intake | 2–3 cups of percolated coffee a day, 2–3 cups of water a day, 1 cup of juice a day. |
| **Food frequency** | |
| Fruit | 1–2 serves daily |
| Vegetables | 3–4 serves daily |
| Dairy | 2 serves daily |
| Cereals | 3–4 serves daily |
| Red meat | 3 serves a week |
| Chicken | 4 serves a week |
| Fish | 1 serve a week |
| Takeaway/fast food | <1 time a week |

**Quality and duration of sleep**
Interrupted sleep. Has difficulty falling asleep due to changeable working hours (sleep latency of approximately 30 minutes); average duration is 6–7 hours.

**Frequency and duration of exercise**
The client has limited opportunities for physical exercise on working days, although does manage to exercise at least 1 hour, three times a week at the gym. Client also engages in incidental exercise (i.e. walking at work) approximately 4–6 hours, three times a week, and sedentary activities less than 2 hours a day.

## Socioeconomic background
The client was born and raised in Northern Ireland, as were her parents. The client and her family – supportive husband and two children, aged 17 and 21 years – also reside in Northern Ireland, in their own home, in a quiet inner city suburb of Belfast. All are practising Catholics. Since completing her flight attendant training program more than 20 years ago, the client has been employed as a flight attendant for an international airline. While she enjoys the occupation, she finds the time spent away from her family distressing at times.

## Physical examination

### Inspection
The bilateral lower legs are pale with no visible pigmentary changes. Thin, superficial varicose veins are evident over the popliteal fossa and calf bilaterally, including four in the left lower leg and two in the right lower leg. Mild bilateral pedal oedema is present up to the ankle; the oedema is worse in the left foot. There is no dyspnoea on exertion, cyanosis, chest deformity or nail clubbing to suggest underlying cardiac disease. Lower limb skin integrity is intact with no lesions or ulcerations.

### Olfaction
Not applicable.

### Palpation
Popliteal, posterior tibial and dorsalis pedis pulses are strong, regular and of equal amplitude bilaterally. No thrills are present over the neck, upper extremity, abdominal and lower extremity pulses or over the auscultatory areas of the heart. The point of maximum impulse (PMI) is located in the fifth intercostal space at the midclavicular

line. The lower limbs and digits are warm. Mild pitting pedal oedema is present up to the ankle bilaterally, but is worse in the left foot. There is no palpable tenderness, numbness or fibrotic or sclerotic changes to the skin of the lower legs. Varicose veins over the bilateral popliteal fossae and calf are palpable.

**Percussion**
Not applicable.

**Auscultation**
There are no audible murmurs over the auscultatory areas of the heart. There are no bruits over the pulse sites of the neck, upper extremities, abdomen or lower extremities.

**Additional signs**
Client is in the ideal weight range (BMI is 24.3 kg/m$^2$, waist circumference is 72 cm). Heart rate is 64 beats per minute and regular, and blood pressure is 135/82.

**Clinical assessment tools**
The mean score for all 10 items on the venous clinical severity score (VCSS) was 6/30. Two points were awarded to each of daily pain, multiple varicose veins and afternoon venous oedema. This score suggests the client has mild venous disease.

## Diagnostics
CAM practitioners can request, perform and/or interpret findings from a range of diagnostic tests in order to add valuable data to the pool of clinical information. While several investigations are pertinent to this case (as described below), the decision to use these tests should be considered alongside factors such as cost, convenience, comfort, turnaround time, access, practitioner competence and scope of practice, and history of previous investigations.

**Pathology tests**
Elevated levels of LDL-C, total cholesterol, triglycerides, homocysteine, apolipopro-tein-B, asymmetric dimethylarginine (ADMA) and/or C-reactive protein (CRP) may be indicative of cardiovascular disease.[5] While these tests have little diagnostic value in CVI, they can be helpful in determining whether a person with lower limb vascular disease also has signs of systemic vascular disease.

**Radiology tests**
Doppler or ultrasound uses sound waves to assess blood flow velocity and direction, as well as blood flow disturbances of major blood vessels, including the veins of the lower limbs. This procedure is particularly useful for identifying the presence of chronic venous insufficiency (evidenced by retrograde venous blood flow), varicose veins and venous occlusion (evidenced by absent venous blood flow).[5]

**Functional tests**
A comprehensive cardiovascular profile identifies a number of lipid-independent risk factors that are related to cardiovascular disease, such as homocysteine, CRP and fibrinogen. The diagnostic value of these tests in CVI is discussed above.

**Invasive tests**
Not applicable.

**Miscellaneous tests**
The presence of arcus senilis, a whitish ring at the perimeter of the cornea, is highly suspicious of hypercholesterolaemia.[6] Even though this sign has little diagnostic value in CVI, it may be useful in determining whether a person with lower limb vascu-lar disease also has signs of systemic vascular disease.

## Diagnosis

Clusters of data extracted from the health history, clinical examination and pertinent diagnostic test results point towards the following differential CAM diagnoses.

- Lower limb heaviness (actual), *secondary to* CVI, *related to* family history (*client's mother has a history of severe leg ulceration, possibly due to CVI*), decreased calf muscle pump activity and increased lower limb venous congestion (*client's occupation requires prolonged periods of standing, which may increase lower limb venous pressure and contribute to the pathogenesis of CVI*).
- Lower limb discomfort (actual), *secondary to* CVI, *related to* family history; decreased calf muscle pump activity and increased lower limb venous congestion.
- Venous leg ulceration (potential), *secondary to* CVI, *related to* family history; decreased calf muscle pump activity and increased lower limb venous congestion.

## Planning

The goals and expected outcomes that best serve the client's needs and are most relevant to the case (as determined by the clinical assessment and CAM diagnoses) are as follows.

Goals
1 Client will be free from leg heaviness (*client is concerned about the way this symptom is affecting her ability to work*).
2 Client will be free from leg discomfort (*client is concerned about the way this symptom is affecting her ability to work*).
3 Client will not develop venous leg ulceration (*client has expressed concern about developing a leg ulcer*).

Expected outcomes
Based on the degree of improvement reported in clinical studies that have used CAM interventions for the management of CVI,[7] the following are anticipated.
1 Client will report a thirty-five per cent reduction in baseline severity of leg heaviness in 7 weeks or by dd/mm/yyyy (measured by a visual analogue scale).
2 Client will report a forty per cent reduction in baseline intensity of leg discomfort in 8 weeks or by dd/mm/yyyy (measured by a 0–10 numerical scale).
3 Client will demonstrate a thirty per cent reduction in baseline severity of venous disease in 8 weeks or by dd/mm/yyyy (measured by VCSS).
4 Client will remain free from venous leg ulceration for 12 months or up to dd/mm/yyyy (according to client history).

## Application

The range of interventions reported in the CAM literature that may be used in the treatment of CVI is appraised below.

Diet
While dietary modification – the modification of fibre, fat, fruit, vegetable and salt intake – plays a key role in the management of cardiovascular disorders, its effectiveness in CVI has not been adequately explored. This is not to say that dietary modification is ineffective, or that it should not be incorporated into a CVI management plan, only that dietary recommendations are not yet supported by high-level evidence.

Lifestyle
**Physical exercise (Level III–1, Strength C, Direction o)**
Physical exercise is likely to improve calf muscle pump function and lower limb venous haemodynamics and thus may be of benefit to people with venous insufficiency. While findings from a small RCT (n = 31 patients with CVI) demonstrated that a supervised calf muscle strength exercise program, together with wearing compression hosiery,

was significantly more effective than control at improving mean venous ejection fraction at 6 months, the intervention was no more effective than control at improving venous reflux, venous severity scores and quality of life.[8] Given that prolonged standing contributes to the pathogenesis of CVI, it is likely that a structured exercise program may still be useful in preventing the onset and/or progression of the disorder.

## Nutritional supplementation

**Ascorbic acid, beta-carotene, copper, glycine, hesperidin, leucine, lysine, quercetin, rutin, selenium and silicon**
These nutrients play an important role in collagen synthesis. Many of them also exhibit actions pertinent to the management of CVI, including antienzymatic, antioxidant and anti-inflammatory effects.[9–11] Still, it is unclear whether monopreparations of these nutrients offer any clinical benefit to people with CVI, because of the paucity of clinical evidence in this area.

## Herbal medicine

**Aesculus hippocastanum (Level I, Strength A, Direction + (for mild to moderate CVI only))**
Horsechestnut seed was traditionally used in Western herbal medicine to treat musculoskeletal, gastrointestinal and venous disorders, including haemorrhoids, varicose veins and leg ulceration. The majority of research to date, which has focused on the vascular effects of the plant, reveals that horsechestnut seed extract (HCSE) and the saponins and sapogenins of the plant inhibit hyaluronidase activity in vitro,[12] scavenge superoxide-anions, increase fibroblast survival,[13] inhibit histamine-induced vascular permeability in vivo and inhibit carageenin-induced paw oedema.[14] These effects are fundamental to the management of venous insufficiency and may explain why a Cochrane review of 17 RCTs found orally administered HCSE (standardised to 50–150 mg aescin daily, for 20 days to 16 weeks) to be more effective than placebo and as effective as other phlebotonic agents at reducing leg pain, pruritus, oedema, leg volume, and ankle and calf girth in individuals with mild to moderate CVI.[7] In severe or advanced CVI, HCSE appears to be less effective.[15]

**Centella asiatica (Level II, Strength B, Direction +)**
Gotu kola is used across several traditional systems of medicine as a treatment for skin complaints.[16] Research to date suggests that the plant may also be suitable for the treatment of vascular disorders. Experimental data demonstrate that *Centella asiatica* flavonoids exhibit free radical scavenging activity in vivo.[17] Clinically, titrated extracts of *C. asiatica* (60–180 mg daily) have been shown in three RCTs to be more effective than placebo at reducing ankle circumference and oedema at 4 weeks,[18] lower leg volume at 6 weeks[19] and leg heaviness and oedema at 8 weeks.[20] While these effects are promising, further investigation is needed regarding the long-term safety and effectiveness of gotu kola in CVI.

**Folia vitis viniferae (Level II, Strength B, Direction +)**
Red vine leaf extract (RVLE) has been shown under experimental conditions to prevent venous endothelial damage from blood platelet and polymorphonuclear granulocyte release products, and to facilitate venular endothelial repair in vitro.[21] These effects can be attributed to the flavonoids quercetin and isoquercitrin. The best available evidence from two RCTs supports these actions; it shows RVLE (360–720 mg daily) to be statistically significantly more effective than placebo at reducing calf circumference and CVI symptoms at 6[22] and 12 weeks.[23] Changes in ankle girth were not consistent across the two studies, however.

**Pinus maritima (Level II, Strength B, Direction +)**
French maritime pine bark extract, or pycnogenol, is not only a powerful scavenger of free radicals,[24] but also an inhibitor of nuclear factor-kappaB and the proinflammatory

cytokine interleukin-1.[25] These effects are fundamental in maintaining and improving venous wall integrity; they also appear to be of benefit in people with CVI. In fact, two RCTs involving a total of 80 patients with CVI found *P. maritima* extract (300 mg daily) to be significantly more effective than placebo at reducing leg heaviness and subcutaneous oedema at 8 weeks.[26,27] Changes in venous haemodynamics were not consistent between studies.

### *Ruscus aculeatus* (Level II, Strength B, Direction +)

Butcher's broom has a long history of use as a treatment for venous disorders.[28] Experimental studies that have explored this action have shown the saponins of *R. aculeatus* to inhibit elastase activity in vitro,[12] and extract of butcher's broom to inhibit histamine-induced vascular permeability in vivo.[29] Butcher's broom also shows clinical promise, with a RCT of 148 women with CVI showing *R. aculeatus* (36.9 mg dried extract twice daily) to be significantly more effective than placebo at reducing leg volume, ankle and leg circumference, and leg heaviness, fatigue and tension at 12 weeks.[30] Further research is required to determine whether butcher's broom is effective in males with CVI.

### Other herbs

*Hamamelis virginiana* (witch hazel) and *Vaccinium myrtillus* (bilberry) have been used traditionally and/or tested under experimental conditions for their anti-inflammatory, antioxidant and venotonic activity,[31] but to date there is insufficient clinical evidence to support or refute the efficacy of these herbal monopreparations in humans with CVI.

## Other

### Reflexology (Level III-1, Strength C, Direction o)

Foot reflexology is based on a theory that stimulating specific zones of the feet, hands and/or ears can generate neurophysiological reflexes or responses in distant organs, glands and tissues. It is reasonable to hypothesise, therefore, that reflexology would be effective in CVI. To test this hypothesis, a single, blind RCT randomly allocated 55 healthy pregnant women with foot oedema to one of three groups: relaxation foot reflexology, lymphatic foot reflexology and rest.[32] Each group received up to four 15-minute treatments. While all groups demonstrated a significant reduction in pain, discomfort and tiredness, there was no statistically significant difference between groups in mean ankle and foot girth measurements. It can be said, then, that the effectiveness of reflexology in venous insufficiency is inconclusive.

### Acupuncture, aromatherapy, chiropractic, homeopathy, massage and osteopathy

There is insufficient clinical evidence to support the use of these therapies in the management of CVI.

## CAM prescription

The CAM interventions that are most appropriate for the management of the presenting case – that is, they target the planned goals, expected outcomes and CAM diagnoses, they are supported by the best available evidence, they are pertinent to the client's needs, and they are most relevant to CAM practice – are outlined below.

### Primary treatments

- Commence oral HCSE, standardised to 50 mg aescin, twice daily (*HCSE reduces lower limb heaviness and pain by improving venous tone and venous flow pressure*).[33]
- Continue using support hosiery while working (*compression stockings that exert an ankle pressure of 10–20 mmHg may help to reduce venous congestion. A meta-analysis of 10 RCTs found support hosiery to be significantly more effective than placebo or no stockings in reducing leg discomfort, including occupation-associated leg discomfort in flight attendants*).[34]

**Secondary treatments**
- Avoid prolonged standing or sitting. When this is unavoidable, maintain regular leg and calf exercises (*calf exercises facilitate lower limb venous drainage, decrease venous congestion and reduce lower limb heaviness and pain; this recommendation is based on theoretical evidentiary support only*).
- Maintain a well-balanced diet (*to improve nutritional intake and protect against lifestyle diseases, consume wholegrain cereals at least five times a day, consume fish at least twice a week and increase vegetable intake by 1–2 serves a day*), and drink at least 5–6 cups of water daily (*to counteract the dehydrating effect of dry aircraft cabin atmosphere*).

Referral
- Refer client to a general practitioner, family physician, vascular specialist or emergency department if the condition deteriorates, if a major complication arises (e.g. cellulitis, venous ulceration) or if a serious pathology is suspected (e.g. DVT).
- Refer client to another CAM practitioner if CVI, or the treatment of CVI, is outside the clinician's area of expertise.

## Review

To determine whether pertinent client goals and expected outcomes have been achieved at follow-up and if any aspects of the client's care need to be improved, consider the factors listed in Table 8.2 (chapter 8), as well as the questions listed below.
- Was there a reduction in the severity of leg heaviness?
- Was there a decrease in the intensity of leg discomfort?
- Was there a reduction in the VCSS?
- Has the client remained free from venous leg ulceration?
- Has the need to rest the legs during long-haul flights reduced?
- Was there an improvement in other CVI symptoms (e.g. oedema, pruritus, leg fatigue)?

# References

1. Beebe-Dimmer JL et al (2004) The epidemiology of chronic venous insufficiency and varicose veins. Annals of Epidemiology, 15: 175–84.
2. Callam M et al (1987). Chronic ulcer of the leg: clinical history. British Medical Journal, 294(6584): 1389–91.
3. Pappas PJ et al (2005) Causes of severe chronic venous insufficiency. Seminars in Vascular Surgery, 18: 30–5.
4. Duque M et al (2005) Itch, pain, and burning sensation are common symptoms in mild to moderate chronic venous insufficiency with an impact on quality of life. Journal of the American Academy of Dermatology, 53(3): 503–7.
5. Van Leeuwen AM. Poelhuis-Leth DJ. (2009) Davis's comprehensive handbook of laboratory and diagnostic tests with nursing implications. 3rd ed. Philadelphia: FA Davis Company.
6. Swartz MH. (2009) Textbook of physical diagnosis: history and examination. 6th ed. Philadelphia: Saunders.
7. Pittler MH. Ernst E. (2006) Horse chestnut seed extract for chronic venous insufficiency. Cochrane Database of Systematic Reviews, (1): CD003230.
8. Padberg FT. Johnston MV. Sisto SA. (2004) Structured exercise improves calf muscle pump function in chronic venous insufficiency: a randomized trial. Journal of Vascular Surgery, 39(1): 79–87.
9. Higdon J. (2003) An evidence-based approach to vitamins and minerals. New York: Thieme.
10. Leach MJ. (2004) A critical review of natural therapies in wound management. Ostomy/Wound Management, 50(2): 36–51.
11. Shils ME et al (2006) Modern nutrition in health and disease. 10th ed. Philadelphia: Lippincott Williams & Wilkins.
12. Facino R et al (1995). Anti-elastase and anti-hyaluronidase activities of saponins and sapogenins from Hedera helix, Aesculus hippocastanum, and Ruscus aculeatus: factors contributing to their efficacy in the treatment of venous insufficiency. Archiv der Pharmazie, 328(10): 720–4.
13. Masaki H et al (1995) Active-oxygen scavenging activity of plant extracts. Biological and Pharmaceutical Bulletin, 18(1): 162–6.
14. Peschen M et al (1998) Increased expression of platelet-derived growth factor receptor alpha and beta and vascular endothelial growth factor in the skin of patients with chronic venous insufficiency. Archives of Dermatological Research, 290(6): 291–7.
15. Leach MJ. Pincombe J. Foster G. (2006) Clinical efficacy of horsechestnut seed extract in the treatment of venous ulceration. Journal of Wound Care, 15(4): 159–67.

16. Bone K. (2003) A clinical guide to blending liquid herbs. St Louis: Churchill Livingstone.
17. Zheng CJ. Qin LP. (2007) Chemical components of Centella asiatica and their bioactivities. Journal of Chinese Integrative Medicine, 5(3): 348–51.
18. De Sanctis MT et al (2001) Treatment of edema and increased capillary filtration in venous hypertension with total triterpenic fraction of Centella asiatica: a clinical, prospective, placebo-controlled, randomized, dose-ranging trial. Angiology, 52(Suppl 2): S55–9.
19. Cesarone MR et al (2001) Microcirculatory effects of total triterpenic fraction of Centella asiatica in chronic venous hypertension: measurement by laser Doppler, TcPO2–CO2, and leg volumetry. Angiology, 52(Suppl 2): S45–8.
20. Pointel JP et al (1987) Titrated extract of Centella asiatica (TECA) in the treatment of venous insufficiency of the lower limbs. Angiology, 38(1 Pt 1): 46–50.
21. Nees S et al (2003) Protective effects of flavonoids contained in the red vine leaf on venular endothelium against the attack of activated blood components in vitro. Arzneimittel-Forschung, 53(5): 330–41.
22. Kalus U et al (2004) Improvement of cutaneous microcirculation and oxygen supply in patients with chronic venous insufficiency by orally administered extract of red vine leaves AS 195: a randomised, double-blind, placebo-controlled, crossover study. Drugs in R&D, 5(2): 63–71.
23. Kiesewetter H et al (2000) Efficacy of orally administered extract of red vine leaf AS 195 (folia vitis viniferae) in chronic venous insufficiency (stages I–II). A randomized, double-blind, placebo-controlled trial. Arzneimittel-Forschung, 50(2): 109–17.
24. Busserolles J et al (2006) In vivo antioxidant activity of procyanidin-rich extracts from grape seed and pine (Pinus maritima) bark in rats. International Journal for Vitamin and Nutrition Research, 76(1): 22–7.
25. Cho KJ et al. (2000) Effect of bioflavonoids extracted from the bark of Pinus maritima on proinflammatory cytokine interleukin-1 production in lipopolysaccharide-stimulated RAW 264.7. Toxicology and Applied Pharmacology, 168(1): 64–71.
26. Arcangeli P. (2000) Pycnogenol in chronic venous insufficiency. Fitoterapia, 71(3): 236–44.
27. Petrassi C. Mastromarino A. Spartera C. (2000) PYCNOGENOL in chronic venous insufficiency. Phytomedicine, 7(5): 383–8.
28. Kraft K. Hobbs C. (2004) Pocket guide to herbal medicine. New York: Thieme.
29. Bouskela E. Cyrino FZ. Marcelon G. (1994) Possible mechanisms for the inhibitory effect of Ruscus extract on increased microvascular permeability induced by histamine in hamster cheek pouch. Journal of Cardiovascular Pharmacology, 24(2): 281–5.
30. Vanscheidt W et al (2002) Efficacy and safety of a Butcher's broom preparation (Ruscus aculeatus L. extract) compared to placebo in patients suffering from chronic venous insufficiency. Arzneimittel-Forschung, 52(4): 243–50.
31. European Scientific Cooperative on Phytotherapy (ESCOP) (2003) ESCOP monographs: the scientific foundation for herbal medicinal products. 2nd ed. Exeter: ESCOP.
32. Mollart L. (2003) Single-blind trial addressing the differential effects of two reflexology techniques versus rest, on ankle and foot oedema in late pregnancy. Complementary Therapies in Nursing and Midwifery, 9(4): 203–8.
33. Guillaume M. Padioleau F. (1994). Veinotonic effect, vascular protection, anti-inflammatory and free radical scavenging properties of Horse chestnut extract. Arzneimittel-Forschung, 44(1): 25–35.
34. Amsler F. Blattler W. (2008) Compression therapy for occupational leg symptoms and chronic venous disorders: a meta-analysis of randomised controlled trials. European Journal of Vascular and Endovascular Surgery, 35(3): 366–72.

# Case 5
# Dysmenorrhoea

## Description of dysmenorrhoea

### Definition
Dysmenorrhoea is defined as cyclic lower abdominal pain that occurs with, or precedes, menstruation.[1] Depending on the aetiology of the condition, dysmenorrhoea may be classified as either primary or secondary. Primary dysmenorrhoea is a functional disorder that has no identifiable pathological aetiology and is typically associated with ovulation. Pain caused by a demonstrable pathology to the pelvic or reproductive structures, however, is referred to as secondary dysmenorrhoea.[1]

### Epidemiology
The prevalence of dysmenorrhoea varies across the globe, affecting between 16.8 and 81 per cent of women.[2] Of the two categories of menstrual pain, primary dysmenorrhoea is the most common, contributing to around ninety per cent of dysmenorrhoeic cases.[3] Primary dysmenorrhoea usually begins during adolescence or the early twenties, generally after regular ovulation is established, and usually after the first three to six menstrual cycles.[4] Unlike the prevalence of secondary dysmenorrhoea, which increases with advancing age, the prevalence of primary dysmenorrhoea diminishes with age and, in some cases, following pregnancy.[4]

### Aetiology and pathophysiology
Primary dysmenorrhoea is caused by abnormal eicosanoid production, specifically, an abnormal increase in endometrium-derived prostaglandin (PG) $F_2\alpha$ and $PGE_2$. These proinflammatory compounds are formed under the influence of progesterone, but can also rise following endometrial shedding, endometrial cell necrosis,[4] excess omega 6 fatty acid intake, low omega 3 fatty acid consumption and/or abnormal fatty acid metabolism.[3,5,6] The PGs implicated in the pathogenesis of dysmenorrhoea exhibit a wide range of effects. $PGF_2\alpha$, for instance, affects the gastrointestinal (GI) tract, causing nausea, vomiting and diarrhoea.[4] $PGF_2\alpha$ is also a potent smooth muscle stimulant and vasoconstrictor, which, in sufficient quantities, can cause uterine ischaemia, myometrial contractions and uterine pain.[3] In contrast, $PGE_2$ is a potent vasodilator and a possible contributor to excessive menstrual bleeding.[4] While the cytokine hypothesis of dysmenorrhoea is theoretically plausible, evidence from clinical studies is mixed.[7,8]

As opposed to the proinflammatory state of primary dysmenorrhoea, the cause of secondary dysmenorrhoea is primarily pathological. Conditions usually associated with secondary dysmenorrhoea include endometriosis, uterine adenomycosis, leiomyomata or fibroids, pelvic adhesions, cervical stenosis, pelvic inflammatory disease, *in situ* intrauterine device and endometrial polyps.[1,4]

Other factors that may increase the severity or duration of dysmenorrhoea are anxiety, low levels of exercise, low fish consumption and cigarette smoking.[1,3] Several studies also report a higher risk of dysmenorrhoea among women with high stress (i.e. occupational or perceived stress) compared to those with low stress.[9,10]

### Clinical manifestations
Dysmenorrhoea typically presents as recurrent, spasmodic lower abdominal or suprapubic pain that is sharp or dull in quality.[4] In many cases, the pain radiates to the lower back or thighs. Some women also report symptomatic improvement following the application of heat to the abdomen or by assuming the fetal position.[4] In primary dysmenorrhoea symptoms usually begin 1–3 days before menses, peak 24 hours after the onset of menstruation and subside 2–3 days later. In secondary dysmenorrhoea, menstrual pain may commence long before menses begins and continue well after menstruation has ceased.[1] It is not uncommon for women with either type of dysmenorrhoea to also experience concomitant nausea, vomiting, diarrhoea, constipation, headache, fatigue, irritability, nervousness, urinary frequency, dizziness, sleeplessness and depression.[1,3]

# Clinical case
*23-year-old woman with primary dysmenorrhoea*

## Rapport

Adopt the practitioner strategies and behaviours highlighted in Table 2.1 (chapter 2) to improve client trust, communication and rapport, as well as the accuracy and comprehensiveness of the clinical assessment.

## Assessment

Once measures have been put into place to build client–practitioner rapport, the clinician can begin the clinical assessment.

Health history
### History of presenting condition
A 23-year-old woman presents to the clinic complaining of dull, spasmodic menstrual pain. The pain is located over the suprapubic region primarily, but at times can radiate to the lower back and is often accompanied by mild nausea, bloating, fatigue and irritability. The pain and concomitant symptoms have been present for the past 7 years and typi-cally follow the same pattern – begin 1 day before menstruation, peak on the first day of menses (pain score = 7/10) and subside 2 days later. The menstrual cycle is regular (cycling every 28–30 days), menstruation volume is moderate and menses duration is generally 4–5 days. There is no mid-cycle bleeding or pain, nor abnormal vaginal or ure-thral discharge, dyspareunia, altered libido or dysuria. Fatigue generally aggravates the symptoms; paracetamol and hot packs to the abdomen provide moderate relief of pain.

### Medical history
**Family history**
Father has hypercholesterolaemia and gastro-oesophageal reflux disease, paternal grandfather has type 2 diabetes mellitus, maternal grandmother has lung cancer.
**Allergies**
Bee venom (anaphylaxis).
**Medications**
Fish oil 1 g daily, paracetamol 1 g 4-hourly as needed.
**Medical conditions**
Severe pneumonia (1989), dysmenorrhoea.
**Surgical or investigational procedures**
Tonsillectomy and adenoidectomy (1993).

### Lifestyle history
**Tobacco use**
Nil.
**Alcohol consumption**
Light social drinker. Consumes 2–3 standard size white wines 3–5 times a year.
**Illicit drug use**
Nil.

| Diet and fluid intake | |
|---|---|
| Breakfast | White toast with butter, coffee. |
| Morning tea | Coffee, banana or carrot cake. |
| Lunch | Leftover dinner, sandwich with white bread, ham, tomato, lettuce and pickles. |
| Afternoon tea | Coffee. |

| Dinner | Chicken or beef and vegetable stirfry with white rice, penne carbonara with mushrooms, focaccia with grilled chicken or roast beef, eggplant, capsicum and lettuce. |
| Fluid intake | 3–4 cups of instant coffee a day, 2–3 cups of water a day. |
| **Food frequency** | |
| Fruit | 0–1 serve daily |
| Vegetables | 2–3 serves daily |
| Dairy | 0–1 serve daily |
| Cereals | 5–6 serves daily |
| Red meat | 6–7 serves a week |
| Chicken | 1–2 serves a week |
| Fish | 0 serves a week |
| Takeaway/fast food | twice a week |

### Quality and duration of sleep
Difficulty falling asleep (sleep latency of approximately 1 hour). Continuous sleep; average duration is 6 hours.

### Frequency and duration of exercise
Has little time for a dedicated exercise program. Drives to work. Engages in incidental exercise (i.e. work-related walking) less than 2 hours a day. Engages in sedentary activities (i.e. desk duties) more than 8 hours a day.

### Socioeconomic background
The client and both parents were born in the US. Since completing her law degree 3 years ago, the client has been employed as a full-time lawyer in a busy law firm in the central business district (CBD), which the client states is very stressful and often requires overtime. The client and her supportive same-sex partner reside in a privately rented apartment in the CBD. This same-sex relationship has led to some hostility between the client and her parents and two siblings. The client has no religious or cultural affiliations.

### Physical examination
Clinical examination of the reproductive system is outside the scope of practice for most CAM practitioners. Thus, the following five elements represent a summary of the clinical examination conducted by the client's physician.

### Inspection
Both breasts are symmetrical, with no visible masses, lesions or discharge. The abdomen is flat. The labia, clitoris, urethral meatus, vaginal orifice, perineum and cervix are unremarkable.

### Olfaction
There are no abnormal odours present.

### Palpation
Both breasts are non-tender, with no palpable masses. The abdomen is soft and non-tender, with no palpable masses. Labia, clitoris, urethral meatus, vagina, perineum and cervix are non-tender. Bimanual examination revealed that the uterus is of normal size, shape and contour, and is non-tender. Rectovaginal examination is unremarkable.

### Percussion
Not applicable.

### Auscultation
Bowel sounds are normoactive in all four quadrants.

**Additional signs**
Client is afebrile (36.7°C, per oral). Blood pressure is 118/64. Client is of normal weight (BMI is 24.1 kg/m$^2$, waist circumference is 71 cm).

**Clinical assessment tools**
The menstrual symptom questionnaire (MSQ) provided an overall score of 72/120, where a score of zero represents no menstrual symptoms and a score of 120 represents frequent and intense menstrual symptoms. The menstrual pain 'often' experienced before and during menses and the concomitant symptoms 'sometimes' experienced during menstruation corroborate the type, frequency and intensity of symptoms reported in the client's history.

## Diagnostics
CAM practitioners may request, perform and/or interpret findings from a range of diagnostic tests in order to add valuable data to the pool of clinical information. While several investigations are pertinent to this case (as described below), the decision to use these tests should be considered alongside factors such as cost, convenience, comfort, turnaround time, access, practitioner competence and scope of practice, and history of previous investigations.

**Pathology tests**

**Fatty acids**
Plasma or red cell fatty acid analysis assesses the concentration of fatty acids within the plasma or erythrocyte, including omega 3, omega 6 and omega 9 polyunsaturated fatty acids, saturated fatty acids and trans fatty acids. Given that the fatty acid composition of plasma and erythrocytes is correlated with the dietary intake of fatty acids,[11] this test can help to determine whether excess omega 6 fatty acid intake and/or low omega 3 fatty acid consumption are contributing factors in dysmenorrhoea.[3,5]

**Hormones and eicosanoids**
Several small studies have compared the plasma concentrations of oxytocin, follicle-stimulating hormone, 17β-estradiol, vasopressin, luteinising hormone, progesterone and PGF$_2\alpha$ in healthy controls to women with primary dysmenorrhoea.[7,12,13] However, findings from these studies have been inconsistent, rendering questionable the value of hormone testing in women with dysmenorrhoea.

**Radiology tests**
Medical imaging, such as CT, MRI, ultrasound and uterosalpingography, may be requested if secondary dysmenorrhoea is suspected, particularly if it is attributed to uterine fibroids, tumours, pelvic inflammatory disease, adhesions or the presence of foreign objects.

**Functional tests**
A female hormone profile measures salivary levels of oestradiol, progesterone, testosterone and dehydroepiandrosterone (DHEA) over a single 28-day menstrual cycle. While saliva is a valid and reliable sample source for hormone analysis,[14] the value of hormone testing in women with dysmenorrhoea is questionable as female hormones appear to play little to no role in the pathogenesis of the condition.

**Invasive tests**
Invasive tests may be required if secondary dysmenorrhoea is suspected. Hysteroscopy, laparoscopy and, in few cases, Papanicolaou testing, can be useful in detecting conditions associated with secondary dysmenorrhoea, such as endometriosis, uterine fibroids, pelvic adhesions and pelvic inflammatory disease.

**Miscellaneous tests**
Not applicable.

## Diagnosis

Clusters of data extracted from the health history, clinical examination and pertinent diagnostic test results point towards the following differential CAM diagnosis.
- Menstrual pain (actual), related to emotional stress (*client works in a stressful occupation, and has reported unresolved family conflict*), high omega 6:omega 3 fatty acid intake (*dietary intake of foods containing omega 3 fatty acid is minimal and the intake of omega 6 fatty acids is relatively high*), and sedentary lifestyle (*client's occupation is largely desk-bound and client engages in very little physical exercise*).

## Planning

The goals and expected outcomes that best serve the client's needs, and are most relevant to the case (as determined by the clinical assessment and CAM diagnoses), are as follows.

Goal
1  Client will demonstrate an improvement in menstrual pain (*client's primary concern is menstrual pain*).

Expected outcomes
Based on the degree of improvement reported in clinical studies that have used CAM interventions for the management of dysmenorrhoea,[15–18] the following are anticipated:
1  Client will demonstrate a fifty per cent reduction in baseline severity of menstrual pain in 7 weeks or by dd/mm/yyyy (measured by 0–10 visual analogue scale).
2  Client will report a thirty per cent decrease in baseline duration of menstrual pain in 8 weeks or by dd/mm/yyyy (measured by symptom diary).
3  Client will demonstrate a fifty per cent reduction in baseline intensity and frequency of menstrual symptoms in 12 weeks or by dd/mm/yyyy (measured by MSQ).

## Application

The range of interventions reported in the CAM literature that may be used in the treatment of dysmenorrhoea are appraised below.

Diet
**Miscellaneous diets (Level I, Strength B, Direction + (low-fat vegetarian diet only))**
According to results from several cross-sectional studies, the dietary consumption of particular foods and nutrients may influence the manifestation of dysmenorrhoea. Low intake of fruit, fish and fibre, for instance, was found to be inversely related to menstrual pain, as was a low omega 3:omega 6 fatty acid intake. The association between egg consumption and dysmenorrhoea was inconsistent, while soy and fat intake were found to have no effect on menstrual symptoms.[19] Some of these findings have been corroborated by data from RCTs.[19] In terms of fat intake, for instance, one trial (n = 30 adults) found neither low dietary fat intake nor a low polyunsaturated fatty acid:saturated fatty acid (P:S) ratio to have an effect on menstrual pain when compared with a high-fat diet or high P:S ratio at 4 months.[20] In a trial of 33 women with moderate to severe dysmenorrhoea, consumption of a low-fat vegetarian diet significantly reduced the duration and intensity of menstrual pain when compared with a normal diet and placebo supplement after two menstrual cycles.[18] Collectively, what these findings suggest is that a low-fat vegetarian diet, an increase in dietary fibre consumption and an increase in omega 3:omega 6 fatty acid intake may be beneficial in alleviating the symptoms of dysmenorrhoea. Further investigation is required to assess the validity of this claim.

## Lifestyle

### Relaxation therapy (Level I, Strength C, Direction o)

Relaxation therapy (RT) describes myriad mind–body techniques that facilitate the relaxation response and moderate sympathetic nervous system activity. In doing so, RT might attenuate the effect of stress on menstrual pain, thereby providing theoretical justification for the use of RT in dysmenorrhoea. Nevertheless, a Cochrane review of three small RCTs (n = 175) of variable duration (i.e. 5–20 weeks) found that RT alone, with biofeedback or with imagery to be no more effective than waiting list controls at improving dysmenorrhoea symptoms (as measured by symptom severity scale), yet when descriptive data were analysed results were mixed.[21] Since these trials are more than 20 years old and the diagnostic criteria and outcome measures are no longer widely used, the validity of these findings is uncertain. Further research in this area is warranted.

## Nutritional supplementation

### Calcium (Level I, Strength B, Direction +)

A 10-year case–control study (n = 3025) nested within the prospective Nurses' Health Study II cohort has shown that women in the highest quintile of dietary calcium intake have a thirty per cent lower risk of developing menstrual symptoms than women in the lowest quintile (p = 0.02).[22] Even though this study is unable to establish a causal relationship between calcium intake and dysmenorrhoea specifically, and mechanistic data explaining this relationship is lacking, evidence from clinical studies is promising.[23] Two RCTs, one using a parallel group design (n = 466)[18] and one a crossover approach (n = 33)[17] found oral calcium carbonate (1.0–1.2 g daily) administered over a period of three menstrual cycles to be significantly superior to placebo in reducing premenstrual and menstrual pain. Research examining the clinical efficacy of other formulations and dosages of supplemental calcium in dysmenorrhoea is now warranted.

### Magnesium (Level I, Strength C, Direction + (pain reduction only))

Magnesium is involved in many enzymatic reactions and physiological processes throughout the body. Low serum magnesium levels have been shown to intensify neuromuscular cell excitability, resulting in increased smooth muscle contractility. High serum levels of magnesium cause smooth muscle relaxation.[24] By decreasing myometrial spasm, magnesium could potentially reduce menstrual pain. A Cochrane review of three small, double-blind, controlled clinical trials (n = 117) has reported mixed results, with two of three trials showing magnesium (variable dosage for 5–6 months) to be more effective than placebo and as effective as vitamin $B_6$ in reducing menstrual pain.[21] Between-group differences in the need for analgesia were inconsistent. While the best available evidence appears to favour the use of magnesium for dysmenorrhoea, the evidence is not strong, suggesting that further investigation is needed.

### Omega 3 fatty acids (Level I, Strength C, Direction o)

The anti-inflammatory effects of essential fatty acids have been reported in numerous populations and clinical studies.[25] Given that heightened inflammatory activity is implicated in the pathogenesis of dysmenorrhoea, it is theoretically plausible that omega 3 fatty acids could attenuate menstrual pain. A Cochrane review of one small double-blind RCT (n = 42 adolescents with dysmenorrhoea) supports this premise; it found fish oil (dose unknown, but containing 1080 mg EPA + 720 mg DHA daily) to be statistically significantly superior to placebo in reducing the Cox menstrual symptom score, a non-standardised aggregate score of the frequency and severity of multiple menstrual symptoms, and analgesic use after 8 weeks of treatment.[26] While the fish oil group reported significantly more adverse effects than the placebo group, only four effects (e.g. nausea, acne exacerbation) were reported in the fish oil group in total, all of which were mild. A more recent, larger and longer double-blind RCT involving 78 adolescents and women with dysmenorrhoea found neither fish oil (2.5 g daily, EPA/DHA content unknown) nor seal oil (2.5 g daily) to be superior to placebo (2.5 g mixed fatty acids daily) in reducing menstrual pain scores at 12 weeks. In the group receiving fish oil (2.5 g daily) and vitamin $B_{12}$ (dose unknown), a statistically significant reduction in menstrual pain was observed when compared with placebo.[27] It must be said, then, that the best available evidence for omega 3 fatty acid supplementation and dysmenorrhoea is inconclusive.

### Pyridoxine (Level I, Strength C, Direction o)

Animal studies have demonstrated enhanced inflammatory activity in the presence of vitamin $B_6$ deficiency.[28] In human studies, plasma pyridoxine and pyridoxal 5-phosphate levels are shown to be similar between women with premenstrual symptoms to those with no or mild premenstrual symptoms.[29–31] Even though biological plausibility is lacking, this has not prevented researchers from examining the clinical efficacy of pyridoxine supplementation in dysmenorrhoea. In a systematic review of one double-blind RCT, orally administered vitamin $B_6$ (200 mg daily for 20 weeks) was shown to be significantly more effective than placebo at reducing menstrual pain and analgesic use in 46 women with dysmenorrhoea,[26] yet in two RCTs involving women with premenstrual symptoms (n = 183), vitamin $B_6$ (50–300 mg daily for 12 weeks) was shown to be no more effective than placebo at reducing abdominal cramping or back pain.[32,33] While differences in patient populations and treatment durations may have contributed to these disparate findings, this may only become clearer with additional research in the area.

### Thiamine (Level II, Strength B, Direction +)

Thiamine is a water-soluble vitamin that plays an important role in carbohydrate metabolism and neurotransmitter biosynthesis. Even though these actions are essential for life, neither of them justifies the use of vitamin $B_1$ in painful or inflammatory conditions such as dysmenorrhoea. In spite of the paucity of mechanistic data in this area, there is good evidence of effectiveness for thiamine in dysmenorrhoea. In a double-blind, randomised placebo-controlled trial involving 556 adolescent girls and young women with moderate to very severe spasmodic dysmenorrhoea, for example, 90 days of thiamine hydrochloride supplementation (100 mg daily) was found to be significantly more effective than placebo in reducing the incidence of menstrual pain.[34] Verification of these findings is needed.

### Vitamin E (Level I, Strength B, Direction +)

Among the many functions of vitamin E, perhaps the most relevant to dysmenorrhoea is its anti-inflammatory activity; in particular, the capacity to reduce the release of proinflammatory cytokines.[35] This mechanism of action is distinctly different from that of the non-steroidal anti-inflammatory drugs (NSAIDs), which suggests that these two anti-inflammatory agents may complement each other in the management of dysmenorrhoea. This does not appear to be the case with an open-label, randomised crossover trial (n = 50 adolescents) that found no statistically significant difference in menstrual pain between groups receiving vitamin E (100 mg daily for 20 days per month, for 2 months) and ibuprofen (400 mg daily at onset of pain for 2 months), to ibuprofen alone (400 mg daily at onset of pain for 2 months).[26,36]

In two RCTs comparing vitamin E to placebo, vitamin E supplementation (200–500 IU for 5 days a month for 2–4 months) was shown to be statistically significantly superior to placebo in reducing the severity and duration of menstrual pain in adolescents with primary dysmenorrhoea (n = 378).[37,38] Since both of these trials were conducted by the same principal researcher, corroboration from independent studies is warranted. In particular, the efficacy of supplemental vitamin E in women with dysmenorrhoea is an area in need of further study.

### Iron, niacin and tryptophan

These minerals demonstrate an array of effects that could affect the outcomes of premenstrual syndrome, although the administration of these nutrients in dysmenorrhoea is not yet supported by rigorous clinical evidence, only by pathophysiologic rationale or experimental research findings.

Herbal medicine

### *Hypericum perforatum* (Level IV, Strength D, Direction o)

St John's wort demonstrates anti-inflammatory and analgesic activity in vivo.[39,40] The administration of hypericum in painful inflammatory conditions, such as dysmenorrhoea, is therefore theoretically justified. Even though several clinical trials have investigated the clinical efficacy of *H. perforatum* in premenstrual syndrome,[41,42] only one of these studies provides sufficient data on the effectiveness of hypericum for menstrual pain.[43] This prospective, open, uncontrolled, observational study reported a statistically significant reduction in cramping pain after the first month of hypericum treatment (300 mg daily for two menstrual cycles) and a non-significant reduction in pain after the second month of treatment when compared with baseline. This inconsistent finding, together with the small size of the trial and the methodological limitations of the study, adds very little to the body of evidence for hypericum and dysmenorrhoea.

### *Oenothera biennis* (Level I, Strength C, Direction o)

Evening primrose oil (EPO) is extracted from the seed of *O. biennis*. The oil is a complex mixture of essential fatty acids, containing around seventy per cent *cis*-linolenic acid (omega 3 fatty acid), nine per cent *cis*-gamma-linolenic acid (omega 6 fatty acid), small amounts of oleic acid (omega 9 fatty acid), and palmitic and stearic acids (saturated fatty acids).[44] Under experimental conditions the oil has been shown to reduce cyclo-oxygenase-derived eicosanoid production, including the generation of $PGE_2$.[45] Thus, while it is possible that EPO could attenuate the pathogenesis of dysmenorrhoea, a systematic review of four small RCTs (n = 105) failed to find any statistically significant difference in premenstrual symptoms between EPO (3–6 g daily for 2–6 menstrual cycles) and placebo.[46] All three controlled trials excluded from the review (because of a lack of evidence of randomisation) found EPO to be superior to placebo in reducing premenstrual symptoms. But the high risk of bias in these latter studies and the uncertainty about the inclusion of pain as an outcome measure in several of these studies adds little strength to the body of evidence for EPO and dysmenorrhoea. A less detailed but more recent review of EPO concluded that the evidence for EPO and premenstrual symptoms was still unconvincing.[23]

### *Vitex agnus castus* (Level V, Strength NA, Direction NA)

Chaste tree is used in traditional Western herbal medicine as a treatment for gynaecological problems, including menstrual pain. Evidence from experimental studies suggests vitex might improve menstrual pain by stimulating mu-opiate receptors and, in doing so, may activate analgesic and mood regulatory pathways.[47] Even though many systematic reviews and clinical trials have shown chaste tree extract to be effective in alleviating a number of premenstrual symptoms,[23,46,48] none have presented specific data on the efficacy of vitex for menstrual pain. Thus, there is no current evidence to show that vitex is effective in treating dysmenorrhoea.

### *Zingiber officinale* (Level III-1, Strength B, Direction +)

Ginger is used in many alternative systems of healing for its anti-inflammatory and circulatory stimulant properties. Under experimental conditions, ginger has been shown to inhibit the synthesis of $PGE_4$ in vivo[49] and leukotriene $B_4$ in vitro,[50] which may be useful in attenuating the pain of dysmenorrhoea. This appears to be the case according to findings from a recent double-blind comparative clinical trial involving 150 university students with primary dysmenorrhoea. The trial found dried ginger rhizome powder (250 mg 4 times a day), when administered for 3 days from the start of menses, to be as effective as ibuprofen and mefenamic acid at reducing the severity of dysmenorrhoea, as well as the need for breakthrough analgesia.[51] The long-term effectiveness of ginger in dysmenorrhoea now warrants further investigation.

## Other herbs

*Alchemilla vulgaris* (ladies mantle), *Angelica sinensis* (dong quai), *Capsella bursa-pastoris* (shepherds purse), *Caulophyllum thalictroides* (blue cohosh), *Chamaelirium luteum* (false unicorn root), *Cimicifuga racemosa* (black cohosh), *Corydalis ambigua* (corydalis), *Dioscorea* spp. (wild yam), *Glycyrrhiza glabra* (licorice), *Hydrastis canadensis* (golden seal), *Leonurus cardiaca* (motherwort), *Matricaria recutita* (German chamomile), *Mentha piperita* (peppermint), *Mitchella repens* (squaw vine), *Paeonia lactiflora* (peony), *Piscidia erythrina* (Jamaican dogwood), *Valeriana officinalis* (valerian), *Viburnum opulus* (cramp bark) and *Viburnum prunifolium* (black haw)

These herbs have been traditionally used and/or tested under experimental conditions for their analgesic, antispasmodic, uterine tonic or anti-inflammatory activity. Herbs, such as *Ginkgo biloba* (maidenhair tree),[52,53] have also been shown under clinical trial conditions to be significantly more effective than placebo in alleviating a number of menstrual symptoms. But there is still insufficient clinical data to support the use of these herbs (as monopreparations) in dysmenorrhoea specifically.

## Other

### Acupuncture (Level I, Strength C, Direction o)

Acupuncture originated in China more than 4000 years ago.[54] Since then, a large traditional evidence base for the therapy has been established. Positive findings from case reports and uncontrolled trials have added to this traditional knowledge, particularly in the area of dysmenorrhoea.[55,56] However, a recent systematic review of 30 RCTs and two controlled clinical trials reported conflicting results for the effectiveness of acupuncture-related therapies in dysmenorrhoea.[57] These inconsistent findings, together with the significant heterogeneity of trials and the low methodological quality of most studies, does not enable any firm conclusions to be made. Evidence from a more recent Cochrane review in this area, which has yet to be completed, may shed further light on the effectiveness of acupuncture in dysmenorrhoea.[58]

### Aromatherapy (Level II, Strength B, Direction +)

Essential oils can generate a range of emotional, psychological and physiological effects that may be useful in the management of dysmenorrhoea. Evidence from a double-blind, randomised placebo-controlled trial lends support to this claim. The trial randomised 67 female college students with moderate to severe menstrual cramps into three groups: aromatherapy abdominal massage (using *Lavandula officinalis*, *Salvia sclarea* and *Rosa centifolia* essential oil (2:1:1) in 5 mL of almond oil), placebo abdominal massage (5 mL of almond oil only) and control (no intervention). After 7 days of treatment, aromatherapy abdominal massage (15 minutes daily) was found to be statistically significantly superior to placebo and control in reducing the severity of menstrual cramps on the first and second days of menstruation.[16] These findings support the use of aromatherapy massage in dysmenorrhoea, although do require replication in much larger studies.

### Chiropractic or osteopathy (Level I, Strength C, Direction o)

Spinal manipulation is often used to treat nervous and musculoskeletal disorders. While spinal manipulation is not considered to be a primary treatment of dysmenorrhoea, it is not outside the scope of chiropractic or osteopathic care. Evidence from a Cochrane review of five RCTs casts doubt on the use of spinal manipulative therapy (SMT) in dysmenorrhoea, with most studies failing to show a statistically significant difference between SMT (i.e. high velocity, low amplitude (HVLA) technique or Toftness technique) and sham SMT for improvement in menstrual pain after 1 to 27 treatments.[59] When SMT was compared with no treatment, improvements in dysmenorrhoea were found to be in favour of spinal manipulation. Even so, the influential effect of expectation bias on these results cannot be discounted.

### Homeopathy, massage and reflexology
There is insufficient clinical evidence supporting the use of these therapies in the management of dysmenorrhoea.

## CAM prescription
The CAM interventions that are most appropriate for the management of the pre-senting case – that is, they target the planned goals, expected outcomes and CAM diagnoses, they are supported by the best available evidence, they are pertinent to the client's needs and they are most relevant to CAM practice – are outlined below.

### Primary treatments
- Commence low-fat, predominantly lacto-ovo-vegetarian diet (*client consumes low levels of omega 3 fatty acids, fruit, vegetables, dietary fibre and fish, and high levels of omega 6 fatty acids, all of which are implicated in the pathogenesis of dysmenorrhoea; consumption of a low-fat vegetarian diet may resolve these dietary imbalances and improve menstrual symptoms*).
- Commence oral calcium carbonate, 1.2 g daily (*client consumes low levels of dietary calcium, which may increase the risk of dysmenorrhoea; calcium supplementation also effectively reduces menstrual pain*).
- Consider aromatherapy abdominal massage (using 2 drops of *Lavandula officinalis* oil, 1 drop of *Salvia sclarea* oil and 1 drop of *Rosa centifolia* essential oil in 5 mL of almond oil) 15 minutes daily for 7 days before the onset of menses (*aromatherapy massage is effective in reducing the severity of menstrual cramps and, together with massage, may also help to reduce emotional stress*).

### Secondary treatments
- Engage in physical exercise, such as swimming, walking or resistance training, at least 30 minutes daily (*stress/anxiety and low levels of exercise can increase the severity and duration of dysmenorrhoea, while commencing a regular exercise program may attenuate the effect of these sustaining factors; this recommendation is based on theoretical evidentiary support only*).

### Referral
- Refer client to general practitioner, family physician or gynaecologist if the condition worsens, if secondary dysmenorrhoea is suspected (such as pelvic inflammatory disease) or if a serious pathology is suspected (such as neoplastic disease).
- Refer client to another CAM practitioner if dysmenorrhoea, or the treatment of dysmenorrhoea, is outside the clinician's area of expertise.

## Review

To determine whether pertinent client goals and expected outcomes have been achieved at follow-up and if any aspects of the client's care need to be improved, consider the factors listed in Table 8.2 (chapter 8), as well as the questions listed below.
- Was there a reduction in the severity of menstrual pain?
- Was there a reduction in the duration of menstrual pain?
- Was there a decrease in the MSQ score?
- Has the need for paracetamol decreased?
- Was there an improvement in other menopausal symptoms (e.g. nausea, bloating, fatigue, irritability)?

# References

1. Porter R et al, editors. (2008). The Merck manual. Rahway: Merck Research Laboratories.
2. Latthe P et al (2006) WHO systematic review of prevalence of chronic pelvic pain: a neglected reproductive health morbidity. BMC Public Health, 6: 177.
3. Harel Z. (2006) Dysmenorrhea in adolescents and young adults: etiology and management. Journal of Pediatric and Adolescent Gynecology, 19(6): 363–71.
4. Beckmann CRB et al (2009) Obstetrics and gynecology. 6th ed. Philadelphia: Lippincott, Williams & Wilkins.

5. Deutsch B. (1995) Menstrual pain in Danish women correlated with low n-3 polyunsaturated fatty acid intake. European Journal of Clinical Nutrition, 49(7): 508–16.

6. Watanabe S et al (2005) Efficacy of γ-linoleic acid for treatment of premenstrual syndrome, as assessed by a prospective daily rating system. Journal of Oleo Science, 54(4): 217–24.

7. Liedman R et al (2008) Reproductive hormones in plasma over the menstrual cycle in primary dysmenorrhea compared with healthy subjects. Gynecological Endocrinology, 24(9): 508–13.

8. Rees MC et al (1984) Prostaglandins in menstrual fluid in menorrhagia and dysmenorrhoea. British Journal of Obstetrics and Gynaecology, 91(7): 673–80.

9. Laszlo KD et al (2008) Work-related stress factors and menstrual pain: a nation-wide representative survey. Journal of Psychosomatic Obstetrics and Gynaecology, 29(2): 133–8.

10. Wang L et al (2004) Stress and dysmenorrhoea: a population based prospective study. Occupational and Environmental Medicine, 61(12): 1021–6.

11. Gibson RS. (2005) Principles of nutritional assessment. Oxford: Oxford University Press.

12. Stromberg P et al (1984) Vasopressin and prostaglandins in premenstrual pain and primary dysmenorrhea. Acta Obstetrica et Gynecologica Scandinavica, 63(6): 533–8.

13. Ylikorkala O. Puolakka J. Kauppila A. (1979) Serum gonadotrophins, prolactin and ovarian steroids in primary dysmenorrhoea. British Journal of Obstetrics and Gynaecology, 86(8): 648–53.

14. Groschl M. (2008) Current status of salivary hormone analysis. Clinical Chemistry, 54: 1759–69.

15. Barnard ND et al (2000) Diet and sex-hormone binding globulin, dysmenorrhea, and premenstrual symptoms. Obstetrics and Gynecology, 95(2): 245–50.

16. Han SH et al (2006) Effect of aromatherapy on symptoms of dysmenorrhea in college students: a randomized placebo-controlled clinical trial. Journal of Alternative and Complementary Medicine, 12(6): 535–541.

17. Thys-Jacobs S et al (1989) Calcium supplementation in premenstrual syndrome: a randomized crossover trial. Journal of General Internal Medicine, 4(3): 183–9.

18. Thys-Jacobs S et al (1998) Calcium carbonate and the premenstrual syndrome: effects on premenstrual and menstrual symptoms. American Journal of Obstetrics and Gynecology, 179(2): 444–52.

19. Fjerbaek A. Knudsen UB. (2007) Endometriosis, dysmenorrhea and diet: what is the evidence? European Journal of Obstetrics Gynecology and Reproductive Biology, 132(2): 140–7.

20. Jones DY. (1987) Influence of dietary fat on self-reported menstrual symptoms. Physiology and Behavior, 40(4): 483–7.

21. Proctor M et al (2007) Behavioural interventions for primary and secondary dysmenorrhoea. Cochrane Database of Systematic Reviews, (3): CD002248.

22. Bertone-Johnson ER et al (2005) Calcium and vitamin D intake and risk of incident premenstrual syndrome. Archives of Internal Medicine, 165(11): 1246–52.

23. Canning S. Waterman M. Dye L. (2006) Dietary supplements and herbal remedies for premenstrual syndrome (PMS): a systematic research review of the evidence for their efficacy. Journal of Reproductive and Infant Psychology, 24(4): 363–78.

24. Kowal A et al (2007) The use of magnesium in bronchial asthma: a new approach to an old problem. Archivum Immunologiae et Therapiae Experimentalis, 55(1): 35–9.

25. Jho DH et al (2004) Role of omega-3 fatty acid supplementation in inflammation and malignancy. Integrative Cancer Therapies, 3(2): 98–111.

26. Proctor M. Murphy PA. (2001) Herbal and dietary therapies for primary and secondary dysmenorrhoea. Cochrane Database of Systematic Reviews, (2): CD002124.

27. Deutch B. Jorgensen EB. Hansen JC. (2000) Menstrual discomfort in Danish women reduced by dietary supplements of omega-3 PUFA and $B_{12}$ (fish oil or seal oil capsules). Nutrition Research, 20(5): 621–30.

28. Lakshmi R et al (1991) Effect of riboflavin or pyridoxine deficiency on inflammatory response. Indian Journal of Biochemistry and Biophysics, 28(5–6): 481–4.

29. Mira M. Stewart PM. Abraham SF. (1988) Vitamin and trace element status in premenstrual syndrome. American Journal of Clinical Nutrition, 47(4): 636–41.

30. Ritchie CD. Singkamani R. (1986) Plasma pyridoxal 5'-phosphate in women with the premenstrual syndrome. Human Nutrition Clinical Nutrition, 40(1): 75–80.

31. van den Berg H et al (1986) Vitamin $B_6$ status of women suffering from premenstrual syndrome. Human Nutrition Clinical Nutrition, 40(6): 441–50.

32. Diegoli MS et al (1998) A double-blind trial of four medications to treat severe premenstrual syndrome. International Journal of Gynaecology and Obstetrics, 62(1): 63–7.

33. Doll H et al (1989) Pyridoxine (vitamin B6) and the premenstrual syndrome: a randomized crossover trial. Journal of the Royal College of General Practitioners, 39(326): 364–8.

34. Gokhale LB. (1996) Curative treatment of primary (spasmodic) dysmenorrhoea. Indian Journal of Medical Research, 103: 227–31.

35. Singh U. Devaraj S. Jialal I. (2005) Vitamin E, oxidative stress, and inflammation. Annual Review of Nutrition, 25: 151–74.

36. Esperanza-Salazar-De-Roldan M. Ruiz-Castro S. (1993) Primary dysmenorrhea treatment with ibuprofen and vitamin E. Revista de Obstetricia y Ginecologia de Venezuela, 53(1): 35–7.

37. Ziaei S et al (2001) A randomised placebo-controlled trial to determine the effect of vitamin E in treatment of primary dysmenorrhoea. BJOG: an international journal of obstetrics and gynaecology, 108(11): 1181–3.

38. Ziaei S. Zakeri M. Kazemnejad A. (2005) A randomised controlled trial of vitamin E in the treatment of primary dysmenorrhoea. BJOG: an international journal of obstetrics and gynaecology, 112(4): 466–9.

39. Abdel-Salam OM. (2005) Anti-inflammatory, antinociceptive, and gastric effects of Hypericum perforatum in rats. Scientific World Journal, 5: 586–95.

40. Kumar V. Singh PN. Bhattacharya SK. (2001) Anti-inflammatory and analgesic activity of Indian Hypericum perforatum L. Indian Journal of Experimental Biology, 39(4): 339–43.

41. Hicks SM et al (2004) The significance of 'nonsignificance' in randomized controlled studies: a discussion inspired by a double-blinded study on St John's wort (Hypericum perforatum L.) for premenstrual symptoms. Journal of Alternative and Complementary Medicine, 10(6): 925–32.

42. Pakgohar M et al (2005) Effect of Hypericum perforatum L. for treatment of premenstrual syndrome. Faslnamahi Giyahani Daruyi, 4(15): 33–42.

43. Stevinson C. Ernst E. (2000) A pilot study of Hypericum perforatum for the treatment of premenstrual syndrome. BJOG: an international journal of obstetrics and gynaecology, 107(7): 870–76.

44. Khare CP. (2007) Indian medicinal plants: an illustrated dictionary. Heidelberg: Springer Verlag.
45. de La Puerta Vazquez R et al (2004) Effects of different dietary oils on inflammatory mediator generation and fatty acid composition in rat neutrophils. Metabolism, 53(1): 59–65.
46. Stevinson C. Ernst E. (2001) Complementary/alternative therapies for premenstrual syndrome: a systematic review of randomised controlled trials. American Journal of Obstetrics and Gynecology, 185(1): 227–35.
47. Webster DE et al (2006) Activation of the mu-opiate receptor by Vitex agnus-castus methanol extracts: implication for its use in PMS. Journal of Ethnopharmacology, 106(2): 216–21.
48. He Z et al (2009) Treatment for premenstrual syndrome with Vitex agnus castus: a prospective, randomized, multi-center placebo controlled study in China. Maturitas, 63(1): 99–103.
49. Shen CL. Hong KJ. Kim SW. (2005) Comparative effects of ginger root (Zingiber officinale Rosc.) on the production of inflammatory mediators in normal and osteoarthrotic sow chondrocytes. Journal of Medicinal Food, 8(2): 149–53.
50. Blumenthal M. (2003) The ABC clinical guide to herbs. Austin: American Botanical Council.
51. Ozgoli G. Goli M. Moattar F. (2009) Comparison of effects of ginger, mefenamic acid, and ibuprofen on pain in women with primary dysmenorrhea. Journal of Alternative and Complementary Medicine: early release.
52. Ozgoli G et al (2009) A randomized, placebo-controlled trial of Ginkgo biloba L. in treatment of premenstrual syndrome. Journal of Alternative and Complementary Medicine, 15(8): 845–51.
53. Tamborini A. Taurelle R. (1993) Value of standardized Gingko biloba (EGb 761) in the management of congestive symptoms of premenstrual syndrome. Revue Francaise de Gynecologie et d'Obstetrique, 88(7–9): 447–57.
54. O'Brien KA. Xue CC. (2003) Acupuncture. In: Robson T, editor. An introduction to complementary medicine. Sydney: Allen & Unwin.
55. Wang XM. (1987) Observations of the therapeutic effects of acupuncture and moxibustion in 100 cases of dysmenorrhea. Journal of Traditional Chinese Medicine, 7(1): 15–17.
56. Zhan C. (1990) Treatment of 32 cases of dysmenorrhea by puncturing hegu and sanyinjiao acupoints. Journal of Traditional Chinese Medicine, 10(1): 33–5.
57. Yang H et al (2008) Systematic review of clinical trials of acupuncture-related therapies for primary dysmenorrhea. Acta Obstetricia and Gynecologica Scandinavica, 87(11): 1114–22.
58. Smith CA et al (2009) Acupuncture for primary dysmenorrhoea (Protocol). Cochrane Database of Systematic Reviews, (3): CD007854.
59. Proctor M et al (2006) Spinal manipulation for primary and secondary dysmenorrhoea. Cochrane Database of Systematic Reviews, (3): CD002119.

# Case 6
# Dermatitis/eczema

## Description of dermatitis/eczema

### Definition
Dermatitis, or eczema, is a superficial inflammatory disorder of the skin that can manifest as an acute, subacute or chronic disorder. Depending on the aetiology of the condition, dermatitis can be classified as either endogenous or exogenous. Endogenous forms include atopic, seborrhoeic, nummular and stasis dermatitis, while exogenous forms include contact and infective dermatitis.

### Epidemiology
Atopic dermatitis affects between ten and twelve per cent of the population, occurring predominantly in children less than 5 years of age.[1] Contact dermatitis affects between 1.5 and 14 per cent of the population and can develop at any age.[2] Infective dermatitis can also occur at any age, while nummular and stasis dermatitis are most likely to occur in middle-aged people and elderly women, respectively.[3]

### Aetiology and pathophysiology
There are many factors that contribute to the pathogenesis of dermatitis. The range of exogenous factors include, but are not limited to, chemicals, cosmetics, detergents, dyes, latex, metal compounds, mineral oils, plants, synthetic fibres, wool, topical drugs, and bacterial or fungal pathogens.[3] Exposure to these agents can produce physiological effects ranging from skin damage and irritation (irritant contact dermatitis) to hypersensitivity reactions (allergic contact dermatitis), depending on individual susceptibility, concentration of the agent and duration of exposure.[4]

Myriad endogenous factors can also facilitate the development of dermatitis, including immunological abnormalities, such as a family history of atopic disease, environmental elements, such as food allergies and psychoemotional influences, such as stress.[4] Patients with endogenous dermatitis may also demonstrate diminished skin itch threshold, reduced ceramide content of the stratum corneum, decreased antimicrobial peptide production of keratinocytes, intestinal *Candida* overgrowth, increased proinflammatory cytokine production and intestinal dysbiosis.[1] For contact dermatitis, an individual's susceptibility to the condition may be increased through excessive water exposure, heat, sweating, low humidity and mechanical stress, such as repeated hand washing.[2]

### Clinical manifestations
The three key manifestations of dermatitis, including erythema, heat and pruritus, are attributed to the underlying inflammatory process of the condition. These symptoms are common across all subtypes of dermatitis, although there are some distinct differences in the presentation of each subtype. Acute dermatitis, for instance, is associated with oedema, vesicle formation, pain, exudation and impaired function. Subacute dermatitis manifests as erosions, scaling, crusting and exfoliation, whereas chronic dermatitis appears as scaling, dryness, thickening and hardening of the skin.[5] As well as the physical manifestations, dermatitis is also associated with a decline in health-related quality of life due to irritability, sleep disturbance and negative self-esteem and self-image.[6]

The clinical presentation of atopic eczema is somewhat more defined than the subtypes. According to Ring's criteria, a diagnosis of atopic eczema may be made if four of the following criteria are present: pruritus, family history of atopy, IgE-mediated sensitisation, stigmata of atopic eczema, age-specific distribution of skin lesions and age-specific morphology.[7]

# Clinical case
*4-year-old boy with neck, cubital fossae and popliteal fossae dermatitis*

## Rapport

Adopt the practitioner strategies and behaviours highlighted in Table 2.1 (chapter 2) to improve client trust, communication and rapport, as well as the accuracy and comprehensiveness of the clinical assessment.

## Assessment

Once measures have been put into place to build client–practitioner rapport, the clinician can begin the clinical assessment.

Health history
### History of presenting condition
The parents of a 4-year-old boy present to the clinic concerned about a rash on their son's neck. The red and pruritic rash to the posterior neck developed 9 months ago, close to the time the client started full-time childcare. Six months ago, the client commenced betamethasone cream (as prescribed by his general practitioner) as there had been no sign of improvement. In the last 3 months, a cubital and popliteal rash has developed. The rash and pruritus are often aggravated by scratching and after the consumption of cow's milk; they improve on the weekends and following the use of hydrocortisone cream. While the condition varies in intensity from mild to severe, it has yet to resolve. There are no radiating symptoms, but the lesion is accompanied by pruritus, irritability, interrupted sleep and frustration.

### Medical history
**Family history**
Mother has a history of childhood dermatitis, maternal grandmother has asthma.
**Allergies**
Penicillin (causes a systemic cutaneous rash).
**Medications**
One per cent hydrocortisone cream twice a day; child multivitamin daily.
**Medical conditions**
Dermatitis and asthma.
**Surgical or investigational procedures**
Bilateral myringotomy and insertion of tympanostomy tubes (2008).

### Lifestyle history
**Tobacco use**
Nil.
**Alcohol consumption**
Nil.
**Illicit drug use**
Nil.

| Diet and fluid intake | |
|---|---|
| Breakfast | Nutri-Grain® cereal with full cream milk. |
| Morning tea | Apple, raisin bread. |
| Lunch | Spaghetti bolognaise, lasagne, vegetable slice, risotto with ham and peas, sandwich with white bread, margarine and jam or peanut butter. |
| Afternoon tea | Fruit, sweet biscuits. |

| Dinner | Beef schnitzel with mashed potato, ham and pineapple pizza, hot chips, roast chicken with roast potato and pumpkin, plain white pasta. |
|---|---|
| Fluid intake | 1 cup of juice daily, 1 cup of water daily, 1 cup of cordial daily, 1 cup of full cream milk daily. |
| **Food frequency** | |
| Fruit | 2–3 serves daily |
| Vegetables | 2–3 serves daily |
| Dairy | 2 serves daily |
| Cereals | 6–7 serves daily |
| Red meat | 2 serves a week |
| Chicken | 3 serves a week |
| Fish | 0–1 serve a week |
| Takeaway/fast food | 2–3 times a week |

**Quality and duration of sleep**
Interrupted sleep; average duration is 10 hours.

**Frequency and duration of exercise**
Engages in active play more than 3 hours a day and sedentary activities (out of child-care) less than 2 hours a day.

### Socioeconomic background
Australian-born with Australian-born Catholic parents. An only child who lives with his parents, who are married, work full time and own their own home. Client attends childcare 5 full days a week, which often upsets him when dropped off in the morning.

Physical examination

### Inspection
The patches to the neck (5 × 10 cm diameter), bilateral antecubital fossae (4 × 4 cm) and bilateral popliteal fossae (4 × 4 cm) are erythemic, with lichenification and excoriation present. There is no exudation, bleeding or ulceration. Finger and toe nails are strong and intact, with no notable markings.

### Olfaction
There is no abnormal odour to the lesions or patient.

### Palpation
The patches are dry, rough and warm. The surrounding skin demonstrates good turgor, moisture and mobility.

### Percussion
Not applicable.

### Auscultation
Subcutaneous crepitus is not detectable.

### Additional signs
Client is afebrile (36.1°C, per axilla).

### Clinical assessment tools
The patient-oriented eczema measure (POEM) provided a baseline score of 12/28, demonstrating moderate eczema severity.

Diagnostics
CAM practitioners may request, perform and/or interpret findings from a range of diagnostic tests in order to add valuable data to the pool of clinical information. While several investigations are pertinent to this case (as described below), the decision to use these tests should be considered alongside factors such as cost, convenience,

comfort, turnaround time, access, practitioner competence and scope of practice, and history of previous investigations.

**Pathology tests**
The radioallergosorbent test (RAST) and enzyme-linked immunosorbent assay (ELISA) may help to determine whether an allergen is responsible for the dermatitis.

**Radiology tests**
Not applicable.

**Functional tests**
Functional skin integrity testing may highlight potential susceptibilities of the skin to dermatitis.

**Invasive tests**
Allergy skin testing may be useful in identifying an allergenic cause of the dermatitis.

**Miscellaneous tests**
Atopic patch testing (APT) may help to isolate an allergenic cause of the dermatitis.

## Diagnosis

Clusters of data extracted from the health history, clinical examination and pertinent diagnostic test results point towards the following differential CAM diagnoses.

- Pruritus (actual), *secondary to* dermatitis, *related to* genetic predisposition (*client has a family history of dermatitis*), heightened inflammatory activity (*dermatitis is relieved following the application of topical corticosteroid cream*), emotional stress (*dermatitis commenced around the time the client started childcare, and improves on the weekends*), contact allergy (*suspicions of contact allergy may be supported by RAST, ELISA or allergy skin testing*), and/or food intolerance (*dermatitis severity intensifies following the consumption of cow's milk; the presence of positive specific IgE to cow's milk (and possibly eggs) should be confirmed by RAST or ELISA testing*).
- Inflamed skin lesions (actual), *secondary to* dermatitis, *related to* genetic predisposition, heightened inflammatory activity, emotional stress, contact allergy, and/or food intolerance.

## Planning

The goals and expected outcomes that best serve the client's needs, and which are most relevant to the presenting case (as determined by the clinical assessment and CAM diagnoses), are as follows.

Goals
1. Client will be free from pruritus (*pruritis is one of the client's/parents, key concerns*).
2. Client will demonstrate an improvement in inflamed skin lesions (*the client and his parents are concerned about the lack of improvement in the cutaneous rash*).

Expected outcomes
Based on the degree of improvement reported in clinical studies that have used CAM interventions for the management of dermatitis,[8–11] the following are anticipated.
1. Client will demonstrate a thirty per cent reduction in baseline pruritus in 4 weeks or by dd/mm/yyyy (measured by pruritis domain of POEM).
2. Client will demonstrate a forty per cent reduction in baseline skin lesion diameter of the neck, popliteal fossae and/or antecubital fossae in 4 weeks or by dd/mm/yyyy (measured in millimetres).
3. Client will demonstrate a forty per cent reduction in baseline dermatitis severity in 4 weeks, or by dd/mm/yyyy (measured by POEM).
4. Client will demonstrate a thirty per cent improvement in baseline sleep quality in 4 weeks or by dd/mm/yyyy (measured by sleeping domain of POEM).

## Application

The range of interventions reported in the CAM literature that may be used in the treatment of dermatitis are appraised below.

### Diet

**Elimination diet (Level I, Strength B, Direction +)**

The effectiveness of the elimination diet in the treatment of dermatitis has been examined in a number of prospective studies and systematic reviews.[8,12,13] The majority of these studies have shown that the elimination of eggs, and possibly cow's milk, from infant diets effectively reduces the severity of dermatitis when the food allergy has been confirmed (i.e. the client has a positive specific IgE to eggs or cow's milk). There is little evidence in support of elemental or general elimination diets, possibly because the presence of food allergy was not established in these studies.

### Lifestyle

**Environmental agents (Level V)**

A number of environmental agents can be implicated in the pathogenesis of exogenous dermatitis. Reducing the level of exposure to these components is a first step to addressing the cause of the condition. The avoidance of topical agents such as cosmetics, medications, mineral oils, moisturisers, perfumes and plant extracts may eliminate some of the more common exogenous triggers of dermatitis. Aerosols, household chemicals, latex, laundry detergents, non-colour-fast dyes, synthetic fibres and wool are among the many textile and cleaning agents that should also be avoided.

**Relaxation therapy (Level II, Strength B, Direction +)**

The relaxation response can be induced by a number of behavioural therapies. In one RCT that involved 137 subjects with atopic dermatitis, autogenic relaxation training, cognitive-behavioural therapy (CBT) and a combined dermatological educational (DE) and CBT program resulted in significantly greater improvements in lesion severity and a significant reduction in topical steroid use when compared with DE or standard dermatological treatment alone.[9]

### Nutritional supplementation

**Ascorbic acid (Level III-2, Strength D, Direction o)**

Even though serum C-reactive protein (CRP) levels (a marker of acute inflammation) have been shown to be inversely related to vitamin C levels in healthy elderly men,[14] findings relating to the clinical effectiveness of ascorbic acid supplementation in atopic disease have been inconsistent. One study demonstrated an inverse relationship between vitamin C content of breastmilk and risk of atopic disease in infants,[15] while two studies found a positive association between perinatal vitamin C intake and risk of atopic eczema in infants at 2 years of age.[16,17]

**Lactobacillus spp. (Level I, Strength A, Direction + (for prevention only))**

Probiotics exhibit local and systemic anti-inflammatory and immunomodulatory activity, although this may be more effective in the prevention of atopic eczema than as a treatment. This is highlighted in a recent meta-analysis of 10 RCTs, which concluded that probiotic supplementation, particularly with the L. rhamnosus strain, reduced the incidence of infant atopic dermatitis by thirty-nine per cent. As a treatment, probiotic supplementation was associated with only a small, statistically non-significant reduction in symptom severity.[18]

**Omega 3 fatty acids (Level I, Strength A, Direction o)**

The anti-inflammatory effects of essential fatty acids have been demonstrated in numerous population and clinical studies.[19] In spite of this, a meta-analysis of 19 placebo-controlled trials found gamma-linolenic acid (GLA) and fish oil were no more effective than placebo at reducing the severity of atopic dermatitis.[20]

### Selenium (Level II, Strength B, Direction o)
The mineral selenium exhibits a number of actions that may facilitate recovery in dermatitis. The inhibition of nuclear factor-kappaB activation in vitro[21] and the enhancement of T-cell function and B-cell activation and proliferation in healthy men[22] are just a few of these effects. Yet in a double-blind RCT of 60 adults, selenium (600 µg daily for 12 weeks) had no statistically significant effect on the severity of atopic dermatitis when compared with placebo.[23]

### Vitamin A (Level I, Strength B, Direction o)
While vitamin A is essential for collagen synthesis, epithelial cell differentiation, antibody production, phagocytosis and intercellular adhesion,[24] these effects have not transpired in clinical research findings. In fact, a Cochrane review of vitamin A and eczema found only one placebo-controlled trial, and it concluded that there was insufficient evidence to support or refute the use of topical vitamin A preparations in the prevention or treatment of napkin dermatitis.[24] The number of case reports that associate topical vitamin A preparations with contact dermatitis should also alert clinicians to the need for caution when using topically administered vitamin A.

### Vitamin E (Level II, Strength C, Direction +)
The tocopherols show some promise as a treatment for dermatitis due to their capacity to decrease the release of proinflammatory cytokines and to reduce monocyte adhesion to endothelial tissue.[25] This is partly supported by findings from a single-blind RCT of 96 subjects with atopic dermatitis. After 8 months of treatment, a greater number of patients receiving vitamin E supplementation (400 IU daily) demonstrated major improvement or complete remission of eczema and a larger reduction in serum IgE levels when compared with those receiving placebo.[26]

### Zinc (Level III, Strength C, Direction o)
The use of zinc in the treatment of dermatitis is controversial. While this mineral has been shown to reduce spontaneous cytokine release and improve T-cell response in healthy elderly subjects,[27] findings from a double-blind placebo-controlled trial of 50 children (1–16 years) found oral zinc sulphate (185.4 mg per day for 8 weeks) to be no more effective than placebo at reducing the severity of atopic dermatitis.[28]

### Iron, quercetin and vitamin D
These nutrients demonstrate an array of effects that could affect the outcomes of dermatitis;[29–31] however, the efficacy of administration of these nutrients in dermatitis is not yet supported by rigorous clinical evidence, only by pathophysiologic rationale or experimental research findings. Given the diversity in organism physiology and metabolism, and the subsequent differences in dosage requirements between species, the translation of experimental data to human subjects is neither reliable nor appropriate.

## Herbal medicine
### Chamomilla recutita (Level II, Strength C, Direction +)
German chamomile exhibits a range of effects that are pertinent to the management of dermatitis, including anti-inflammatory, antibacterial, immunostimulant and mild sedative activity. The clinical efficacy of topically administered chamomile ointment, specifically, the proprietary product Kamillosan, has also been examined in a number of comparative trials and shown to be as effective as 0.25 per cent hydrocortisone, yet superior to 0.75 per cent fluocortin butyl ester and 5 per cent bufexamac in patients with eczema of the hands, forearms and lower legs after 3–4 weeks,[32] more effective than 0.5 per cent hydrocortisone cream and placebo in patients with atopic dermatitis after 2 weeks[33] and superior to 0.1 per cent hydrocortisone acetate and Kamillosan ointment base in subjects with experimentally induced toxic contact dermatitis.[34] The methodological limitations of these trials suggest further research is needed.

### Centella asiatica (Level IV, Strength D, Direction +)

Gotu kola is used in traditional Western herbal medicine for its anti-inflammatory and vulnerary activity. One of the constituents of the plant, madecassol, has been shown to be more effective than controls at reducing the severity of acute radiation dermatitis in rats. This could be attributed to the anti-inflammatory effect of the plant.[35] The topical application of a C. asiatica extract and essential oil formulation in 20 adults also prevented wound infection in seventy-five per cent of contaminated wounds at 6 weeks, while healing sixty-four per cent of all acute and chronic wounds.[36] The absence of blinding and a suitable control in this study and the lack of specific clinical data on the efficacy of gotu kola in dermatitis suggest further investigation is required.

### Glycyrrhiza glabra (Level II, Strength B, Direction +)

Licorice has a long history of use as an anti-inflammatory and demulcent agent. This use is partly supported by a double-blind RCT of 60 patients with atopic dermatitis that found the topical application of a two per cent licorice gel for 2 weeks to be more effective than one per cent licorice gel in reducing the scores for erythema, oedema and pruritus ($p<0.05$).[37] Without a suitable control, it remains uncertain whether licorice offers any clinical benefit over and above the placebo effect.

### Hypericum perforatum (Level II, Strength B, Direction +)

St John's wort plays an important role in the treatment of integumentary disease due to its vulnerary, anti-inflammatory and analgesic properties. Building on this traditional evidence are findings from a double-blind RCT of 21 patients with mild to moderate atopic dermatitis. The study found that five per cent hypericum cream (standardised to 1.5 per cent hyperforin) applied twice daily for 4 weeks significantly reduced the intensity of eczematous lesions ($p<0.05$), as well as skin colonisation with Staphylococcus aureus ($p = 0.06$), when compared with placebo.[11]

### Other herbs

Albizia lebbeck (albizia), Aloe barbadensis (aloe vera), Arctium lappa (burdock), Azadirachta indica (neem leaf) and Echinacea spp. (echinacea) have all been traditionally used as antiallergic, antimicrobial, anti-inflammatory and/or immunostimulant agents. Even so, there are insufficient clinical data to support their use in dermatitis.

## Other

### Aromatherapy (Level III-1, Strength D, Direction o)

Essential oils exhibit a range of physiological, emotional and psychological effects that may be useful in the overall treatment of dermatitis. To test this assumption, a small RCT set out to compare the efficacy of counselling and massage with essential oils to counselling and massage without essential oils in eight children with atopic dermatitis. After 8 weeks of daily therapy, improvements in dermatitis were evident, although the differences between groups were not statistically significant.[38]

### Homeopathy (Level II, Strength C, Direction +)

Homeopathic medicine has long been used as a treatment of acute and chronic integumentary disorders. While good clinical evidence is lacking for many of these conditions, the evidence supporting the use of homeopathy in the management of dermatitis is promising, though not convincing. One small RCT of 29 patients showed the administration of a homeopathic complex for 10 weeks to be significantly more effective than placebo at improving seborrheic dermatitis.[39] A prospective multicentre cohort study of 118 children has also found 12 months of homeopathic treatment to be as effective as conventional treatment at reducing dermatitis symptoms and disease-related quality of life.[10]

### Massage (Level III-1, Strength D, Direction +)

Psychosocial stress can be an exacerbating factor in endogenous dermatitis. Thus, therapies that induce the relaxation response may be helpful in managing this form of dermatitis. One therapy that may be of particular benefit is massage. In a controlled clinical trial of 20 children suffering from atopic eczema, for instance, parent-admin-istered massage, 20 minutes daily for 4 weeks, significantly ($p<0.05$) reduced ery-thema, lichenification, scaling, excoriation and pruritus, compared with the control, which demonstrated significant improvement only on the scaling measure.[40]

**Acupuncture, chiropractic, osteopathy and reflexology**
There is a paucity of clinical evidence to support the use of these therapies in the management of dermatitis.

CAM prescription
The CAM interventions that are most appropriate for the management of the pre-senting case – that is, they target the planned goals, expected outcomes and CAM diagnoses, they are supported by the best available evidence, they are pertinent to the client's needs and they are most relevant to CAM practice – are outlined below.

**Primary treatments**
- Commence audiotape or parent-directed relaxation therapy, at least 10 minutes three times a week. The approach should focus on the relaxation of specific body parts, while also using autosuggestion (*meditation induces the relaxation response and may help to reduce levels of emotional stress, a known facilitator of dermatitis; in doing so, meditation may help to reduce the severity of dermatitis, as well as the need for topical corticosteroid medication*).
- Commence elimination diet (*if an allergy to foods, such as dairy and eggs, is con-firmed by RAST or ELISA testing, have the client avoid the consumption of these allergenic foods as elimination may diminish the severity of dermatitis*).
- Administer *Hypericum perforatum* five per cent cream (standardised to five per cent hyperforin) to lesions twice daily (*St John's wort, which has vulnerary and anti-inflammatory properties, may be beneficial in reducing the severity of eczematous lesions*).

**Secondary treatments**
- Consider individualised, classical homeopathic treatment (*homeopathy may help in addressing several of the client's expected outcomes, namely, quality of life (i.e. sleep quality), and dermatitis symptoms (i.e. pruritus)*).

Referral
- Refer client to a general practitioner, family physician, dermatologist or emer-gency department if the condition deteriorates, if serious pathology is sus-pected (e.g. pemphigus, squamous cell carcinoma), or if a serious complication arises (e.g. adverse drug reaction, cellulitis).
- Refer client to another CAM practitioner if dermatitis, or the treatment of der-matitis, is outside the clinician's area of expertise.
- Liaise with the general practitioner about the client's overall management plan.

## Review

To determine whether pertinent client goals and expected outcomes have been achieved at follow-up and if any aspects of the client's care need to be improved, consider the factors listed in Table 8.2 (chapter 8), as well as the questions listed below.
- Was there a reduction in the overall POEM score?
- Was there an improvement in the pruritus and sleeping domains of POEM?
- Was there a reduction in lesion size to the neck, popliteal fossae and/or ante-cubital fossae?
- Did any new lesions develop?
- Is the client less irritable?
- Has the need for hydrocortisone cream decreased?

# References

1. Hogan PA. (2005) Atopic dermatitis. In: Marks R, editor. Dermatology. 2nd ed. Sydney: Australasian Medical Publishing Company.
2. Nixon RL. Frowen KE. (2005) Contact dermatitis and occupational skin disease. In: Marks R, editor. Dermatology. 2nd ed. Sydney: Australasian Medical Publishing Company.
3. Porter R et al, editors. (2008). The Merck manual. Rahway: Merck Research Laboratories.
4. Graham-Brown R. Burns T. (2007) Lecture notes on dermatology. 9th ed. Oxford: Blackwell.
5. Buchanan P. Courtenay M. (2006) Prescribing in dermatology. Cambridge: Cambridge University Press.
6. Lewis-Jones S. (2006) Quality of life and childhood atopic dermatitis: the misery of living with childhood eczema. International Journal of Clinical Practice, 60(8): 984–92.
7. Ring J. Przybilla B. Ruzicka T. (2006) Handbook of atopic eczema. 2nd ed. Berlin: Springer-Verlag.
8. Bath-Hextall FJ. Delamere FM. Williams HC. (2008) Dietary exclusions for established atopic eczema. Cochrane Database of Systematic Reviews, (1): CD005203.
9. Ehlers A. Stangier U. Gieler U. (1995) Treatment of atopic dermatitis: a comparison of psychological and dermatological approaches to relapse prevention. Journal of Consulting and Clinical Psychology, 63(4): 624–35.
10. Keil T et al (2008) Homoeopathic versus conventional treatment of children with eczema: a comparative cohort study. Complementary Therapies in Medicine, 16(1): 15–21.
11. Schempp CM et al (2003) Topical treatment of atopic dermatitis with St. John's wort cream: a randomized, placebo controlled, double blind half-side comparison. Phytomedicine, 10(Suppl 4): 31–7.
12. Fiocchi A et al (2004) Dietary treatment of childhood atopic eczema/dermatitis syndrome (AEDS). Allergy, 59(S78): 78–85.
13. Norrman G et al (2007) Significant improvement of eczema with skin care and food elimination in small children. Acta Paediatrica, 94(10): 1384–8.
14. Wannamethee SG et al (2006) Associations of vitamin C status, fruit and vegetable intakes, and markers of inflammation and hemostasis. American Journal of Clinical Nutrition, 83(3): 567–74.
15. Hoppu U et al (2005) Vitamin C in breast milk may reduce the risk of atopy in the infant. European Journal of Clinical Nutrition, 59(1): 123–8.
16. Laitinen K et al (2005) Evaluation of diet and growth in children with and without atopic eczema: follow-up study from birth to 4 years. British Journal of Nutrition, 94(4): 565–74.
17. Martindale S et al (2005) Antioxidant intake in pregnancy in relation to wheeze and eczema in the first two years of life. American Journal of Respiratory and Critical Care Medicine, 171(2): 121–8.
18. Lee J. Seto D. Bielory L. (2008) Meta-analysis of clinical trials of probiotics for prevention and treatment of pediatric atopic dermatitis. Journal of Allergy and Clinical Immunology, 121(1): 116–21.
19. Jho DH et al (2004) Role of omega-3 fatty acid supplementation in inflammation and malignancy. Integrative Cancer Therapies, 3(2): 98–111.
20. van Gool CJ. Zeegers MP. Thijs C. (2004) Oral essential fatty acid supplementation in atopic dermatitis-a meta-analysis of placebo-controlled trials. British Journal of Dermatology, 150(4): 728–40.
21. Vunta H et al (2007) The anti-inflammatory effects of selenium are mediated through 15-deoxy-Delta12, 14-prostaglandin J2 in macrophages. Journal of Biological Chemistry, 282(25): 17964–73.
22. Hawkes WC. Kelley DS. Taylor PC. (2001) The effects of dietary selenium on the immune system in healthy men. Biological Trace Element Research, 81(3): 189–213.
23. Fairris GM et al (1989) The effect on atopic dermatitis of supplementation with selenium and vitamin E. Acta Dermato-Venereologica, 69(4): 359–62.
24. Davies MW. Dore AJ. Perissinotto KL. (2005) Topical vitamin A, or its derivatives, for treating and preventing napkin dermatitis in infants. Cochrane Database of Systematic Reviews, (4): CD004300.
25. Singh U. Devaraj S. Jialal I. (2005) Vitamin E, oxidative stress, and inflammation. Annual Review of Nutrition, 25: 151–74.
26. Tsoureli-Nikita E et al (2002) Evaluation of dietary intake of vitamin E in the treatment of atopic dermatitis: a study of the clinical course and evaluation of the immunoglobulin E serum levels. International Journal of Dermatology, 41(3): 146–50.
27. Kahmann L et al (2008) Zinc supplementation in the elderly reduces spontaneous inflammatory cytokine release and restores T cell functions. Rejuvenation Research, 11(1): 227–37.
28. Ewing CI et al (1991) Failure of oral zinc supplementation in atopic eczema. European Journal of Clinical Nutrition, 45(10): 507–10.
29. Giulietti A et al (2007) Monocytes from type 2 diabetic patients have a pro-inflammatory profile. 1,25-dihydroxyvitamin D(3) works as anti-inflammatory. Diabetes Research and Clinical Practice, 77(1): 47–57.
30. Muthian G. Bright JJ. (2004) Quercetin, a flavonoid phytoestrogen, ameliorates experimental allergic encephalomyelitis by blocking IL-2 signaling through JAK-STAT pathway in T lymphocyte. Journal of Clinical Immunology, 24(5): 542–52.
31. Shaheen SO et al (2004) Umbilical cord trace elements and minerals and risk of early childhood wheezing and eczema. European Respiratory Journal, 24(2): 292–7.
32. Aertgeerts P et al (1985) Comparative testing of Kamillosan cream and steroidal (0.25% hydrocortisone, 0.75% fluocortin butyl ester) and non-steroidal (5% bufexamac) dermatologic agents in maintenance therapy of eczematous diseases. Zeitschrift fur Hautkrankheiten, 60(3): 270–7.
33. Patzelt-Wenczler R. Ponce-Poschl E. (2000) Proof of efficacy of Kamillosan(R) cream in atopic eczema. European Journal of Medical Research, 5(4): 171–5.
34. Nissen HP. Biltz H. Kreysel HW. (1988) Profilometry, a method for the assessment of the therapeutic effectiveness of Kamillosan ointment. Zeitschrift fur Hautkrankheiten, 63(3): 184–90.
35. Chen YJ et al (1999) The effect of tetrandrine and extracts of centella asiatica on acute radiation dermatitis in rats. Biological and Pharmaceutical Bulletin, 22(7): 703–6.

36. Morisset R et al (1987). Evaluation of the healing activity of Hydrocotyle tincture in the treatment of wounds. Phytotherapy Research, 1(3): 117–21.
37. Saeedi M. Morteza-Semnani K. Ghoreishi MR. (2003) The treatment of atopic dermatitis with licorice gel. Journal of Dermatological Treatment, 14(3): 153–7.
38. Anderson C. Lis-Balchin M. Kirk-Smith M. (2000) Evaluation of massage with essential oils on childhood atopic eczema. Phytotherapy Research, 14(6): 452–6.
39. Smith SA. Baker AE. Williams JH. (2002) Effective treatment of seborrheic dermatitis using a low dose, oral homeopathic medication consisting of potassium bromide, sodium bromide, nickel sulfate, and sodium chloride in a double-blind, placebo-controlled study. Alternative Medicine Review, 7(1): 59–67.
40. Schachner L et al (1998) Atopic dermatitis symptoms decreased in children following massage therapy. Pediatric Dermatology, 15(5): 390–5.

# Case 7
# Irritable bowel syndrome

## Description of irritable bowel syndrome

Definition
Irritable bowel syndrome (IBS) is a chronic, functional bowel disorder characterised by abnormal defecation, visceral hypersensitivity and altered bowel motility. Depending on the prevailing stool pattern of the condition, IBS may be classified as IBS with constipation (IBS-C), IBS with diarrhoea (IBS-D), mixed IBS (IBS-M) or unclassified IBS (IBS-U).[1]

Epidemiology
Between four and thirty-five per cent of the world's population is affected by IBS. Much of this variation can be explained by geographical variability, with higher prevalence rates observed in China and Western countries, and lower rates noted in South Africa and Thailand.[1] Onset of IBS typically occurs in the teens or second decade of life; incidence peaks in the third and fourth decades of life and falls in the sixth and seventh decades.[1] Race does not appear to be a factor in the incidence of IBS, though the condition does more commonly affect women than men, at a ratio of 3:1.[2]

Aetiology and pathophysiology
IBS appears to be a disease of multifactorial aetiology. While the primary cause is still not known, a number of factors have been shown to precipitate or aggravate the condition. These triggers include psychosocial stress (e.g. parental rejection, history of abuse, increased life stressors), anxiety, infectious gastroenteritis, diet (e.g. food intolerance), medication (e.g. antibiotics, hormone replacement therapy) and the act of eating.[1–3]

Even though the cause of IBS is not yet known, many theories have attempted to explain the pathophysiological basis of the disease. It is postulated that exposure to the triggers mentioned above, together with genetic predisposition, contributes to the development of chronic enteric inflammation and/or small intestinal bacterial overgrowth. These pathological changes may be responsible for local neuronal degeneration and immune dysfunction, and the subsequent development of visceral hypersensitivity (which may cause abdominal and/or rectal discomfort) and altered bowel motility (a possible cause of constipation, diarrhoea and nausea).[1,3]

Clinical manifestations
People with IBS often present with an array of gastrointestinal, psychological and/or systemic symptoms of varying intensity and frequency. Non-specific symptoms such as fatigue, chronic headache and sleep disturbances may be accompanied by psychological manifestations that include poor concentration, anxiety and depression. An individual may also complain of dyspepsia, flatulence, mucorrhoea, rectal sensitivity, nausea, abdominal bloating, left lower quadrant tenderness and periodic constipation and/or diarrhoea.[2] According to the Rome III criteria for the diagnosis of IBS, the defining feature is the presence of colicky pain or continuous dull ache to the lower abdomen or left lower abdominal quadrant for at least 3 days a month in the past 3 months (with the onset of symptoms occurring at least 6 months prior), which is associated with at least two of the following: a change in stool consistency, a change in the frequency of defecation and/or improvement post defecation.[1]

# Clinical case
*32-year-old woman with irritable bowel syndrome*

## Rapport

Adopt the practitioner strategies and behaviours highlighted in Table 2.1 (chapter 2) to improve client trust, communication and rapport, as well as the accuracy and comprehensiveness of the clinical assessment.

## Assessment

Once measures have been put into place to build client–practitioner rapport, the clinician can begin the clinical assessment.

### Health history
**History of presenting condition**

A 32-year-old woman presents to the integrative healthcare clinic complaining of a 6-month history of lower abdominal discomfort and loose bowel actions. The client is initially referred to the clinic's general practitioner, who diagnoses irritable bowel syndrome with diarrhoea (IBS-D). The client is commenced on loperamide as a short-term measure, and is then referred onto the clinic's CAM practitioner for further care. Her pain, located in the left lower quadrant of the abdomen, is described as dull and colicky, non-radiating, moderately intense (pain score = 5/10) and of 3–4 hours duration. The pain began 6 months ago after completion of a second course of oral antibiotics for severe infectious gastroenteritis. Since then, the pain has occurred at least once every 2 weeks and is often accompanied by loose bowel actions (stools are described as brown in colour and mushy in texture), flatulence, mucorrhoea and abdominal bloating. These symptoms are embarrassing and inconvenient for the client when at work. The symptoms are aggravated by emotional stress and ameliorated after defecation. Interstate or international travel, use of aperients and the consumption of sugar-free or artificially sweetened foods have been excluded as potential causes of the IBS symptoms.

### Medical history
**Family history**

Mother has asthma and generalised anxiety disorder, father has hypertension.

**Allergies**

Peanuts (causes anaphylaxis).

**Medications**

Loperamide hydrochloride 8–16 mg as needed, Microgynon 20 (ethinyloestradiol and levonorgestrel) once daily.

**Medical conditions**

Appendicitis (2004), irritable bowel syndrome.

**Surgical or investigational procedures**

Laparoscopic appendicectomy (2004).

### Lifestyle history
**Tobacco use**

Nil.

**Alcohol consumption**

Social drinker. 2–3 standard-size rum and colas every 2–3 weeks.

**Illicit drug use**

Nil.

| Diet and fluid intake | |
|---|---|
| Breakfast | Coffee, wheat biscuits (breakfast cereal) with full-cream milk. |
| Morning tea | Coffee, 2–3 sweet biscuits, muesli bar. |
| Lunch | Vegetarian pasty, white bread roll with lettuce, tomato and cheese, sandwich with white bread, ham, cheese and tomato, cola. |
| Afternoon tea | Coffee. |
| Dinner | White pasta with Neapolitan or carbonara sauce, chicken Kiev or cordon bleu with cauliflower, broccoli and green beans, omelette with ham and cheese. |
| Fluid intake | 3–4 cups of instant coffee a day, 2–3 cups of water a day, 375 mL cola 1–2 days a week. |
| **Food frequency** | |
| Fruit | 0–1 serve daily |
| Vegetables | 2–3 serves daily |
| Dairy | 2–3 serves daily |
| Cereals | 5–6 serves daily |
| Red meat | 3–4 serves a week |
| Chicken | 2 serves a week |
| Fish | 0–1 serve a week |
| Takeaway/fast food | once a week |

### Quality and duration of sleep

Difficulty falling asleep (sleep latency is less than 1 hour), continuous sleep; average duration is 6–7 hours.

### Frequency and duration of exercise

Client states she has limited time available for physical exercise. Walks 20–30 minutes, 1–2 times a week. Drives to work. Engages in incidental exercise (e.g. work-related walking, cleaning) less than 3 hours a day. Engages in sedentary activities (e.g. desk-bound activities) more than 6 hours a day.

### Socioeconomic background

The client is English-born with a German-born father and Dutch-born mother. The client is a non-practising Christian with no firm cultural affiliations. Since completing her teaching degree 11 years ago she has been employed as a full-time secondary school teacher, which she enjoys but often finds very stressful. The client has no children and is living with her partner in a de facto relationship in a small unit in the outer suburbs. Her partner and family are all supportive; she has a group of very close friends.

## Physical examination

### Inspection

The oral cavity is unremarkable. There is no evidence of goitre or proptosis. Abdomen is flat with no visible masses, herniation, discolouration or lesions. A 3-cm scar is evident over the right lower quadrant. The client denies the presence of haemorrhoids, anal bleeding, pruritis ani and anal or perineum discomfort. Client reports her stools to be generally brown in colour, mushy in texture (with a Bristol stool chart rating of 6) and often coated in small amounts of clear to pale white mucus.

### Olfaction

There is no evidence of halitosis or other abnormal body odours. According to the client, flatus can be foul-smelling, whereas stools generally are not.

## Palpation
Abdomen is soft with no palpable masses. Mild left lower quadrant tenderness is evident (pain score = 4/10). Rebound tenderness, Murphy's sign, Rovsing's sign and voluntary guarding are absent.

## Percussion
Percussive tones over the abdomen are unremarkable.

## Auscultation
Bowel sounds are normoactive in all four quadrants.

## Additional signs
Client is afebrile (36.3°C, per oral) and of normal weight (weight is 70.5 kg, BMI is 22.2 kg/m$^2$, waist circumference is 69 cm). Weight has remained stable over the past 6 months, ranging between 69 and 72 kg. Blood pressure is 128/74.

## Clinical assessment tools
The score for all 34 items on the irritable bowel syndrome quality of life (IBS-QoL) measure was 47/100, which indicates the client has moderate quality of life. A higher score would indicate better quality of life, while a lower score would indicate poorer quality of life.

## Diagnostics
CAM practitioners may request, perform and/or interpret findings from a range of diagnostic tests in order to add valuable data to the pool of clinical information. While several investigations are pertinent to this case (as described below), the decision to use these tests should be considered alongside factors such as cost, convenience, comfort, turnaround time, access, practitioner competence and scope of practice, and history of previous investigations.

## Pathology tests
### Carbohydrate breath test
This test examines carbohydrate malabsorption (specifically, lactose and/or fructose malabsorption), orocecal transit time and small intestinal bacterial overgrowth.[4] This test may be indicated if carbohydrate malabsorption is a suspected cause of IBS symptoms.

### Faecal analysis
This test assesses a number of stool characteristics, including appearance, colour, occult blood, epithelial cells, leucocytes, carbohydrates, fat, meat fibres and trypsin.[5] It may also help to exclude colorectal carcinoma, malabsorption, inflammatory bowel disease or intestinal infection as potential causes of IBS symptoms.

### Radioallergosorbent test (RAST) and enzyme linked immunosorbent assay (ELISA)
RAST and ELISA quantify the presence of IgE in client serum.[5] These tests may be required if food allergy is a suspected cause of IBS.

## Radiology tests
The diagnosis of IBS is generally based on clinical examination alone. Where other conditions are suspected of masquerading as IBS, such as diverticulosis or colorectal carcinoma, a CT, MRI or lower GI series may be indicated.

## Functional tests
A comprehensive digestive stool analysis (CDSA) obtains data on enzymatic digestion, fatty acid absorption, microbiological balance and metabolic markers of disease. This test may be warranted if intestinal dysbiosis, intestinal candidiasis, malabsorption and/or indigestion cannot be excluded as potential causes of IBS symptoms.[6]

## Invasive tests
Invasive tests are not usually required for a diagnosis of IBS. When serious underlying pathology is a suspected cause of the IBS symptoms, certain tests may be indicated, for example, small bowel biopsies can be performed to rule out coeliac disease and a

colonoscopy and/or sigmoidoscopy may be indicated if colorectal carcinoma, inflammatory bowel disease or diverticulosis are suspected.

**Miscellaneous tests**
Not applicable.

## Diagnosis

Clusters of data extracted from the health history, clinical examination and pertinent diagnostic test results point towards the following differential CAM diagnoses.

- Left lower quadrant pain (actual), *secondary to* irritable bowel disease, *related to* emotional stress (*the client states that the IBS symptoms are aggravated by stress – the client has a stressful occupation*), food sensitivity (*if supported by an elimination diet and/or RAST testing*), and infectious gastroenteritis (*an episode of severe infectious gastroenteritis preceded the onset of IBS symptoms*).
- Diarrhoea (actual), *secondary to* irritable bowel disease, *related to* emotional stress, food intolerance and infectious gastroenteritis.

## Planning

The goals and expected outcomes that best serve the client's needs, and which are most relevant to the presenting case (as determined by the clinical assessment and CAM diagnoses), are as follows.

Goals
1 Client will demonstrate an improvement in left lower quadrant pain (*client is concerned about the abdominal pain*).
2 Client will report reduced episodes of diarrhoea (*client has expressed concern about the loose bowel actions*).
3 Client will demonstrate an improvement in IBS-specific quality of life (*client has expressed concern about the embarrassment and social inconvenience of IBS*).

Expected outcomes
Based on the degree of improvement reported in clinical studies that have used CAM interventions for the management of IBS,[7–12] the following are anticipated.
1 Client bowel actions will be formed in 8 weeks or by dd/mm/yyyy (measured by bowel activity chart and determined by Bristol stool chart).
2 Client will have one bowel action daily at 8 weeks or by dd/mm/yyyy (measured by bowel activity chart).
3 Client will report a thirty-five per cent reduction in baseline frequency of lower abdominal discomfort in 9 weeks or by dd/mm/yyyy (measured by IBS activity chart).
4 Client will report a fifty per cent reduction in baseline severity of lower abdominal discomfort in 9 weeks or by dd/mm/yyyy (measured by 0–10 numerical pain scale).
5 Client will demonstrate a fifteen per cent improvement in baseline IBS-specific quality of life in 12 weeks or by dd/mm/yyyy (measured by IBS-QoL).

## Application

The range of interventions reported in the CAM literature that may be used in the treatment of IBS is appraised below.

Diet
**Elimination diet (Level I, Strength B, Direction +)**
Food intolerance is implicated in the pathogenesis of IBS. The elimination of offending foods from the diet could potentially lead to an improvement in IBS symptoms and a reduction in symptom recurrence. In a systematic review of seven open label, single-arm studies (n = 386), between 12.5 per cent and 67 per cent of patients

treated with an elimination diet demonstrated remission of IBS symptoms within 4 to 21 days.[13] Double-blind challenges identified milk, wheat and eggs as the most frequent causes of IBS symptom exacerbation. While these studies have major methodological limitations, they are supported by data from three rigorously designed clinical trials (n = 562). These studies have shown the elimination diet to be superior to a sham elimination diet in reducing IBS symptom severity and global rating score at 12 weeks[8] and as effective as disodium cromoglycate (1.5 g daily) at improving IBS symptoms at 4 weeks.[14] When elimination diet and disodium cromoglycate (250 mg 4 times a day for 16 weeks) are used together, they are shown to be significantly more effective than diet alone in reducing IBS symptoms.[15] Foods most frequently excluded from the elimination diets were milk, wheat, eggs, cashew nuts, tomato, yeast and potato. In spite of these favourable outcomes, the heterogeneity in diets across studies makes the clinical application of these findings difficult. Replicating studies using individualised elimination diets (i.e. by eliminating foods for which the patient has elevated IgG antibodies), such as that reported by Atkinson et al,[7] would produce findings that are directly applicable to CAM practice and would help to improve consumer and practitioner confidence in this intervention.

**High-fibre diet (Level I, Strength C, Direction + (for soluble fibre only))**
Dietary fibre is essential for maintaining gastrointestinal (GI) tract function, specifically, fibre increases faecal volume, decreases GI transit time, decreases bowel lumen pressure, promotes the growth of beneficial bowel flora, generates lactate to acidify the colon lumen and generates short-chain fatty acids to stimulate mucosal cell proliferation and provide energy for colonic cells.[16] Each of these functions can help to attenuate the pathophysiological processes and the symptoms of IBS. Evidence from a systematic review of 12 RCTs (n = 591) adds support to this claim, but only for certain types of fibre. When compared with placebo, for instance, soluble fibre (isphagula and psyllium) showed significant improvement in abdominal pain and global IBS symptoms, whereas insoluble fibre (10–30 g wheat bran daily) had no significant effect on IBS manifestations.[8] It is probable, then, that IBS may be more responsive to soluble than insoluble fibre. Given that wheat intolerance is a common trigger of IBS,[13] and most of the studies included in this systematic review neither listed wheat intolerance or coeliac disease as an exclusion criterion, nor investigated the presence of wheat intolerance, it is also possible that wheat intolerance could have confounded these results, which means that the comparative efficacy of different types of fibre warrants further investigation.

## Lifestyle

**Meditation (Level II, Strength B, Direction +)**
Meditation is a mind–body therapy that uses a range of methods, such as mindfulness, breathing, concentration, visualisation, mantras and/or affirmations, to bring about inner tranquillity and/or improve self-awareness. Given that stress and anxiety aggravate IBS, meditation may be a suitable treatment option for people with the condition. This assumption was tested in a small RCT of 13 adults with IBS. The study found relaxation response meditation (15 minutes twice daily for 6 weeks) to be significantly superior to waiting list control at reducing the composite score of IBS abdominal symptoms.[10] Even so, given the small size of the study, these findings should be interpreted with caution.

**Relaxation therapy (Level I, Strength C, Direction + (for overall IBS symptom score only))**
The relaxation response can be induced by a number of behavioural therapies. In so doing, these therapies may help to attenuate the effect of stress and anxiety on IBS. A recent Cochrane review of 10 RCTs examined the effect of relaxation therapy and stress management on the symptoms of IBS. The review found a small but statistically

significant benefit from relaxation therapy and stress management on overall IBS symptom score when compared with usual care or waiting list control, although changes in abdominal pain and quality of life were not consistent across studies.[17] The low methodological quality, small sample sizes and considerable heterogeneity of the trials prevents any firm conclusions being made about the effectiveness of relaxation therapy for IBS.

### Yoga (Level II, Strength C, Direction + (for bowel symptoms only))

Yoga is an ancient Indian practice that integrates stretching, exercise, posture and breathing with meditation. As these techniques are likely to induce a relaxation response, yoga may be helpful in alleviating the symptoms of IBS. Two RCTs have examined the effectiveness of yoga in people with IBS. The first trial, which enrolled 22 adult males with diarrhoea-predominant IBS, found yoga (i.e. yogic poses and right-nostril breathing, twice a day for 8 weeks) to be as effective as the antidiarrhoeal loperamide (2–6 mg daily) at reducing bowel symptoms and state anxiety.[18] In a trial of 25 adolescents with IBS, yoga (i.e. video-guided yogic poses and breathing, 10 minutes daily for 4 weeks) was found to be no more effective than waiting list control at reducing functional disability, anxiety and emotion-focused avoidance.[11] The inconsistencies in these study findings, the uncertainty about the effect of meditation in adult females and the small size of these trials highlights the need for further research in this area.

## Nutritional supplementation

### Flaxseed (Level III-1, Strength C, Direction +)

The seeds of *Linium usitatissimum*, or flax, are a good source of dietary fibre, protein, lignans, alpha-linolenic acid (omega 3 fatty acid), linoleic acid (omega 6 fatty acid) and oleic acid (omega 9 fatty acid).[19] The anti-inflammatory effects of these fatty acids, together with the mucilaginous effect of the seed, suggest flaxseed may be useful in the management of IBS. A single-blind RCT involving 55 patients with constipation-dominant IBS supports this claim. The trial found roughly ground, partly defatted flaxseed (6–24 g daily), when administered for 3 months, to be statistically significantly more effective than psyllium (6–24 g daily) at improving constipation, abdominal pain and bloating.[20] Replication of these results may provide practitioners with the confidence to select this intervention as a treatment for IBS-C.

### Prebiotics (Level II, Strength B, Direction o)

Prebiotics are non-digestible substances (typically, carbohydrates or soluble fibre) that stimulate the growth of bowel flora. In so doing, these substances help to maintain microbial balance in the GI tract. Few prebiotics have been investigated for their effectiveness in IBS. Fructo-oligosaccharides (FOS) are one exception. In a multicentre, double-blind RCT of 96 patients with IBS, FOS powder (20 g daily for 12 weeks) was found to improve abdominal distension, rumbling, flatulence and pain in fifty-eight per cent of patients; the difference between the FOS and placebo groups was not statistically significant.[21]

### Probiotics (Level I, Strength A, Direction +)

Probiotics are live microbial dietary supplements. These agents are essential for minimising pathogen growth, synthesising vitamins, manufacturing short-chain fatty acids, modulating local immune and inflammatory responses, and maintaining intestinal epithelial integrity.[22] Much of the research on probiotics and IBS has focused on the effectiveness of two microbial species – *Lactobacillus spp.* and *Bifidobacterium spp.* A systematic review and meta-analysis of 14 RCTs (n = 1225) found probiotic treatment for 4–26 weeks to be significantly more effective than placebo at improving abdominal pain (in seven trials), flatulence (in five trials), bloating (in four trials) and global IBS symptoms (in seven trials).[9] Even though these outcomes are positive, the clinical application of these findings may be difficult due to the disparate dosages, treatment durations, types of microbial strains and combinations of strains used across studies.

**Beta-carotene, magnesium, selenium, vitamin B complex and vitamin C**
These exhibit a range of effects that are relevant to the management of IBS, including anti-inflammatory, anxiolytic, immunomodulating and spasmolytic activity, yet there is insufficient clinical evidence to justify the administration of these agents in individuals with IBS.

Herbal medicine
*Curcuma longa* **(Level III-1, Strength D, Direction +)**
Turmeric is a culinary spice, an approved food colouring agent and a medicinal plant. In Ayurvedic, Chinese, Thai and Western herbal medicine the plant has been used for the treatment of pyrexia, menstrual irregularity, jaundice and pain. Turmeric has also been used as a treatment for digestive disorders, which, together with the anti-inflammatory,[23] antispasmodic,[24] immunomodulatory[25] and antimicrobial activity of the plant (and its active constituents), highlight a potential role for turmeric in the management of IBS. While a partially blinded, randomised, two-dose, pilot study involving 192 otherwise healthy adults with IBS found turmeric extract (72 mg or 144 mg daily for 8 weeks) to be effective in reducing IBS prevalence, abdominal discomfort and IBS quality of life,[26] a placebo effect cannot be ruled out given the absence of a placebo control and the similar efficacy of the two turmeric doses.

*Cynara scolymus* **(Level III-1, Strength C, Direction +)**
Globe artichoke, or artichoke leaf extract (ALE), is used in Western herbal medicine as a hepatoprotective, cholagogue, choleretic, hypolipidaemic and diuretic, primarily for the treatment of hepatic and biliary complaints. Recent studies suggest *C. scolymus* may also be useful for conditions affecting the GI tract, such as IBS. A postmarketing surveillance study, for instance, found ALE (1920 mg daily for 6 weeks) reduced IBS symptoms in 279 adults with IBS.[27] A subanalysis of an open, two-dose clinical study found that ALE (320 mg or 640 mg for 8 weeks) was also effective at improving IBS incidence, bowel function and quality of life.[28] Both of these studies have major methodological shortcomings and, as such, do not allow for any conclusions to be made about the efficacy of globe artichoke in IBS.

*Mentha piperita* **(Level I, Strength A, Direction +)**
Peppermint has a long history of use as an antiemetic, antimicrobial, carminative and antispasmodic. In fact, peppermint oil and its main constituent menthol have been shown in a number of different animal studies to reduce experimentally induced spasm of GI smooth muscle,[29] an effect that has been attributed to the calcium antagonist effect of menthol. These findings are congruent with those reported in human studies, with a meta-analysis of four well-designed RCTs (n = 392) finding peppermint oil (450–748 mg daily for 4–12 weeks) to be significantly superior to placebo at improving abdominal pain and global IBS symptoms.[8] The number needed to treat to prevent one patient having persistent symptoms was half that reported for conventional antispasmodics.

*Plantago* **spp. (Level I, Strength A, Direction +)**
The seed husks of psyllium and isphagula are classified as water-soluble fibres because they form a mucilagenous gel when exposed to water.[30] This acts as an effective stool bulking agent that may be useful for the management of constipation and diarrhoea, both of which are characteristic symptoms of IBS. Evidence from a recent meta-analysis of six well-designed RCTs (n = 321) found psyllium (6.4 g daily for 8 weeks) and isphagula husk (unknown dose for 4–12 weeks) to be statistically significantly more effective than placebo at reducing abdominal pain and global IBS symptoms.[9] The number needed to treat to prevent one patient having persistent symptoms was similar to that reported for conventional antispasmodics.

**Other herbs**
*Filipendula ulmaria* (meadowsweet), *Foeniculum vulgare* (fennel), *Glycyrrhiza glabra* (licorice), *Matricaria recutita* (chamomile), *Melissa officinalis* (lemon balm),

*Paeonia lactiflora* (peony), *Ulmus rubra* (slippery elm) and *Viburnum opulus* (cramp bark) are traditionally used as carminative, spasmolytic and/or demulcent agents, but there is insufficient clinical evidence to support or refute the efficacy of these herbal monopreparations in humans with IBS.

## Other

### Acupuncture (Level I, Strength C, Direction o)

Acupuncture originated in China more than 4000 years ago.[31] Since then, the therapy has established a large traditional evidence base; however, in the case of IBS, the best available evidence is not convincing. In a Cochrane review of six RCTs/quasi-RCTs (n = 464),[32] as well as a more recent clinical trial (n = 43),[33] acupuncture treatment for 4–24 weeks was found to be no more effective than sham acupuncture, psychotherapy, a Chinese polyherbal or orthodox medication at improving general wellbeing, global IBS symptoms, symptom recurrence, abdominal pain, defecation difficulties, diarrhoea or bloating. Yet when acupuncture was combined with psychotherapy, a significant improvement in IBS symptoms and symptom recurrence was observed when compared with psychotherapy alone.[32] Similarly, significant improvements in IBS symptom severity scores were observed among patients receiving acupuncture and usual general practice (GP) care when compared to usual GP care alone.[34] This suggests that an integrative approach to IBS may be more effective than acupuncture alone in the management of this condition.

### Osteopathy (Level II, Strength B, Direction +)

Osteopathic medicine applies a range of manipulative techniques in order to facilitate recovery of neuromusculoskeletal complaints. Given that the aetiology of IBS has a neurological basis, osteopathic manipulation may have a place in the management of this disorder. Evidence from two RCTs supports this assumption. One RCT involving 39 IBS patients found 6 months of osteopathic treatment to be significantly more effective than standard care at reducing IBS severity and change in overall symptom improvement. Changes in mean symptom scores were not significantly different between groups.[35] By contrast, an RCT of 61 IBS patients found 10 weeks of osteopathic manipulation to be superior to sham osteopathy in improving the incidence and intensity of abdominal pain, constipation, diarrhoea and abdominal distension.[13] Even though these outcomes are promising they are not conclusive. Hence, larger, long-term studies are now required to strengthen the evidence in this area.

### Reflexology (Level II, Strength C, Direction o)

Reflexology is a tactile therapy that induces neurophysiological reflexes or responses in distant glands, tissues and organs by stimulating specific zones of the feet, hands and/or ears. Several uncontrolled open-label studies have reported improvements in constipation following reflexology treatment,[36,37] which suggests that reflexology could be effective in alleviating the symptoms of IBS. When foot reflexology (six 30-minute sessions over 10 weeks) was administered to patients with IBS under single-blind RCT conditions, it was found to be no more effective than light foot massage at reducing abdominal pain, constipation or diarrhoea or bloatedness.[38] Given the small scale of the study (n = 34) and the potential confounding effect of the massage control, the value of reflexology in IBS should not be dismissed until larger, more rigorously designed trials are conducted in this area.

### Aromatherapy, chiropractic and homeopathy

There is insufficient clinical evidence to support the use of aromatherapy, chiropractic and homeopathy in the management of IBS.

## CAM prescription

The CAM interventions that are most appropriate for the management of the presenting case – that is, they target the planned goals, expected outcomes and CAM diagnoses, they are supported by the best available evidence, they are pertinent to the client's needs and they are most relevant to CAM practice – are outlined below.

## Primary treatments

- Commence elimination diet. Have, for example, the client avoid the consumption of potentially allergenic foods, artificial colours, flavours and/or preservatives for 1 week. After a 1-week elimination period, ask client to reintroduce a new food every 2 days and monitor the recurrence of IBS-related signs and symptoms. The presence or absence of any adverse reactions during these oral food challenges should be recorded in a food and lifestyle diary, and reviewed at the next consultation. The foods identified as being associated with IBS symptoms should be eliminated from the diet (*client may be consuming foods that are contributing to the manifestation of IBS symptoms; eliminating the consumption of these dietary components may lessen the frequency and/or severity of IBS symptoms*).
- Commence relaxation response meditation, 15 minutes twice a day (*IBS symptoms are aggravated by stress, meditation induces the relaxation response and effectively improves IBS abdominal symptoms*).
- Consider one of the following biological interventions:
  - encapsulated enteric-coated peppermint oil, 0.2 mL three times a day (*peppermint oil is effective in reducing abdominal pain and global IBS symptoms; however, given that peppermint oil might increase the oral bioavailability of some medications,[39] the client should be counselled to disclose the use of this intervention with her physician and pharmacist to avoid the possibility of a herb–drug interaction*)
  - psyllium husk, 6.4 g daily (*psyllium husk is effective in reducing abdominal pain and global IBS symptoms*)
  - *Lactobacillus* spp. or *Bifidobacterium* spp. supplement, $1 \times 10^9$ colony forming units/g twice a day (*probiotics are effective in decreasing abdominal pain, flatulence, abdominal bloating and global IBS symptoms*)
  - Consider individualised osteopathic treatment series, with treatment sessions occurring at least every 2 weeks (*osteopathy is effective in reducing the incidence and intensity of abdominal pain, diarrhoea and abdominal distension*).

## Secondary treatment

- Consider integrated yoga program (which is inclusive of yoga postures and yoga breathing), 30 minutes twice daily (*IBS symptoms are aggravated by stress; yoga induces the relaxation response and may improve IBS symptoms*).

## Referral

- Refer client to a general practitioner, family physician or gastroenterologist if the condition deteriorates or if another pathology is suspected (e.g. bowel cancer, inflammatory bowel disease, diverticulosis).
- Refer client to another CAM practitioner if IBS, or the treatment of IBS, is outside the clinician's area of expertise.
- Liaise with the general practitioner about the client's overall management plan.

## Review

To determine whether pertinent client goals and expected outcomes have been achieved at follow-up, and if any aspects of the client's care need to be improved, consider the factors listed in Table 8.2 (chapter 8) as well as the questions listed below.

1. Are bowel actions formed on most occasions?
2. Is the client defecating only once a day?
3. Was there a reduction in the frequency of lower abdominal discomfort?
4. Was there a reduction in the severity of lower abdominal discomfort?
5. Did the client experience an increase in IBS-specific quality of life?
6. Has the need for loperamide reduced?

# References

1. Padovei M. Kuo B. (2006) Irritable bowel syndrome: a practical review. Southern Medical Journal, 99(11): 1235–42.
2. Porter R et al, editors. (2008). The Merck manual. Rahway: Merck Research Laboratories.
3. McQuaid KR. (2008) Gastrointestinal disorders. In: McPhee SJ, Papadakis MA, editors. Current medical diagnosis and treatment 2009. 46th ed. New York: McGraw-Hill.
4. Saad RJ. Chey WD. (2007) Breath tests for gastrointestinal disease: the real deal or just a lot of hot air? Gastroenterology, 133(6): 1763–6.
5. Van Leeuwen AM. Poelhuis-Leth DJ. (2009) Davis's comprehensive handbook of laboratory and diagnostic tests with nursing implications. 3rd ed. Philadelphia: FA Davis Company.
6. Genova Diagnostics. (2008) Comprehensive digestive stool analysis. Asheville: Genova Diagnostics.
7. Atkinson W et al (2004) Food elimination based on IgG antibodies in irritable bowel syndrome: a randomised controlled trial. Gut, 53(10): 1459–64.
8. Ford AC et al (2008) Effect of fibre, antispasmodics, and peppermint oil in the treatment of irritable bowel syndrome: systematic review and meta-analysis. British Medical Journal, 337: a2313.
9. Hoveyda N et al (2009) A systematic review and meta-analysis: probiotics in the treatment of irritable bowel syndrome. BMC Gastroenterology, 9: 15.
10. Keefer L. Blanchard EB. (2001) The effects of relaxation response meditation on the symptoms of irritable bowel syndrome: results of a controlled treatment study. Behaviour Research and Therapy, 39(7): 801–11.
11. Kuttner L et al (2006) A randomized trial of yoga for adolescents with irritable bowel syndrome. Pain Research and Management, 11(4): 217–23.
12. Muller A et al (2006) Osteopathy as a promising short-term strategy for irritable bowel syndrome: a randomized controlled trial. Osteopathische Medizin, 7(3): 20–1.
13. Niec AM. Frankum B. Talley NJ. (1998) Are adverse food reactions linked to irritable bowel syndrome? American Journal of Gastroenterology, 93(11): 2184–90.
14. Stefanini GF et al (1995) Oral cromolyn sodium in comparison with elimination diet in the irritable bowel syndrome, diarrheic type. Multicenter study of 428 patients. Scandinavian Journal of Gastroenterology, 30(6): 535–41.
15. Leri O et al (1997) Management of diarrhoeic type of irritable bowel syndrome with exclusion diet and disodium cromoglycate. Inflammopharmacology, 5(2): 153–8.
16. Gropper SS. Smith JL. Groff JL. (2008) Advanced nutrition and human metabolism. 5th ed. Belmond: Cengage Learning.
17. Zijdenbos IL et al (2009) Psychological treatments for the management of irritable bowel syndrome. Cochrane Database of Systematic Reviews, (1): CD006442.
18. Taneja I et al (2004) Yogic versus conventional treatment in diarrhea-predominant irritable bowel syndrome: a randomized control study. Applied Psychophysiology and Biofeedback, 29(1): 190–33.
19. Braun L. Cohen M. (2007) Herbs and natural supplements: an evidence-based guide. 2nd ed. Sydney: Elsevier Australia.
20. Tarpila S et al (2004) Efficacy of ground flaxseed on constipation in patients with irritable bowel syndrome. Current Topics in Nutraceuticals Research, 2(2): 119–25.
21. Olesen M. Gudmand-Hoyer E. (2000) Efficacy, safety, and tolerability of fructooligosaccharides in the treatment of irritable bowel syndrome. American Journal of Clinical Nutrition, 72(6): 1570–5.
22. Lee YK. Salminen S. (2009) Handbook of probiotics and probiotics. 2nd ed. Oxford: Wiley.
23. Lantz RC et al (2005) The effect of turmeric extracts on inflammatory mediator production. Phytomedicine, 12(6–7): 445–52.
24. Itthipanichpong C et al (2003) Antispasmodic effects of curcuminoids on isolated guinea-pig ileum and rat uterus. Journal of the Medical Association of Thailand, 86(Suppl 2): S299–309.
25. Xia X et al (2006) Ethanolic extracts from Curcuma longa attenuates behavioral, immune, and neuroendocrine alterations in a rat chronic mild stress model. Biological and Pharmaceutical Bulletin, 29(5): 938–44.
26. Bundy R et al (2004) Turmeric extract may improve irritable bowel syndrome symptomology in otherwise healthy adults: a pilot study. Journal of Alternative and Complementary Medicine, 10(6): 1015–18.
27. Walker AF. Middleton RW. Petrowicz O. (2001) Artichoke leaf extract reduces symptoms of irritable bowel syndrome in a post-marketing surveillance study. Phytotherapy Research, 15(1): 58–61.
28. Bundy R et al (2004b) Artichoke leaf extract reduces symptoms of irritable bowel syndrome and improves quality of life in otherwise healthy volunteers suffering from concomitant dyspepsia: a subset analysis. Journal of Alternative and Complementary Medicine, 10(4): 667–9.
29. Grigoleit HG. Grigoleit P. (2005) Pharmacology and preclinical pharmacokinetics of peppermint oil. Phytomedicine, 12(8): 612–16.
30. Jalili T. Medeiros DM. Wildman REC. (2006) Dietary fiber and coronary heart disease. In: Wildman REC, editor. Handbook of nutraceuticals and functional foods. 2nd ed. Boca Raton: CRC Press.
31. O'Brien KA. Xue CC. (2003) Acupuncture. In: Robson T, editor. An introduction to complementary medicine. Sydney: Allen & Unwin.
32. Lim B et al (2006) Acupuncture for treatment of irritable bowel syndrome. Cochrane Database of Systematic Reviews, (4): CD005111.
33. Schneider A et al (2006) Acupuncture treatment in irritable bowel syndrome. Gut, 55(5): 649–54.
34. Reynolds JA. Bland JM. MacPherson H. (2008) Acupuncture for irritable bowel syndrome an exploratory randomised controlled trial. Acupuncture in Medicine, 26(1): 8–16.
35. Hundscheid HW et al (2007) Treatment of irritable bowel syndrome with osteopathy: results of a randomized controlled pilot study. Journal of Gastroenterology and Hepatology, 22(9): 1394–8.
36. Bishop E et al (2003) Reflexology in the management of encopresis and chronic constipation. Paediatric Nursing, 15(3): 20–1.
37. Kunz B. Kunz K. (2003) Findings in research about safety, efficiency, mechanism of action, and cost effectiveness of reflexology (revised). Albuquerque: RRP Press.
38. Tovey P. (2002) A single-blind trial of reflexology for irritable bowel syndrome. British Journal of General Practice, 52(474): 19–23.
39. Wacher VJ. Wong S. Wong HT. (2001) Peppermint oil enhances cyclosporine oral bioavailability in rats: Comparison with D-α-tocopheryl poly(ethylene glycol) 1000) succinate (TPGS) and Ketoconazole. Journal of Pharmaceutical Sciences, 91(1): 77–90.

# Case 8
# Migraine

## Description of migraine

### Definition
Migraine is a complex neurovascular disorder characterised by episodic headaches. The two major categories of migraine are classic migraine (i.e. migraine with aura) and common migraine (i.e. migraine without aura). Other variants of the disorder are chronic migraine (i.e. producing ≥15 attacks per month), hemiplegic migraine (i.e. associated with defects to chromosomes 1, 2 and 19) and basilar artery migraine (i.e. caused by verte-brobasilar ischaemia).[1,2]

### Epidemiology
Migraine typically begins in adolescence. The prevalence of the condition increases from this point, peaking around age 40 and declining thereafter. In the US, migraine affects around eighteen per cent of women and six per cent of men.[3] The higher prevalence rate reported in the female population is evident across all age groups, except for the prepubescent period, in which migraine is relatively more common in males. Migraine is also more prevalent among Caucasians, particularly Europeans and Americans; it is least prevalent in the African and Asian populations.[3]

### Aetiology and pathophysiology
The aetiology and pathophysiology of migraine are complex and still not completely understood. Genetic predisposition is likely to be a contributing factor, although not all cases have a familial tendency.[4] Even though specific causes of migraine have yet to be established, a number of triggers have been identified. Intrinsic triggers, such as oestrogen fluctuation, brain serotonin depletion, temporomandibular joint dysfunction, emotional stress, excessive or inadequate sleep and neck pain, as well as extrinsic triggers such as tyramine-containing foods (i.e. cheese, red wine, choco-late, preserved meats), monosodium glutamate, weather changes (such as increased temperature or elevated barometric pressure), head trauma, hormone therapy, oral contraceptive use, strong odours, intense or flashing light and skipped meals, have all been associated with the onset of migraine.[1,2,5] It is also suggested that nutritional deficiency, specifically, magnesium deficiency, could play a role in the pathogenesis of migraine.[6-8]

Genetic predisposition and/or risk factors as yet unknown may lower an individual's threshold to these triggers, upon exposure to which, susceptible individuals may experience a reduction in cerebral blood flow, which, in some people, may manifest as an aura. The cortical spreading depression (CSD) of blood flow from the occipital lobe to other regions of the cerebral cortex, which may be preceded by brain sero-tonin depletion, triggers the diffuse activation of perivascular trigeminal sensory nerves.[5] These impulses are transmitted to the trigeminal nucleus caudalis of the brainstem and from there to the periaqueductal grey matter, sensory thalamus and sensory cortex. The stimulation of these regions results in the manifestation of pain.[2,4]

There are several deviations from this theory, however. Some argue that the pain of migraine is simply a rebound vasodilatatory response to CSD. Others propose that the activation of the trigeminovascular system increases neuropeptide release, which results in painful inflammation to the dura mater and cranial vessels.[1] Still others have also indicated that migraine may be the result of mitochondrial dysfunction and a subsequent impairment in cellular oxygen metabolism.[9] While researchers do not completely agree on the pathophysiology of migraine, there is general agreement that migraine is a neuro-vascular disorder.

## Clinical manifestations

The International Headache Society (IHS) defines migraine as a repeated, episodic headache of 4–72 hours duration that is characterised by any two of the following: unilateral distribution, throbbing quality, moderate or severe intensity and/or worsened by movement. To complete the IHS criteria, the pain also should be accompanied by nausea and vomiting, or photophobia and phonophobia.[4] It is not unusual for individuals with migraine to also experience osmophobia, poor concentration, blurred vision, clumsiness, localised weakness, numbness or tingling, irritability and scalp tenderness.[1,2]

In cases of classic migraine, the headache is preceded by a temporary neurological disturbance known as an aura. This phenomenon typically presents as a visual defect (e.g. bright zigzags, scintillating lights), but may also manifest as a sensory or motor disturbance (e.g. paraesthesias, dysarthria, ataxia, confusion).[2] Hemiplegic migraine generally presents as unilateral weakness, and basilar artery migraine as focal weakness, vertigo, ataxia and altered consciousness.[1] The symptoms of migraine are often aggravated by bright lights, noise, strong odours and physical activity, and are somewhat relieved following seclusion in a dark, quiet environment.[1]

---

## Clinical case
*35-year-old woman with classic migraine*

### Rapport

Adopt the practitioner strategies and behaviours highlighted in Table 2.1 (chapter 2) to improve client trust, communication and rapport, as well as the accuracy and comprehensiveness of the clinical assessment.

### Assessment

Once measures have been put into place to build client–practitioner rapport, the clinician can begin the clinical assessment.

Health history

**History of presenting condition**

A 35-year-old woman is referred to the clinic for complementary management of migraine. The client was diagnosed with classic migraine at the age of 17 years and has, in conjunction with her general practitioner, been managing the condition with Mersyndol Forte® (paracetamol, codeine phosphate and doxylamine succinate) and metoclopramide, and, in severe cases, with pethidine and metoclopramide. The headaches, which occur every 3–6 weeks, are preceded by a visual aura, specifically, bright zigzags, and typically last 4–6 hours. The client describes the migraine as pulsating, non-radiating and unilateral. In most cases, the pain is of moderate intensity (pain score = 6/10). The pain is almost always accompanied by nausea, photophobia, phonophobia and blurred vision, and, infrequently, by vomiting. Bright light and emotional stress often trigger the condition, but not always. The onset of migraine is not associated with the consumption of any particular foods or with any stages of the menstrual cycle. Physical activity, bright light and noise aggravate the condition. While the client obtains moderate relief of symptoms from the aforementioned analgesics and from seclusion in a dark, quiet room, these strategies are only palliative. The client is now seeking alternative treatment options to decrease the frequency and intensity of migraine in order to improve her quality of life.

**Medical history**

**Family history**

Mother suffers from migraine headaches, grandfather has Parkinson's disease.

**Allergies**
Nil.

**Medications**
Mersyndol Forte® 2 tablets 4-hourly as needed, metoclopramide 10 mg 4-hourly as needed, 1 multivitamin daily.

**Medical conditions**
Classic migraine, tension headaches.

**Surgical or investigational procedures**
Bilateral carpal tunnel release (2002).

## Lifestyle history

**Tobacco use**
Nil.

**Alcohol consumption**
Consumes one standard glass of red wine 6–7 times a week.

**Illicit drug use**
Nil.

| Diet and fluid intake | |
| --- | --- |
| Breakfast | Black tea, white English muffin with butter. |
| Morning tea | Apple, banana, orange. |
| Lunch | White wrap with lettuce, cheese, chicken and avocado, quiche with mixed green salad. |
| Afternoon tea | Black tea, mixed nuts (e.g. almonds, cashews, Brazil nuts). |
| Dinner | Grilled whiting or chicken breast with steamed carrots, beans and potato au gratin, cream of chicken soup or potato and leek soup with white bread. |
| Fluid intake | 2–4 cups of black tea a day, 2–3 cups of water a day. |
| **Food frequency** | |
| Fruit | 1–2 serves daily |
| Vegetables | 2–4 serves daily |
| Dairy | 2–3 serves daily |
| Cereals | 3–4 serves daily |
| Red meat | 0–1 serve a week |
| Chicken | 3 serves a week |
| Fish | 1–2 serves a week |
| Takeaway/fast food | 0–1 time a week |

**Quality and duration of sleep**
Interrupted sleep; has difficulty falling asleep (sleep latency of approximately 1–1.5 hours); average duration is 5–6 hours.

**Frequency and duration of exercise**
Drives to work. Walks the dog 1–2 times a week for 20 minutes. Engages in incidental exercise (e.g. cleaning, gardening, shopping) less than 3 hours a day and sedentary activities (e.g. desk-bound activities, television) more than 7 hours a day.

## Socioeconomic background

The client was born in Canada, as was her mother. Her father was born in France. Upon completing her social work degree 13 years ago, the client moved interstate and took up residence in an inner city apartment. The client has seen very little of her parents and siblings since the move, which upsets her at times. The client works in a general hospital as a senior social worker and, while she enjoys her chosen career and the company of her work colleagues during and outside normal working hours, the work is very demanding and stressful. The client is single with no children and there are no notable religious or cultural beliefs to report.

## Physical examination

### Inspection
Client is alert, cooperative, appropriately dressed, well-groomed and maintains good attention and eye contact. No anomalies in coordination, posture or gait are evident during standing, sitting or ambulation. Cranial nerves I to XII are grossly intact, with extraocular muscles intact. Pupils are equal and reactive to light and accommodation, and face, palate and neck and shoulder muscles are symmetrical. There is no sign of muscular atrophy to the neck, back, shoulders, upper limbs or lower limbs.

### Olfaction
There is no loss of smell or perception of abnormal odours. There is no abnormal odour to the client.

### Palpation
Paranasal sinuses are non-tender. There is no tenderness to the head, neck, spine or shoulders. Range of motion of the neck, spine and shoulders is unremarkable. Peripheral sensory examination is intact to light touch and pinprick.

### Percussion
All deep tendon reflexes are normal.

### Auscultation
The client expresses concerns about the migraine headaches in a calm, clear, well-paced and articulate manner. There is no evidence of obsessions, compulsions, delusions, paranoid thoughts or impaired memory recall and retention. Client is oriented to time, place and person.

### Additional signs
Client is afebrile (36.4°C, per oral), weight is high-normal (BMI is 24.8 kg/m$^2$, waist circumference is 75 cm) and blood pressure is high-normal (138/86).

### Clinical assessment tools
Client responses to the 14 items in the migraine-specific quality of life questionnaire (MSQ v.2.1) show migraine headaches have a moderate impact on the client's quality of life. Specifically, migraine was shown to have a modest impact on role restriction (55/100), role prevention (73/100) and emotional functioning (62/100); higher scores were indicative of greater function.

## Diagnostics
CAM practitioners can request, perform and/or interpret findings from a range of diagnostic tests in order to add valuable data to the pool of clinical information. While several investigations are pertinent to this case (as described below), the decision to use these tests should be considered alongside factors such as cost, convenience, comfort, turnaround time, access, practitioner competence and scope of practice, and history of previous investigations.

### Pathology tests

#### Magnesium deficiency test
Magnesium deficiency may be implicated in the pathogenesis of migraine.[6–8] Intracellular and/or extracellular magnesium concentration may be measured using a range

of different specimens – hair, erythrocytes, serum, urine and faeces. While some authorities indicate that erythrocytic magnesium concentration may be more sensitive than other methods in measuring magnesium levels,[10] there has been little rigorous research to substantiate this argument. In fact, studies suggest that hair magnesium may be a more sensitive measure of magnesium concentration than erythrocytic magnesium, and serum magnesium the least sensitive.[11] Thus, assessing hair or erythrocytic magnesium concentration may help to determine whether magnesium deficiency is a contributing factor in this condition.

**Radiology tests**
X-ray, CT, MRI and/or PET are indicated only if the migraine is believed to be caused by an underlying condition, such as stroke, chronic sinusitis, vertebral anomaly, or space-occupying lesion.

**Functional tests**
Not applicable.

**Invasive tests**
Invasive tests are not usually required for a diagnosis of migraine unless serious underlying pathology is a suspected cause of the migraine, in which case a lumbar puncture may be performed to rule out conditions such as encephalitis or meningitis.

**Miscellaneous tests**
Electroencephalogram (EEG) measures the electrical activity of the brain by placing electrodes on an individual's scalp. The abnormal frequency, characteristics and amplitude of these brain wave patterns, either at rest or following stimulation, may indicate the presence and location of epilepsy. An EEG may be indicated if epilepsy is believed to be masquerading as migraine.[12]

## Diagnosis

Clusters of data extracted from the health history, clinical examination and pertinent diagnostic test results point towards the following differential CAM diagnosis.
- Headache (actual), *secondary to* classic migraine, *related to* genetic predisposition (*client's mother has a history of migraine*), emotional stress (*client is employed in a stressful occupation, and is often upset by the lack of contact with her family*), inadequate sleep (*client reports poor-quality sleep, including an interrupted sleep pattern, long sleep latency and short sleep duration*), bright lights (*client identifies bright lights as being a trigger of migraine*), magnesium deficiency (*magnesium deficiency may predispose a person to migraine attacks; the client regularly consumes alcohol and caffeine, which can decrease magnesium absorption and increase urinary excretion; this should be confirmed by measuring hair/red blood cell (RBC) magnesium concentration*), and food intolerance (*client frequently consumes high tyramine-containing foods such as red wine and cheese – these foods may trigger migraine attacks in susceptible individuals*).

## Planning

The goals and expected outcomes that best serve the client's needs, and are most relevant to this case (as determined by the clinical assessment and CAM diagnoses), are as follows.

Goals
1 Client will report an improvement in migraine headaches (*client is seeking a reduction in the frequency and intensity of migraine attacks*).

2 Client will demonstrate an improvement in migraine-specific quality of life (*client is seeking an improvement in her quality of life*).

## Expected outcomes

Based on the degree of improvement reported in clinical studies that have used CAM interventions for the management of migraine,[13–17] the following are anticipated:

1 Client will demonstrate a forty-five per cent reduction in the baseline frequency of migraine attacks in 13 weeks or by dd/mm/yyyy (measured by headache diary).
2 Client will report a forty per cent decrease in baseline duration of migraine headaches in 13 weeks or by dd/mm/yyyy (measured by a 0–10 numerical pain scale).
3 Client will exhibit a forty per cent increase in baseline migraine-specific quality of life in 13 weeks or by dd/mm/yyyy (measured by MSQ).

## Application

The range of interventions reported in the CAM literature that may be used in the treatment of migraine are appraised below.

### Diet

**Low antigenic diet (Level II, Strength C, Direction + (for oligoantigenic diet only))**
Tyramine-containing foods, such as cheese, red wine, chocolate and preserved meats, and food additives such as monosodium glutamate, are considered to be key dietary triggers of migraine headache.[1,2] Even though many studies have explored the relationship between these triggers and the onset of migraine, the evidence is not convincing. Several dietary studies have, for instance, reported a large reduction in migraine frequency during the consumption of an oligoantigenic diet and the provocation of migraine attacks following double-blind challenges with suspected dietary triggers.[18–20] These findings should be considered with caution given the small size of the studies and the lack of corroborating evidence from larger trials.

Several controlled clinical trials have also demonstrated an increased incidence of migraine attacks following the consumption of low tyramine-containing red wine[21] and aspartame[22] when compared with controls, but many studies have failed to find a statistically significant difference in migraine frequency in groups receiving tyramine,[23] chocolate[24] or a low vasoactive amine diet[25] when compared with controls. This is corroborated by findings from a systematic review of 10 RCTs exploring the relationship between oral ingestion of biogenic amines and food intolerance reactions.[26] The discrepancies between these research findings and those reported in the professional literature need to be resolved to minimise clinician confusion about the best practice care of migraine.

### Lifestyle

**Guided imagery (Level II, Strength B, Direction o)**
Guided imagery is a mind–body technique that requires an individual to visualise images and/or imagine tastes, smells, sensations and sounds in order to induce relaxation, facilitate healing and/or alter behaviours and thoughts. This suggests that guided imagery could help to reduce migraine frequency by alleviating emotional stress, a known trigger of migraine. Two RCTs have explored this hypothesis, with mixed results. The trial by Brown[27] compared two different guided imagery approaches to a subconscious reconditioning control (5 × 1-hour sessions over 4 weeks) in 39 adults with migraine headache. The improvement in composite headache score (i.e. changes in headache frequency, duration, intensity and headache-free days) at 4 weeks significantly favoured guided imagery over control. Ilacqua[28] found no statistically significant difference between guided imagery, psychosynthetic approach or biofeedback and control in reducing migraine activity after six sessions

of training. Subjects receiving guided imagery or mind–body therapy did report an increased capacity to cope with pain, as well as a reduced perception of pain when compared with subjects receiving control. Even so, changes in medication use between groups were not statistically significant in either study. The evidence of effectiveness for guided imagery and migraine can thus be said to be inconclusive.

### Meditation (Level II, Strength C, Direction +)

Meditation is a mind–body therapy that uses a diverse range of techniques, such as mindfulness, breathing, concentration, visualisation, mantras and/or affirmations, to bring about inner tranquillity and/or improve self-awareness. A 1985 report of three cases highlighted the possible benefit of meditation in reducing migraine headache,[29] but it was not until more recently that the use of meditation for migraine was examined under randomised controlled conditions. The RCT compared the effects of three meditative techniques – spiritual meditation, internally focused secular meditation and externally focused secular meditation – to muscle relaxation in 83 meditation naïve migraine sufferers. After 4 weeks of treatment for 20 minutes a day, spiritual meditation was found to be statistically significantly more effective than the other three interventions in reducing headache frequency and pain tolerance, but not headache severity.[30] Whether other forms of meditation are any more effective than spiritual meditation in improving migraine symptoms is yet to be determined.

### Relaxation therapy (Level I for children, Level II for adults, Strength C, Direction +)

Relaxation therapy describes a collection of mind–body techniques that induce the relaxation response, which in turn lessens sympathetic nervous system activity. Utilising these techniques in the management of migraine has been an area of much study over the past three decades, most of which has been conducted in children,[31,32] though a few clinical trials were conducted in adults.[33,34] Evidence from these trials is generally consistent. It indicates that relaxation therapy either alone (e.g. progressive muscle relaxation, breathing exercises) or in combination with other behavioural techniques (e.g. stress management, biofeedback, cognitive training) is significantly superior to controls (e.g. metoprolol, physical therapy, waiting list, attention control, neutral writing) in reducing migraine severity, particularly headache frequency, immediately after treatment and at follow-up. Although the best available evidence is in favour of relaxation therapy, the real challenge for clinicians, given the heterogeneous treatment durations, outcome measures and treatment combinations used, will be to apply these findings to clinical practice.

### Yoga (Level II, Strength B, Direction +)

Yoga is an ancient Indian practice that integrates stretching, exercise, posture and breathing with meditation. Given that these techniques are likely to induce a relaxation response, yoga may be helpful in alleviating stress-induced migraine. Two RCTs have examined the effectiveness of yoga in people with common migraine (n = 72)[14] and migraine or tension headache (n = 20).[16] Both trials reported a statistically significant improvement in headache activity (i.e. migraine intensity and frequency) and symptomatic medication use following yoga therapy when compared with controls at 3–4 months. Both studies are, though, considered to be at moderate risk of bias because of insufficient detail relating to allocation concealment and intention-to-treat analysis.

## Nutritional supplementation

### Coenzyme Q10 (Level II, Strength B, Direction +)

Defective energy metabolism, secondary to mitochondrial dysfunction, is implicated in the pathogenesis of migraine.[9] Thus, substances that improve mitochondrial function, such as CoQ10, may play a role in migraine prevention. Several open-label trials suggest CoQ10 supplementation (150 mg daily for 3 months) may be effective in reducing the frequency and duration of attacks in people with migraine;[35,36] evidence from a double-blind RCT corroborates these findings.[37] The trial involving

42 migraine sufferers found that CoQ10 supplementation (300 mg daily) for 3 months was significantly more effective than placebo in reducing migraine frequency and duration, and the number of days with nausea. In fact, the percentage of subjects in each group whose degree of improvement in attack frequency reached or exceeded 50 per cent was 47.6 per cent for the CoQ10 group and 14.4 per cent for the placebo group. These positive findings now require replication in larger trials.

### Magnesium (Level II, Strength B, Direction + (for magnesium citrate and magnesium oxide only))

Magnesium is involved in many enzymatic reactions and physiological processes throughout the body. While its role in migraine is not clear, it is suggested that migraine may be a magnesium deficiency disease, with several studies demonstrating comparatively lower levels of brain,[7] salivary, serum[6,8] and red blood cell magnesium[8] in migraine sufferers than non-migraine sufferers. It is plausible, therefore, that magnesium supplementation may improve the symptoms of migraine. According to findings from three double-blind RCTs (n = 201 adults), this appears to be the case, with oral magnesium citrate (600 mg daily) found to be statistically significantly more effective than placebo in reducing migraine frequency.[15,17,38] In terms of improving migraine severity, the evidence is mixed. Studies using other forms of magnesium have produced contrasting results. One RCT, involving 118 children and adolescents with migraine, found magnesium oxide supplementation (253.5–760.5 mg daily) for 16 weeks to be superior to placebo in reducing migraine severity, but no more effective than placebo in decreasing migraine frequency.[39] An RCT (n = 69 adults) using magnesium aspartate (486 mg daily for 12 weeks) reported no significant difference in the frequency or duration of migraine between those receiving magnesium and those on placebo.[40] What these findings reveal is that supplementation with oral magnesium citrate is likely to be effective in migraine prophylaxis and that magnesium oxide may be effective in the treatment of migraine.

### Niacin (Level I, Strength C, Direction +)

Vitamin $B_3$ is responsible for a wide range of biological functions. Several of these actions are particularly relevant to migraine management, namely, the ability to dilate intracranial vessels and to maintain adequate mitochondrial energy metabolism.[41] Weak evidence from a systematic review of three case reports suggests that orally administered niacin (300–500 mg of variable duration) may reduce headache frequency in people with a history of migraine.[41] Despite these findings, all studies were small, lacked controls and were at high risk of bias, which limits any conclusions that can be drawn.

### Riboflavin (Level II, Strength B, Direction + (in adults only))

Vitamin $B_2$ is a water-soluble vitamin that plays an important role in cellular respiration, a function that may help to improve mitochondrial energy efficiency and, in so doing, may address the underlying mitochondrial dysfunction associated with migraine.[9] Several studies have examined the clinical effectiveness of riboflavin for migraine prophylaxis, with the best available evidence arising from two double-blind RCTs. The first trial found oral riboflavin (400 mg daily for 12 weeks) to be significantly superior to placebo in reducing headache frequency and duration in 55 adults with migraine.[42] In children (n = 48), riboflavin supplementation (200 mg daily for 4 weeks) was found to be no more effective than placebo at improving migraine frequency, severity and duration, analgesic use and days with nausea and vomiting.[43] Although the latter study indicates riboflavin may not be effective in preventing migraine in children, it is possible that the short treatment duration and lower dose of riboflavin could have influenced the outcomes of the study.

### Omega 3 fatty acids (Level II, Strength B, Direction o)

Neurogenic inflammation and subsequent neurogenic vasodilatation are believed to be contributing factors in the pathophysiology of migraine headache.[44] Anti-inflammatory agents, such as omega 3 fatty acids,[45] may help to attenuate neurogenic inflammation and, in turn, prevent the onset of migraine. In spite of this theoretically plausible hypothesis, evidence from two double-bind RCTs fails to support this theory. Both trials showed oral supplementation of omega 3 fatty acids (2–6 g daily for 8–16 weeks) to be no more effective than placebo (olive oil) in reducing migraine frequency, severity, duration or analgesic use in adults (n = 196)[46] and adolescents (n = 27)[47] with a history of migraine. These findings should be interpreted with caution as the effect of olive oil in migraine headaches cannot be dismissed as just a placebo effect.

## Quercetin and vitamin C
These nutrients exhibit actions that are considered desirable in the management of migraine, in particular, anti-inflammatory activity. In theory, pyridoxine may also help to reduce migraine symptoms by improving serotonin synthesis. Even so, there is insufficient clinical evidence to justify the administration of these nutrients in people with migraine.

## Herbal medicine
### *Petasites vulgaris* (Level I, Strength B, Direction + (for adults only))
Butterbur was traditionally used as a treatment for gastrointestinal, respiratory and urogenital complaints. Evidence of anti-inflammatory and vasodilatory activity in experimental studies suggest this herb may be useful in migraine prophylaxis.[13] Evidence from a systematic review of three RCTs (n = 365) concluded that butterbur root extract (100–150 mg daily for 12–16 weeks) was superior to placebo in reducing the frequency of migraine attacks in adults.[13] A more recent trial, which involved 58 primary school children, found butterbur to be no more effective than placebo or music therapy at reducing attack frequency at 12 weeks. Interestingly, both butterbur and music therapy demonstrated a statistically significant reduction in attack frequency when compared with placebo at 8 weeks follow-up.[48] While the results are promising for adult migraine sufferers, larger trials of longer duration are required before any firm conclusions can be drawn about the efficacy of butterbur in childhood migraine.

### *Tanacetum parthenium* (Level I, Strength B, Direction o)
Feverfew has long been used in the treatment and prevention of migraine headaches. Its use is supported by data from experimental studies that have shown the plant to exhibit analgesic,[49] anti-inflammatory[50] and vasodilator activity.[51] Findings from a Cochrane review of five RCTs (n = 343), and results from a more recent double-blind RCT (n = 170), are mixed in terms of change in global migraine scores, migraine frequency and severity, and nausea and vomiting.[52,53] Between study differences in feverfew dosage, method of preparation (including the use of $CO_2$ extracts, dried extracts and ethanolic extracts) and treatment duration (4–24 weeks) also do not allow for the pooling of results, which indicates that the effectiveness of feverfew in the prevention and/or treatment of migraine is inconclusive.

## Other herbs
Even though *Chelidonium majus* (greater celandine), *Harpagophytum procumbens* (devil's claw), *Oenothera biennis* (evening primrose), *Paeonia lactiflora* (peony), *Piscidia erythrina* (Jamaican dogwood), *Tabebuia avellanedae* (pau d'arco), *Tilia* spp. (lime blossom), *Valeriana officinalis* (valerian) and *Verbena officinalis* (vervain) have all been used traditionally and/or tested under experimental conditions for their analgesic, sedative and/or anti-inflammatory activity, there is insufficient clinical data to support their use (as monopreparations) in the prevention or treatment of migraine.

## Other
### Acupuncture (Level I, Strength B, Direction +)
Acupuncture originated in China more than 4000 years ago.[54] This ancient therapy has long been used as a treatment for many acute and chronic conditions, including migraine. Its use as a treatment for migraine is supported by a Cochrane review of

22 RCTs involving 4419 participants. The review found acupuncture treatment to be significantly superior to acute treatment or routine care in reducing headache frequency, headache days and headache scores 3–4 months after randomisation, as effective as prophylactic drug treatment in reducing analgesic use and migraine attacks, and significantly superior to prophylactic drug treatment in improving migraine days and intensity 2–6 months after randomisation. Comparisons with routine care and prophylactic drug treatment could, though, be biased due to inadequate blinding and high dropout rates, respectively. When true acupuncture was compared with sham acupuncture, no statistically significant difference in participant outcomes was observed.[55] Given that, in several of the trials, the sham acupuncture technique could not be distinguished from true acupuncture suggests that the sham intervention may not have been physiologically inert, which might have confounded the results.

### Chiropractic (Level II, Strength B, Direction +)

Chiropractic manipulation is generally prescribed for the treatment of musculoskeletal and nervous disorders, including migraine. Three RCTs have explored the effectiveness of chiropractic manipulation in migraine prevention, two of which were reported in a systematic review of the literature.[56] Two of the trials found chiropractic spinal manipulative therapy (SMT) for 8 weeks to be significantly more effective than control in improving migraine frequency, duration, disability and medication use (n = 127)[57] and as effective as amitriptyline in reducing headache index scores (n = 218).[58] Findings from the latter study should be interpreted with caution as the trial may not have been adequately powered to test for therapeutic equivalence.[56] The third RCT (n = 85) measured changes in migraine frequency, duration and disability in groups receiving SMT performed by a chiropractor, SMT provided by a physiotherapist or medical practitioner, or mobilisation control performed by a physiotherapist or medical practitioner.[59] No statistically significant differences were found between groups after 6 months of treatment, rendering the effectiveness of chiropractic SMT for migraine inconclusive, although findings from two of the three trials are promising.

### Homeopathy (Level I, Strength C, Direction + (for non-classical treatment only))

Homeopathy is a system of medicine that uses highly diluted and potentised remedies to influence the body's vital force and restore balance. The therapy can be used to treat a wide range of acute and chronic conditions, including migraine. According to a systematic review of three RCTs (n = 193) on homeopathy and migraine, results from clinical trials have been inconsistent.[60] For the two trials that used individualised homeopathic prescriptions, homeopathic treatment (over a 4-month period) was found to be no more effective than placebo in reducing the frequency, intensity and severity of migraine, or the level of medication required. The remaining trial, which administered a single dose of 30c potency four times over a 2-week period, found homeopathy to be significantly superior to placebo in reducing migraine frequency, intensity and severity; it also reduced the need for medication. At first glance, these findings suggest that individualised homeopathic treatment is ineffective for migraine, yet the low quality of these trials and the poor reporting of study procedures and results do not allow for any conclusions to be made.

### Massage (Level II, Strength B, Direction +)

Massage is the systematic manipulation of soft tissues of the body. This tactile therapy may be particularly helpful for migraine as it can help reduce anxiety and pain by stimulating parasympathetic nervous system activity, and elevate serotonin and endorphin release.[61] Findings from two RCTs (n = 74) show that massage therapy (either 45 minutes a week for 6 weeks or 30 minutes twice a week for 5 weeks) elevates urinary serotonin levels and lowers salivary cortisol levels, but more importantly, significantly improves migraine frequency and sleep quality when compared with controls.[62,63] Changes in migraine intensity and analgesic use were not consistent across studies. While these findings indicate massage may be of benefit to people suffering from migraine, evidence from much larger trials is still needed.

### Reflexology (Level IV, Strength D, Direction +)
The stimulation of specific zones of the feet, hands and/or ears to trigger neuro-physiological reflexes or responses in distant tissues, glands and organs is a guiding principle of reflexology. While evidence from a preliminary study suggests reflexology may be effective in reducing levels of perceived stress,[64] and thus may have a role in the management of migraine, rigorous clinical evidence is lacking. The best available evidence regarding the use of reflexology in migraine comes from a prospective, uncontrolled exploratory study.[65] Even though the study found individualised reflexology treatment for up to 6 months to be effective at reducing the incidence of headache and the level of analgesic use in 220 randomly selected patients with migraine or tension headache, the trial had major methodological limitations. The absence of a control intervention and blinding, for instance, meant the risk of bias was particularly high.

### Aromatherapy and osteopathy
There is insufficient clinical evidence supporting the use of these therapies in the management of migraine.

## CAM prescription
The CAM interventions that are most appropriate for the management of the presenting case – that is, they target the planned goals, expected outcomes and CAM diagnoses, they are supported by the best available evidence, they are pertinent to the client's needs and they are most relevant to CAM practice – are outlined below.

### Primary treatments
- Commence integrated yoga program (which is inclusive of yoga postures, yoga breathing, breathing practices, relaxation practices and meditation), aiming for 60 minutes, 5 days a week (*emotional stress is a probable trigger of the client's migraine headaches; yoga reduces emotional stress, and effectively decreases the intensity and frequency of migraine headaches*).
- Commence oral magnesium supplement, containing 600 mg magnesium citrate and 500 mg magnesium oxide, daily (*magnesium deficiency is a probable cause of the client's migraine headaches. A combined magnesium supplement will help to resolve the magnesium deficiency and reduce the severity and frequency of migraine*).
- Commence oral butterbur root extract, 100 mg daily (*butterbur effectively reduces migraine frequency, which may help to improve migraine-associated quality of life*).

### Secondary treatments
- Reduce consumption of tea (to 1–2 cups a day) (*magnesium deficiency is a probable cause of the client's migraine headaches and caffeinated beverages promote urinary losses of magnesium*).
- Minimise exposure to bright lights by wearing sunglasses where possible (*bright lights are a known trigger of the client's migraine headaches; minimising exposure to this trigger may reduce the frequency of migraine attacks, a recommendation based on theoretical evidentiary support only*).
- Establish good sleep hygiene: set times for settling and rising, avoid alcohol, caffeine or heavy meals before settling, develop a relaxing bedtime routine (e.g. mood lighting, yoga, relaxation music) (*inadequate sleep is a trigger of the client's migraine headaches; improving sleep hygiene may help to reduce sleep latency and improve sleep duration, and thus help to reduce the frequency of migraine, this recommendation being based on theoretical evidentiary support only*).

- Commence elimination diet. Have client avoid, for example, the consumption of potentially reactive foods and foods containing tyramine, artificial colours, flavours and/or preservatives for 1 week. After a 1-week elimination period, ask client to reintroduce a new food every 2 days and monitor the recurrence of migraine-related signs and symptoms. The presence or absence of any adverse reactions during these oral food challenges should be recorded in a food and lifestyle diary, and reviewed at the next consultation. The foods identified as being associated with migraine should be eliminated from the diet (*client consumes foods that may be implicated in the pathogenesis of migraine; eliminating the consumption of these dietary triggers may lessen the frequency and/or severity of migraine attacks*).
- Increase consumption of magnesium-containing foods, such as wholegrains, pumpkin seeds, nuts and spinach (*magnesium deficiency is a probable cause of the client's migraine headaches; increasing the consumption of dietary magnesium may help to sustain magnesium levels in the long term, a recommendation that is based on theoretical evidentiary support only*).

Referral
- Refer client to a general practitioner, family physician, neurologist or emergency department if the condition deteriorates, if serious pathology is suspected (such as a space-occupying lesion or trans-ischaemic attack) or if a serious complication arises (such as an ischaemic stroke).
- Refer client to another CAM practitioner if migraine, or the treatment of migraine, is outside the clinician's area of expertise.
- Liaise with the general practitioner about the client's overall management plan.

## Review

To determine whether pertinent client goals and expected outcomes have been achieved at follow-up and if any aspects of the client's care need to be improved, consider the factors listed in Table 8.2 (chapter 8), as well as the questions listed below.
1  Was there a decrease in the frequency of migraine attacks?
2  Was there a reduction in the intensity of migraine headaches?
3  Was there an improvement in migraine-specific quality of life?
4  Has the need for Mersyndol Forte,® pethidine and/or metoclopramide decreased?
5  Was there an improvement in other migraine-associated symptoms, such as nausea, vomiting, photophobia, phonophobia, blurred vision?

# References

1. Porter R et al, editors. (2008). The Merck manual. Rahway: Merck Research Laboratories.
2. Simon RP. Greenberg DA. Aminoff MJ. (2009) Clinical neurology. 7th ed. New York: McGraw-Hill.
3. Bigal ME. Lipton RB. (2008) The epidemiology and burden of headaches. In: Morris L, editor. Comprehensive review of headache medicine. New York: Oxford University Press.
4. Goadsby PJ. (2006) Recent advances in understanding migraine mechanisms, molecules and therapeutics. Trends in Molecular Medicine, 13(1): 39–44.
5. Schwedt TJ. (2008) Serotonin and migraine: the latest developments. Cephalalgia, 27(11): 1301–7.
6. Gallai V et al (1992) Serum and salivary magnesium levels in migraine: Results in a group of juvenile patients. Headache, 32(3): 132–5.
7. Ramadan NM et al (1989) Low brain magnesium in migraine. Headache, 29(9): 590–3.
8. Soriani S et al (1995) Serum and red blood cell magnesium levels in juvenile migraine patients. Headache, 35(1): 14–16.
9. Bianchi A et al (2004) Role of magnesium, coenzyme Q10, riboflavin, and vitamin $B_{12}$ in migraine prophylaxis. Vitamins and Hormones, 69: 297–312.
10. Stargrove MB. Treasure J. McKee DL. (2008) Herb, nutrient and drug interactions. St Louis: Mosby Elsevier.
11. Kozielec T. Starobrat-Hermelin B. (1997) Assessment of magnesium levels in children with attention deficit hyperactivity disorder (ADHD). Magnesium Research, 10(2): 143–8.
12. Pagana KD. Pagana TJ. (2008) Mosby's diagnostic and laboratory test reference. 9th ed. St Louis: Elsevier Mosby.

13. Giles M et al (2005) Butterbur: an evidence-based systematic review by the natural standard research collaboration. Journal of Herbal Pharmacotherapy, 5(3): 119–43.

14. John PJ et al (2007) Effectiveness of yoga therapy in the treatment of migraine without aura: a randomized controlled trial. Headache, 47(5): 654–61.

15. Koseoglu E et al (2008) The effects of magnesium prophylaxis in migraine without aura. Magnesium Research, 21(2): 101–8.

16. Latha M. Kaliappan KV. (1992) The efficacy of yoga therapy in the treatment of migraine and tension headaches. Journal of the Indian Academy of Applied Psychology, 13(2): 95–100.

17. Peikert A et al (1996) Prophylaxis of migraine with oral magnesium: results from a prospective, multi-center, placebo-controlled and double-blind randomized study. Cephalalgia, 16(4): 257–63.

18. Guariso G et al (1993) Migraine and food intolerance: a controlled study in pediatric patients. Medical & Surgical Pediatrics, 15(1): 57–61.

19. Egger J et al (1983) Is migraine a food allergy? A double-blind controlled trial of oligoantigenic diet treatment. Lancet, 2(8355): 865–9.

20. Mansfield LE et al (1985) Food allergy and adult migraine: double-blind and mediator confirmation of an allergic etiology. Annals of Allergy, 55(2): 126–9.

21. Littlewood JT et al (1988) Red wine as a cause of migraine. Lancet, 1(8585): 558–9.

22. Koehler SM. Glaros A. (1988) The effect of aspartame on migraine headache. Headache, 28(1): 10–14.

23. Ryan JRE. (1974) A clinical study of tyramine as an etiological factor in migraine. Headache, 14(1): 43–8.

24. Marcus DA et al (1997) A double-blind provocative study of chocolate as a trigger of headache. Cephalalgia, 17(8): 855–62.

25. Salfield SA et al (1987) Controlled study of exclusion of dietary vasoactive amines in migraine. Archives of Disease in Childhood, 62(5): 458–60.

26. Jansen SC et al (2003) Intolerance to dietary biogenic amines: a review. Annals of Allergy, Asthma and Immunology, 91(3): 233–40.

27. Brown JM. (1984) Imagery coping strategies in the treatment of migraine. Pain, 18(2): 157–67.

28. Ilacqua GE. (1994) Migraine headaches: coping efficacy of guided imagery training. Headache, 34(2): 99–102.

29. Lovell-Smith HD. (1985) Transcendental meditation and three cases of migraine. New Zealand Medical Journal, 98(780): 443–5.

30. Wachholtz AB. Pargament KI. (2008) Migraines and meditation: does spirituality matter? Journal of Behavioral Medicine, 31(4): 351–66.

31. Eccleston C et al (2009) Psychological therapies for the management of chronic and recurrent pain in children and adolescents. Cochrane Database of Systematic Reviews, (2): CD003968.

32. Osterhaus SO et al (1993) Effects of behavioral psychophysiological treatment on schoolchildren with migraine in a nonclinical setting: predictors and process variables. Journal of Pediatric Psychology, 18(6): 697–715.

33. D'Souza PJ et al (2008) Relaxation training and written emotional disclosure for tension or migraine headaches: a randomized, controlled trial. Annals of Behavioral Medicine, 36(1): 21–32.

34. Marcus DA et al (1998) Nonpharmacological treatment for migraine: incremental utility of physical therapy with relaxation and thermal biofeedback. Cephalalgia, 18(5): 266–72.

35. Hershey AD et al (2007) Coenzyme Q10 deficiency and response to supplementation in pediatric and adolescent migraine. Headache, 47(1): 73–80.

36. Rozen TD et al (2002) Open label trial of coenzyme Q10 as a migraine preventive. Cephalalgia, 22(2): 137–41.

37. Sandor PS et al (2005) Efficacy of coenzyme Q10 in migraine prophylaxis: a randomized controlled trial. Neurology, 64(4): 713–15.

38. Taubert K. (1994) Magnesium in migraine: results of a multicenter pilot study. Fortschritte der Medizin, 112(24): 328–30.

39. Wang F et al (2003) Oral magnesium oxide prophylaxis of frequent migrainous headache in children: a randomized, double-blind, placebo-controlled trial. Headache, 43(6): 601–10.

40. Pfaffenrath V et al (1996) Magnesium in the prophylaxis of migraine: a double-blind placebo-controlled study. Cephalalgia, 16(6): 436–40.

41. Prousky J. Seely D. (2005) The treatment of migraines and tension-type headaches with intravenous and oral niacin (nicotinic acid): systematic review of the literature. Nutrition Journal, 4: 3.

42. Schoenen J. Jacquy J. Lenaerts M. (1998) Effectiveness of high-dose riboflavin in migraine prophylaxis: a randomized controlled trial. Neurology, 50(2): 466–70.

43. MacLennan SC et al (2008) High-dose riboflavin for migraine prophylaxis in children: a double-blind, randomized, placebo-controlled trial. Journal of Child Neurology, 23(11): 1300–4.

44. Peroutka SJ. (2005) Neurogenic inflammation and migraine: implications for the therapeutics. Molecular Interventions, 5(5): 304–11.

45. Jho DH et al (2004) Role of omega-3 fatty acid supplementation in inflammation and malignancy. Integrative Cancer Therapies, 3(2): 98–111.

46. Pradalier A et al (2001) Failure of omega-3 polyunsaturated fatty acids in prevention of migraine: a double-blind study versus placebo. Cephalalgia, 21(8): 818–22.

47. Harel Z et al (2002) Supplementation with omega-3 polyunsaturated fatty acids in the management of recurrent migraines in adolescents. Journal of Adolescent Health, 31(2): 154–61.

48. Oelkers-Ax R et al (2008) Butterbur root extract and music therapy in the prevention of childhood migraine: an explorative study. European Journal of Pain, 12(3): 301–13.

49. Jain NK. Kulkarni SK. (1991) Antinociceptive and anti-inflammatory effects of Tanacetum parthenium L. extract in mice and rats. Journal of Ethnopharmacology, 68(1–3): 251–9.

50. Kwok BH et al (2001) The anti-inflammatory natural product parthenolide from the medicinal herb Feverfew directly binds to and inhibits IkappaB kinase. Chemistry and Biology, 8(8): 759–66.

51. Barsby RW et al (1992) Feverfew extracts and parthenolide irreversibly inhibit vascular responses of the rabbit aorta. Journal of Pharmacy and Pharmacology, 44(9): 737–40.

52. Diener HC et al (2005) Efficacy and safety of 6.25 mg t.i.d. feverfew CO2-extract (MIG-99) in migraine prevention: a randomized, double-blind, multicentre, placebo-controlled study. Cephalalgia, 25(11): 1031–41.

53. Pittler MH. Ernst E. (2004) Feverfew for preventing migraine. Cochrane Database of Systematic Reviews, (1): CD002286.

54. O'Brien KA. Xue CC. (2003) Acupuncture. In: Robson T, editor. An introduction to complementary medicine. Sydney: Allen & Unwin.

55. Linde K et al (2009) Acupuncture for migraine prophylaxis. Cochrane Database of Systematic Reviews, (1): CD001218.
56. Bronfort G et al (2001) Efficacy of spinal manipulation for chronic headache: a systematic review. Journal of Manipulative and Physiological Therapeutics, 24(7): 457–66.
57. Tuchin PJ. Pollard H. Bonello R. (2000) A randomized controlled trial of chiropractic spinal manipulative therapy for migraine. Journal of Manipulative and Physiological Therapeutics, 23(2): 91–5.
58. Nelson CF et al (1998) The efficacy of spinal manipulation, amitriptyline and the combination of both therapies for the prophylaxis of migraine headache. Journal of Manipulative and Physiological Therapeutics, 21(8): 511–19.
59. Parker GB. Tupling H. Pryor DS. (1978) A controlled trial of cervical manipulation of migraine. Australian and New Zealand Journal of Medicine, 8(6): 589–93.
60. Owen JM. Green BN. (2004) Homeopathic treatment of headaches: a systematic review of the literature. Journal of Chiropractic Medicine, 3(2): 45–52.

61. Moyer CA. Rounds J. Hannum JW. (2004) A meta-analysis of massage therapy research. Psychological Bulletin, 130(1): 3–18.
62. Hernandez-reif M et al (1998) Migraine headaches are reduced by massage therapy. International Journal of Neuroscience, 96(1–2): 1–11.
63. Lawler SP. Cameron LD. (2006) A randomized, controlled trial of massage therapy as a treatment for migraine. Annals of Behavioral Medicine, 32(1): 50–9.
64. Lee YM. (2006) Effect of self-foot reflexology massage on depression, stress responses and immune functions of middle aged women. Taehan Kanho Hakhoe Chi, 36(1): 179–88.
65. Launso L. Brendstrup E. Arnberg S. (1999) An exploratory study of reflexological treatment for headache. Alternative Therapies in Health and Medicine, 5(3): 57–65.

# Case 9
# Osteoarthritis

## Description of osteoarthritis

Definition
Osteoarthritis (OA) is a degenerative joint disease characterised by biochemical, cellular and structural changes to the articular cartilage, joint space and subchondral bone. The diarthrodial joints of the body, including the knees, hips and hands, are the most commonly affected. Depending on the aetiology of OA, the condition can be classified as either primary OA (idiopathic aetiology) or secondary OA. Secondary OA can be further defined as traumatic, metabolic, neuropathic, inflammatory or anatomic.[1]

Epidemiology
The prevalence of OA increases with advancing age. The prevalence rate of symptomatic OA in people under the age of 45 years, for example, is five per cent. Between the ages of 45 and 64 years, the prevalence rate increases to more than ten per cent, and over 75 years of age, to more than thirty per cent.[2] In radiological prevalence surveys, the prevalence rate of OA is much higher (i.e. more than fifty per cent of people over 65 years of age),[3] and in autopsy studies, even higher again (sixty to seventy per cent of people aged between 70 and 80 years).[4] The disease is also more prevalent in women than men, particularly radiologically confirmed hand and knee OA, with the female:male ratio varying between 1.5 and 4.0 across studies.[4]

Aetiology and pathophysiology
Many risk factors are associated with the pathogenesis of OA. Increasing age, female sex, ethnicity, congenital joint abnormalities and family history are some of the major non-modifiable risk factors of OA. The modifiable risk factors include obesity, repetitive joint loading (e.g. repetitive squatting, kneeling, lifting), trauma (e.g. fractures, dislocations, joint surgery, meniscal or cruciate ligament tears), diet (e.g. low vitamin D, vitamin C and fruit intake, and elevated omega 6 fatty acid intake), and quadricep weakness.[4] Several pathological conditions are also associated with the development of OA, including metabolic disease (e.g. haemochromatosis, hypothyroidism, Wilson's disease), joint inflammation or infection, neuropathy (e.g. Charcot's arthropathy) and cartilage disorders (e.g. rheumatoid arthritis, chondrocalcinosis).[5] All of these factors impair the integrity of joint tissue, causing direct damage to joint tissues, impairing repair processes or increasing joint susceptibility to injury.[4]

An initial insult to the joint stimulates chondrocyte activity, but at the same time triggers the release of inflammatory mediators from the synovium into the cartilage.[5] While the chondrocytes attempt to repair the tissue by increasing the production of proteoglycans and collagen, they do so in opposition to the actions of the inflammatory mediators and proteolytic enzymes, which cause cartilage degradation. When the equilibrium between proteoglycan synthesis and degradation shifts towards net degradation, damage to articular cartilage occurs. Over time, subchondral bone becomes exposed, eburnated, sclerotic and stiff, which results in osseous infarction and subchondral cyst formation. In an attempt to protect the subchondral bone and to stabilise the joint, the body produces osteophytes.[6] But instead of protecting the tissue, these spurs cause joint immobility and pain, and in some cases, synovitis. Eventually, joint mobility diminishes to such an extent that menisci fissure, supportive muscles weaken and periarticular tendons and ligaments become stressed, resulting in tendinitis and contractures.[5]

Clinical manifestations
OA is a progressive disease and, as such, may not present with any clinical manifestations in the early stages of development. Eventually, the client may begin to

experience deep, aching arthralgia in one or several joints, particularly the hips, knees and hands. This pain is often aggravated by exercise, weight-bearing activity and changing weather, and alleviated with rest.[7] As the disease progresses, joint stiffness develops, which is generally worse in the morning and after prolonged periods of rest. Further loss of articular cartilage results in reduced joint mobility, joint tenderness and crepitus. In the later stages of the disease, the client may experience joint instability and/or locking, muscle contractures and spasms. The structural changes to articular tissue, synovial thickening and joint effusion may also lead to joint enlargement.[5] The pain and functional impairment associated with this disease also contribute to significant disability and reduced quality of life.[2]

---

# Clinical case
*69-year-old woman with bilateral knee osteoarthritis*

## Rapport

Adopt the practitioner strategies and behaviours highlighted in Table 2.1 (chapter 2) to improve client trust, communication and rapport, as well as the accuracy and comprehensiveness of the clinical assessment.

## Assessment

Once measures have been put into place to build client–practitioner rapport, the clinician can begin the clinical assessment.

### Health history
**History of presenting condition**
A 69-year-old woman presents to the clinic complaining of bilateral knee pain, stiffness and reduced mobility secondary to OA. The knee pain is described as a constant deep dull ache of varying intensity. The pain is worse on rising in the morning (pain score = 6/10), after a period of walking (5/10) and in damp weather (5/10), but is alleviated with rest (3/10), ibuprofen (2/10) and cold packs (2/10). Bilateral knee stiffness accompanies the pain, which is worse after prolonged rest. The pain does not radiate and there are no concomitant symptoms. The client began to experience the pain approximately 5–6 years ago, but the pain has now reached the point where the client requires oral ibuprofen 400 mg three times a day. The client is reluctant to continue with this medication long term and is now seeking alternative treatment options.

### Medical history
**Family history**
Mother had severe OA, father had ischaemic heart disease.
**Allergies**
Nil known.
**Medications**
Perindopril 4 mg mane, Salbutamol inhaler as needed, ibuprofen 400 mg three times a day (self-prescribed), paracetamol 1 g 4-hourly as needed, vitamin B complex 1 daily.
**Medical conditions**
Hypertension, mild intermittent asthma, bilateral knee OA.
**Surgical or investigational procedures**
Appendicectomy (1972), cholecystectomy (1976).

### Lifestyle history
**Tobacco use**
Ceased smoking 20 years ago (inhaled up to 20 cigarettes a day).

**Alcohol consumption**
Social drinker. Drinks 1–2 glasses of white wine per week.
**Illicit drug use**
Nil.

| Diet and fluid intake | |
| --- | --- |
| Breakfast | Toasted white bread with marmalade, black tea. |
| Morning tea | Scones, or sweet biscuits or cake, black tea. |
| Lunch | Braised steak or beef sausages or roast chicken with boiled potato, cabbage and peas, battered butterfish with potato chips. |
| Afternoon tea | Sweet biscuits, black tea. |
| Dinner | Sandwich with white bread, ham and/or cheese. |
| Fluid intake | 2–3 cups of water a day, 2–3 cups of tea a day. |
| **Food frequency** | |
| Fruit | 0–1 serve daily |
| Vegetables | 2–3 serves daily |
| Dairy | 0–1 serve daily |
| Cereals | 6–7 serves daily |
| Red meat | 4 serves a week |
| Chicken | 3 serves a week |
| Fish | 1 serve a week |
| Takeaway/fast food | 0 times a week |

**Quality and duration of sleep**
Continuous sleep. Has difficulty falling asleep; average duration is 5–6 hours.
**Frequency and duration of exercise**
Client finds it difficult to engage in physical exercise programs due to arthralgia, but
can mobilise moderate distances with a cane. Client engages in incidental exercise
(e.g. gardening, laundry, cleaning, cooking) less than 3 hours a day and sedentary
activities more than 6 hours a day.

**Socioeconomic background**
The client was born in England and both parents (who are now deceased) were born
in Scotland. The client is a retired registered nurse who lives with her husband in
a small unit in a secure retirement village in a quiet agricultural community. The
retirement village provides regular social events, which the client enjoys. Both of
the client's sons are supportive; they visit at least once a fortnight. The client is
also a volunteer for a number of local groups and is particularly active in the local
Anglican church.

Physical examination
**Inspection**
Client mobilises with a single cane, partially weight-bearing on each leg. Gait is staggered and the expression of discomfort is observed in her face. On closer examination, there is mild swelling and enlargement to both knees, but no evidence of
erythema, bruising, deformity, tophi or scarring. Active range of motion is reduced in
both knees. Other major articulations (i.e. hips, shoulders, elbows, ankles and wrists)
are unremarkable.

**Olfaction**
There are no abnormal odours present.

## Palpation

Palpable tenderness and mild non-pitting oedema is present to both knees. Local skin temperature is unremarkable. Passive range of motion (ROM) is reduced in both knees, with knee flexion reduced to 105° (right) and 100° (left). Bent knee hip flexion is also reduced to 110° bilaterally. Mild bilateral quadricep weakness is also noted. ROM of other major articulations (i.e. shoulders, elbows, ankles and wrists) is unremarkable.

## Percussion

Not applicable.

## Auscultation

Joint crepitus and friction rubs are absent.

## Additional signs

Client is afebrile (36.2°C, per oral), hypertensive (138/85) and obese (BMI is 33.8 kg/m$^2$, waist circumference 101 cm).

## Clinical assessment tools

The short form Arthritis Impact Measurement Scale 2 (AIMS2) revealed a score of 68/120 (AIMS2 score ranges from 0, which is high impact, to 120, low impact). This indicates that the client's arthritis has a moderate impact on physical activity, social function and activities of daily living. The lowest scores (or highest impact) were noted for mobilisation and mood.

## Diagnostics

CAM practitioners can request, perform, and/or interpret findings from a range of diagnostic tests in order to add valuable data to the pool of clinical information. While several investigations are pertinent to this case (as described below), the decision to use these tests should be considered alongside factors such as cost, convenience, comfort, turnaround time, access, practitioner competence and scope of practice, and history of previous investigations.

## Pathology tests

### C-reactive protein (CRP)

CRP is a marker of inflammatory activity. The use of CRP in OA has not yet been established as there is a lack of consistent evidence to show that CRP is a valid and/or reliable marker of OA activity or a suitable predictor of OA incidence.[8,9]

### Plasma/red cell fatty acid analysis

This test assesses the concentration of fatty acids within the plasma or erythrocyte, including omega 3, omega 6 and omega 9 polyunsaturated fatty acids, saturated fatty acids and trans fatty acids. Given that high dietary omega 6 fatty acid intake may be associated with a higher risk of developing bone marrow lesions in the knee,[10] this test may help to determine whether increased omega 6 fatty acid consumption is a contributing factor in knee OA.

## Radiology tests

Plain film X-rays and, less commonly, ultrasound, CT and MRI, are able to detect structural changes in the joint space, articular cartilage and subchondral bone. This is useful in providing radiographic confirmation of OA.[11]

## Functional tests

Not applicable.

## Invasive tests

It is not routine practice to use invasive tests in the diagnosis of OA. When there are suspicions of serious pathology, arthroscopy and/or arthrocentesis may be indicated.

**Miscellaneous tests**
Not applicable.

## Diagnosis

Clusters of data extracted from the health history, clinical examination and pertinent diagnostic test results point towards the following differential CAM diagnoses.

- Bilateral knee arthralgia (actual), *secondary to OA, related to* genetic pre-disposition (*client has a family history of OA*), chronic inflammation (*knee pain is relieved by non-steroidal anti-inflammatory drugs and cold packs*), elevated omega 6 fatty acid intake (*client frequently consumes baked goods and fried foods that are generally high in omega 6 fatty acids; suspicions of high omega 6 fatty acid intake may be supported by plasma/red cell fatty acid analysis*), obesity (*obesity is a risk factor for OA – the client's BMI and waist circumference are in the obesity range*), low vitamin C and fruit intake (*the client typically consumes less than fifty per cent of the recommended daily intake of fruit*) and/or proteoglycan degradation (*non-steroidal anti-inflammatory drugs inhibit the synthesis of human cartilage matrix in vitro,[12] which is likely to accelerate the rate of degeneration of articular cartilage in OA*).
- Bilateral knee stiffness (actual), *secondary to OA, related to* genetic predisposition, chronic inflammation, elevated omega 6 fatty acid intake, obesity, low vitamin C and fruit intake, and/or proteoglycan degradation.
- Impaired physical mobility (actual), *secondary to OA, related to* genetic predisposition, chronic inflammation, elevated omega 6 fatty acid intake, obesity, low vitamin C and fruit intake, and/or proteoglycan degradation.

## Planning

The goals and expected outcomes that best serve the client's needs, and that are most relevant to the presenting case (as determined by the clinical assessment and CAM diagnoses), are as follows.

Goals
1 Client will experience an improvement in knee pain (*this is the first concern expressed by the client*).
2 Client will report a reduction in knee stiffness (*this is the second concern voiced by the client*).
3 Client will demonstrate an improvement in physical mobility (*this is the third concern reported by the client*).

Expected outcomes
Based on the degree of improvement reported in clinical studies that have used CAM interventions for the management of OA,[13–19] the following are anticipated.
1 Client will report a thirty per cent reduction in baseline severity of bilateral knee pain in 6 weeks or by dd/mm/yyyy (as measured by 0–10 numerical pain score).
2 Client will report a thirty-five per cent reduction in baseline severity of bilateral knee stiffness in 14 weeks or by dd/mm/yyyy (as measured by 0–10 numerical pain score).
3 Client will demonstrate a thirty-five per cent increase in baseline mobility in 18 weeks or by dd/mm/yyyy (as measured by short form AIMS2 score).

## Application

The range of interventions reported in the CAM literature that may be used in the treatment of OA are appraised below.

Diet
OA is an inflammatory disorder, thus it is conceivable that the consumption of foods and/or nutrients with demonstrable anti-inflammatory activity may play a role in the management of the disease. In a 10-year longitudinal cohort study, a positive

association was observed between dietary intake of omega 6 polyunsaturated fatty acids and risk of bone marrow lesions in the non-osteoarthritic knee joint,[12] while an inverse association was reported between dietary intake of vitamin C and fruit, and bone marrow lesions.[12] Neither of these nutrients was found to be associated with statistically significant changes in cartilage volume. In spite of these encouraging results, it is uncertain whether the increased consumption of fruit and foods containing vitamin C, and the reduced intake of omega 6 fatty acid-containing foods, is of any benefit in the secondary prevention of OA.

### Dairy and tea consumption (Level III-3, Strength C, Direction +)
There is some evidence to suggest that the consumption of milk and tea could be of benefit to people with joint inflammation. A cross-sectional study of 655 individuals with symptomatic knee OA found lower rates of symptomatic OA among people consuming higher intakes of milk and tea.[20] Whether different types of milk (e.g. cow versus goat) and tea (e.g. black versus green) confer different levels of benefit to people with knee OA is an area in need of further research.

### Low-calorie diet (Level II, Strength B, Direction +)
Many risk factors are associated with the pathogenesis of OA. One risk factor that is amenable to dietary modification is obesity, which makes effective weight reduction an important goal in OA management. Evidence from two controlled clinical trials shows low-energy diets (with and without exercise) are significantly more effective than control diets at reducing body fat, but more importantly, are significantly more effective than controls in improving functional outcomes in obese individuals with OA.[21,22] These improvements may be attributed to a reduction in joint load, as well as to a decrease in systemic inflammatory activity.[23]

Lifestyle

### Relaxation therapy (Level II, Strength B, Direction +)
The relaxation response can be induced by a number of behavioural therapies, such as progressive muscle relaxation, guided imagery and autogenic training. Many RCTs have examined the effect of these therapies on pertinent OA outcomes. Results from three small trials have shown progressive muscle relaxation (PMR), hypnosis and guided imagery plus PMR to be significantly more effective than controls at improving OA-related pain,[24,25] immobility,[24] quality of life[26] and analgesic use[25] over 8–12 weeks; there was no statistically significant difference between hypnosis and PMR.[25] Further research is needed to examine the comparative effectiveness of other relaxation therapies.

### Tai chi (Level I, Strength B, Direction +)
Tai chi is an ancient Chinese therapy generally used as a meditative technique, soft martial art or form of physical exercise. In many ways, the physical and psychological benefits of tai chi are similar to those of exercise.[27,28] Evidence from a systematic review of five RCTs and seven non-randomised controlled clinical trials is not convincing, with tai chi (for 6–24 weeks) failing to demonstrate consistent improvements in pain or physical function in people with OA.[29] Findings from recent trials have been more favourable, with 12 weeks of Sun-style tai chi demonstrating significant symptomatic improvements in people with OA when compared with controls.[15,18] The weight of the evidence seems to be in favour of tai chi, although further investigation is still warranted.

### Yoga (Level II, Strength B, Direction +)
Yoga is an ancient Indian practice that integrates stretching, exercise, posture and breathing with meditation. Because aerobic exercise and stretching improve the symptoms of OA as well as the person's functional capacity,[30,31] it is possible that yoga could also offer some benefit to individuals suffering from this condition. Findings from two small trials lend support to this claim. An RCT of 25 patients with hand OA found yoga (once weekly for 8 weeks) to be significantly more effective

than no treatment at reducing joint tenderness, finger range of motion and activity-induced hand pain.[32] In an uncontrolled pilot study, yoga (once weekly for 8 weeks) was found to be effective at reducing Western Ontario and McMaster Universities Osteoarthritis Index (WOMAC) pain, WOMAC physical function, and Arthritis Impact Measurement Scale 2 (AIMS2) effect in 11 patients with knee OA.[33] Given the methodological limitations of the latter study, and the small size of both trials, no firm conclusions can yet be made about the effectiveness of yoga for OA.

## Nutritional supplementation

### Chondroitin sulfate (Level I, Strength B, Direction o)

Chondroitin sulfate is a sulfated glycosaminoglycan (GAG), an important component of cartilage. In addition to this structural function, chondroitin sulfate serves to protect articular cartilage by reducing inflammatory and proteolytic enzyme activity, and by stimulating proteoglycan and hyaluronic acid synthesis.[34] Not surprisingly, more than 22 controlled trials have examined the clinical efficacy of chondroitin sulfate in OA. A meta-analysis of 20 of these clinical trials (n = 3846) found chondroitin sulfate (administered orally or intramuscularly) to be more effective than controls at reducing joint pain.[35] But due to the high degree of statistical heterogeneity of trials, the analysis was limited to three studies with large sample sizes and an intention-to-treat analysis (representing forty per cent of the total sample size). The revised analysis demonstrated that chondroitin sulfate was neither clinically nor statistically more effective than controls in improving the pain of OA. Larger trials that use more rigorous methodology are now needed in this area.

### Glucosamine (Level I, Strength C, Direction + (for Rotta preparations))

Glucosamine is an amino sugar and an important precursor of glycosaminoglycans (GAGs), a key constituent of articular cartilage. Glucosamine also inhibits proteolytic enzyme activity,[36] reduces inflammation[37] and stimulates proteoglycan synthesis.[38] Even though these properties are fundamental to attenuating the pathogenesis of OA, the best available evidence is not conclusive. A Cochrane meta-analysis of 25 RCTs (n = 4963) found glucosamine (administered orally or parenterally) to be significantly superior to controls at improving OA pain and function using the Lequesne index, but non-superior to controls using WOMAC pain, function or stiffness subscales.[39] When studies with inadequate allocation concealment were omitted from the analysis, glucosamine failed to show any benefit for pain. When glucosamine preparations were compared, those manufactured by Rotta Pharm were found to be significantly more effective than placebo at reducing pain and functional limitation. Non-Rotta preparations were no more effective than placebo at improving these outcomes; the increased severity of OA in these studies and the use of formulations other than glucosamine sulfate may have contributed to these results.

### Methylsulfonylmethane (MSM) (Level I, Strength B, Direction o)

MSM is an organic sulfur compound that has been shown to downregulate nuclear factor kappaB signalling and to reduce tissue necrosis factor-alpha (TNF-$\alpha$), interleukin-6, prostaglandin (PG) $E_2$ and nitric oxide release in lipopolysaccharide-stimulated murine macrophages.[40] This anti-inflammatory effect is not corroborated by data from human studies, with a meta-analysis of three double-blind, placebo controlled RCTs (including one for MSM and two for a similar compound, dimethyl sulfoxide (DMSO)) concluding that DMSO/MSM supplementation for 3–12 weeks is neither statistically nor clinically more effective than placebo in reducing knee OA pain.[41] Changes in mobility, physical function and stiffness were also inconsistent across the three studies.

### *Perna canaliculus* (Level I, Strength C, Direction + (for pain only))

New Zealand green-lipped mussel (NZGLM) is a species of mollusc with high omega 3 fatty acid content. These fatty acids are believed to be responsible for the anti-inflammatory properties of the mussel. In animal and in vitro studies, NZGLM has been shown to inhibit cyclo-oxygenase (COX) activity, $PGE_2$, TNF-α, interleukin (IL)-1, IL-2, IL-6, IL-12 and leukotriene $B_4$ production, and swelling in several models of inflammation.[42] In mechanistic studies, NZGLM supplementation failed to produce significant changes in blood levels of thromboxane $B_2$, $PGE_2$, IL-1β and TNF-α in human subjects after 6 weeks.[43] Even so, a systematic review of three placebo-controlled RCTs reported significant improvements in OA pain after 6 months of NZGLM supplementation in two of three trials.[44] Changes in joint mobility, physical and functional activity, and patient global assessment were not statistically significantly different between groups at 24 weeks, which suggests that more rigorously designed trials of NZGLM are needed.

### S-adenosyl-L-methionine (Level I, Strength B, Direction +)

The coenzyme SAMe exhibits a range of activities considered beneficial to the management of OA. Specifically, SAMe demonstrates anti-inflammatory activity in vivo and a cartilage regenerating effect in vitro.[45] According to a meta-analysis of 11 RCTs, these effects appear to translate into clinical practice. The review found orally administered SAMe (600–1200 mg daily, for 10–84 days) to be as effective as non-steroidal anti-inflammatory drugs (NSAIDs) at reducing OA pain and functional limitation,[46] but with comparatively fewer adverse effects. Yet in studies comparing SAMe to placebo, no statistically or clinically significant effects were observed for pain (n = 2 RCTs) or functional impairment (n = 3 RCTs).[47] A major limitation of these studies is their short duration; hence, longer trials are required to ascertain if long-term supplementation of SAMe is a safe and effective treatment option for OA.

### Vitamin C (Level II, Strength B, Direction +)

Serum CRP levels (a marker of acute inflammation) have been shown to be inversely related to vitamin C levels in healthy elderly men,[48] suggesting that vitamin C may play a role in the regulation of inflammation and, possibly, in the management of OA. A double-blind, crossover RCT has shown that supplementation with calcium ascorbate (1 g) for 14 days was significantly more effective than placebo at improving pain (p = 0.008) and OA severity (p = 0.04) in 133 patients with radiographically verified symptomatic OA of the hip and/or knee.[49] Investigation into the long-term effectiveness of vitamin C supplementation in OA, as well as the effect of different dosages, forms and chelating agents, is now required.

### Vitamin E (Level II, Strength C, Direction o)

The tocopherols may attenuate the pathogenesis of OA by inhibiting the release of proinflammatory cytokines and by reducing monocyte adhesion to endothelial tissue.[50] Data from four double-blind RCTs have not been consistent though. Results from two earlier and comparatively smaller trials found that supplementation with vitamin E (400–1200 IU daily, for 6–12 weeks) was significantly more effective than placebo at reducing knee pain, hip pain and analgesic use,[51] and as effective as diclofenac (50 mg three times a day) at improving knee and/or hip pain, knee circumference and joint mobility.[52] In contrast, results from two larger, more recent studies found that vitamin E supplementation (500 IU daily, for 6 months to 2 years) was no more effective than placebo at reducing knee OA symptoms or improving cartilage loss.[53,54] While the weight of the evidence does not support the use of vitamin E in OA, there are some areas warranting further investigation, particularly the efficacy of higher dose vitamin E and the comparative efficacy of natural versus synthetic tocopherols.

### Vitamin K (Level I, Strength C, Direction o)

One of the pathological signs of OA is cartilage calcification. Vitamin-K-dependent matrix gla protein (MGP) is responsible for opposing the mineralisation of cartilage,[55] which could explain why people with lower plasma phylloquinone (vitamin K) levels have a higher risk of developing hand OA.[56] It seems plausible, then, that vitamin K supplementation would reduce the risk or progression of OA. In a 3-year RCT of 378 otherwise healthy older adults, vitamin K (500 µg daily) plus multivitamin was found to be no more effective than control (multivitamin) at reducing hand OA prevalence, joint space narrowing and osteophyte formation.[57] A subgroup analysis of the data did find that those deficient in vitamin K at baseline, who achieved sufficient concentrations of the vitamin at follow-up, demonstrated a forty-seven per cent reduction in joint space narrowing (p = 0.02). This finding should be interpreted with caution as subgroup analyses are not always reliable. The finding does highlight an important area for future research though.

### Calcium, omega 3 fatty acids and selenium
These nutrients are cited in the general literature as being useful for the treatment of OA. Yet, it is not clear if these nutrients offer any clinical benefit to people with OA due to the paucity of clinical evidence in this area.

## Herbal medicine
### *Boswellia serrata* (Level I, Strength B, Direction +)
Frankincense has long been used as an anti-inflammatory herb in Ayurvedic medicine and, more specifically, as a treatment for arthritis. Data from experimental studies support this action, with the boswellic acids in frankincense gum resin shown to inhibit 5-lipo-oxygenase (LOX) and COX activity, as well as the subsequent release of pro-inflammatory mediators.[58] The traditional use of frankincense is further supported by findings from three clinical trials, including two well-designed double-blind placebo controlled trials, and one open label RCT. The oral administration of *B. serrata* resin extract (100–999 mg daily for 8–24 weeks) was found to be as effective as valdecoxib (an NSAID)[19] and significantly more effective than placebo[13,17] at improving OA knee pain and function. Whether these effects can be replicated in people with hip or hand OA is not yet clear.

### *Capsicum annuum* (Level II, Strength B, Direction +)
Across the globe chilli is commonly used as a culinary herb, but in traditional herbal medicine it is used as a circulatory stimulant and decongestant. Capsaicin, the pungent principle of chilli, also exhibits analgesic activity by depleting stores of substance P from sensory neurons.[59] When administered topically to OA joints (at 0.025–0.075 per cent concentration, four times a day for 4–12 weeks) capsaicin cream demonstrates statistically significant superiority to placebo in reducing joint pain and tenderness. These effects are consistently reported across five RCTs in a total sample of 430 people with OA.[60–64]

### *Harpagophytum procumbens* (Level I, Strength B, Direction + (for pain only))
Devil's claw is used in traditional South African medicine as a bitter tonic, vulnerary and analgesic for childbirth. In traditional Western herbal medicine, the plant is prescribed for the treatment of musculoskeletal complaints, specifically, inflammatory disorders such as arthritis.[65] Even though devil's claw has been shown in a number of experimental studies to modulate inflammatory activity by inhibiting COX, LOX, $PGE_2$, TNF-$\alpha$, IL-1$\beta$ and IL-6, reported effects are conflicting.[66] Findings from a systematic review of four double-blind, placebo-controlled RCTs in this area are a little more promising.[67] In most studies, *H. procumbens* extract (960–2400 mg for 3–20 weeks) was found to be more effective than placebo at reducing OA pain. Individual studies also found devil's claw to be significantly more effective than placebo at improving OA-associated mobility and stiffness, although these findings have yet to be replicated.

### *Pinus maritima* (Level II, Strength B, Direction + (for some outcomes))
Under experimental conditions, French maritime pine bark extract (or pycnogenol) exhibits free radical scavenging[67] and anti-inflammatory activity.[69] The latter has been attributed to the inhibition of nuclear factor-kappaB and the proinflammatory cytokine interleukin-1.[68] Under RCT conditions, pycnogenol (100–150 mg for 3 months) statistically significantly improves total WOMAC score, walking distance and stiffness when compared with placebo in people with knee OA.[69–71] People receiving pycnogenol also require less breakthrough analgesic medication than people receiving placebo.

Changes in WOMAC pain subscore and WOMAC physical function subscore were not consistent across studies.

### Zingiber officinale (Level I, Strength C, Direction o)

Ginger is used in many alternative systems of healing for its anti-inflammatory and circulatory stimulant properties. Under experimental conditions, ginger has been shown to inhibit the synthesis of $PGE_4$ and nitric oxide in porcine chondrocytes[72] and leukotriene $B_4$ in vitro.[73] While both of these effects may be useful in reducing the pain and inflammation of OA, this has yet to be demonstrated conclusively in humans. According to a recent systematic review, orally administered monopreparations of ginger (1.5–3.0 g per day) were found to be no more effective than placebo at reducing the severity of OA joint pain in two of three RCTs, and statistically significantly inferior to Ibuprofen in one of two trials. In relation to disability and functional capacity, ginger was found to be statistically significantly superior to placebo in one of two trials, and significantly inferior to Ibuprofen in one trial.[74] Given the inconsistencies in these findings, no firm conclusions can yet be made about the effectiveness of ginger as a treatment for OA.

### Other herbs

Although *Apium graveolens* (celery seed), *Curcuma longa* (turmeric), *Solidago virgaurea* (goldenrod), *Tanacetum parthenium* (feverfew) and *Zanthoxylum americanum* (prickly ash) have all been used traditionally and/or tested under experimental conditions for their anti-inflammatory, analgesic and/or antirheumatic activity, there are insufficient clinical data to support the use of these herbal monopreparations in OA.

## Other

### Acupuncture (Level I, Strength B, Direction +)

Acupuncture originated in China more than 4000 years ago.[75] This ancient therapy has long been used as a treatment for a number of acute and chronic complaints, including musculoskeletal disorders such as OA. The effectiveness of acupuncture in OA has also been extensively studied. Evidence from several systematic reviews and meta-analyses indicate that acupuncture treatment (including manual and electro-acupuncture) is significantly more effective than sham acupuncture and usual care at reducing pain and improving function in people with OA of the hip, knee and thumb, but particularly the knee.[14,76] Findings from more recent RCTs have, however, been inconsistent,[77–79] which suggests that current systematic reviews need updating.

### Aromatherapy (Level II, Strength B, Direction o)

Essential oils can generate a range of emotional, psychological and physiological effects, which may be helpful in the management of OA. Although no well-designed studies have investigated the effect of aromatherapy in people with OA, one double-blind RCT has tested the effectiveness of essential oil massage in 59 elderly patients with non-specific moderate to severe knee pain.[80] Patients were randomised to three groups: essential oil massage (0.5 per cent orange oil and 1 per cent ginger oil in olive oil carrier), placebo massage (carrier oil only) or control (no massage). Patients received six 30–35 minute massage or control sessions over 3 weeks. Differences between groups for changes in knee pain intensity, stiffness level, physical function and quality of life were not statistically significant. Whether outcomes would be different in people with OA or by using different blends or higher concentrations of essential oils remains to be seen.

### Chiropractic (Level II, Strength C, Direction +)

Chiropractic manipulation is generally prescribed for the treatment of nervous and musculoskeletal disorders, including OA. It was not until a few years ago that the effectiveness of this treatment in OA was rigorously examined. In a RCT published in 2006, 252 patients with lower back pain secondary to OA were randomly assigned to chiropractic care (including flexion or distraction and spinal manipulation) plus moist heat or moist heat only, for 20 treatment sessions over 6–10 weeks.[81] Compared with the control group, chiropractic care and moist heat were found to be more effective at reducing back pain and increasing spinal ROM. Patients receiving chiropractic care also demonstrated greater improvements in several activities of daily living than people in the control group. Due to the likely introduction of observer bias from inadequate investigator blinding, these findings should be interpreted with caution.

### Homeopathy (Level I, Strength B, Direction +)
Homeopathy is a system of medicine that uses highly diluted and potentised remedies to influence the body's vital force and restore homeostasis. As such, the therapy can be used to treat a wide range of acute and chronic conditions, including OA. Data from a 2001 systematic review of four RCTs (n = 406)[16] and a 2002 controlled clinical trial (n = 80)[82] have been promising, with four of the five studies showing homeopathic or combined allopathic-homeopathic medicines (administered intra-articularly, orally and topically) to be at least as effective as, if not superior to, conventional treatment at reducing pain and joint tenderness in people with OA. These results should be interpreted with caution though, as the study designs and treatments do not accurately reflect classical homeopathic practice.

### Massage (Level II, Strength B, Direction +)
Massage is the systematic manipulation of soft tissues of the body. This tactile therapy may be particularly helpful for musculoskeletal disorders as it can help reduce anxiety, depression and pain by stimulating parasympathetic nervous system activity, as well as elevating serotonin and endorphin release.[83] An RCT involving 68 adults with radiographically confirmed OA of the knee set out to test whether standard full-body Swedish massage (twice-weekly 1-hour sessions for 4 weeks, then once-weekly sessions for 4 weeks) was able to improve knee pain and function when compared to control (delayed intervention).[84] The group receiving massage demonstrated greater improvements in pain, stiffness, physical functional disability and WOMAC global score than people in the control group. The difference between groups was statistically significant (p<0.008). While these outcomes are promising, further research is needed to improve the strength of the evidence.

### Thermotherapy (Level I, Strength C, Direction + (for some outcomes))
Thermotherapy, or the application of heat or cold to an affected body part, is generally indicated in conditions characterised by pain, oedema and/or inflammation. Given that these manifestations typically present in OA, it is probable that thermotherapy may be of some benefit to people with this disorder. A systematic review of the literature identified three RCTs on thermotherapy and OA.[85] Treatments included ice massage and cold or hot pack application. Ice massage (five 20-minute sessions per week for 2 weeks) was found to be significantly more effective than control at improving quadriceps strength, knee ROM and time to walk 15 metres (p<0.001). No benefit was detected for knee oedema. In terms of knee pain, the difference between ice pack application (three treatment sessions per week for 3 weeks) and control was only marginally significant (p = 0.06). When cold and hot pack applications were compared (20 minutes, 10 sessions), cold was found to be significantly superior at reducing knee oedema (p=0.04). While heat therapy was not found to be effective in this review, a more recent RCT indicates that moist heat rather than dry heat might be effective in arthritis. The study of 37 female patients with knee OA found that the continuous application of a heat or steam-generating sheet to the knee for 4 weeks was significantly more effective than a dry heat-generating sheet at improving total WOMAC score and gait ability score.[86] Studies examining the comparative effectiveness of these treatments are now needed.

### Osteopathy and reflexology
There is insufficient clinical evidence to support the use of osteopathy and reflexology in the management of OA.

## CAM prescription

The CAM interventions that are most appropriate for the management of the presenting case – that is, they target the planned goals, expected outcomes and CAM diagnoses, they are supported by the best available evidence, they are pertinent to the client's needs and they are most relevant to CAM practice – are outlined below.

### Primary treatments

- Commence low-energy diet (4500 kJ daily) (*client consumes around 7000 kJ daily; decreasing daily energy intake to 4500 kJ may be beneficial in reducing client obesity, joint load and inflammatory activity, as well as improving mobility and OA pain*)
- Consider one of the following biological interventions:
  - oral *Boswellia serrata* resin extract (containing a minimum of thirty per cent boswellic acids), 125 mg twice daily (*this anti-inflammatory herb is shown to be effective in improving OA knee pain and function*)
  - oral S-adenosyl-L-methionine (SAMe), 300 mg twice daily for 2 weeks, then reduce to 200 mg twice daily (*SAMe is shown to be as effective as NSAIDs in reducing OA pain and functional limitation, possibly by reducing inflammatory activity and improving cartilage regeneration*)
- Consider one of the following CAM therapies:
  - acupuncture treatment series (*manual or electro-acupuncture is effective in improving OA knee pain and function*)
  - homeopathic treatment series (*oral or topical administration of combination homeopathic formulations may be useful in reducing OA joint pain and tenderness*)
  - consider Sun-style tai chi, 60 minutes twice a week (*tai chi may help to improve OA knee pain, stiffness and ROM, as well as physical mobility*).

### Secondary treatments

- Consider increasing the consumption of oily fish (to 2 serves a week), fruit (to 2 serves a day) and vegetables (to 5 serves a day), and decreasing the intake of baked goods and fried foods (to no more than once a day) (*increasing the consumption of foods high in vitamin C and omega 3 fatty acids may offer some protection against the progression of OA; this is based on theoretical evidentiary support only*).

### Referral

- Refer client to a general practitioner, family physician, orthopaedic specialist or emergency department if the condition deteriorates, if serious pathology is suspected (e.g. metastatic carcinoma, multiple myeloma) or if a serious complication arises (e.g. infectious arthritis, nerve compression).
- Refer client to another CAM practitioner if OA, or the treatment of OA, is outside the clinician's area of expertise.
- Liaise with the general practitioner about the client's overall management plan.

## Review

To determine whether pertinent client goals and expected outcomes have been achieved at follow-up and if any aspects of the client's care need to be improved, consider the factors listed in Table 8.2 (chapter 8), as well as the questions listed below.

- Was there a reduction in bilateral knee pain and stiffness?
- Was there an improvement in knee flexion?
- Was there an improvement in the AIMS2 score?
- Has the need for ibuprofen decreased?
- Is the client's gait less staggered?
- Was there a reduction in body mass index or waist circumference?
- Has knee tenderness and/or swelling diminished?

# References

1. Sharma L. Kapoor D. (2006) Epidemiology of osteoarthritis. In: Moskowitz RW, editor. Osteoarthritis: diagnosis and medical/surgical management. 4th ed. Philadelphia: Lippincott, Williams & Wilkins.
2. Australian Bureau of Statistics (ABS). (2006) Musculoskeletal conditions in Australia: a snapshot, 2004 (Cat. No. 4823.0.55.001). Canberra: ABS.
3. March LM. Bagga H. (2004) Epidemiology of osteoarthritis in Australia. Medical Journal of Australia, 180: S6–10.
4. Arden N. Nevitt MC. (2006) Osteoarthritis: epidemiology. Best Practice and Research Clinical Rheumatology, 20(1): 3–25.
5. Porter R et al, editors. (2008) The Merck manual. Rahway: Merck Research Laboratories.
6. Freemont AJ. (2006) Pathophysiology of osteoarthritis. In: Arden N, editor. Osteoarthritis handbook. London: Taylor & Francis.
7. Lippincott Williams & Wilkins. (2008) Professional guide to diseases. 9th ed. Philadelphia: Lippincott, Williams & Wilkins.
8. Engstrom G et al (2009) C-reactive protein, metabolic syndrome and incidence of severe hip and knee osteoarthritis: a population-based cohort study. Osteoarthritis and Cartilage, 17(2): 168–73.
9. Matsubara T et al (2006) Investigation of serum C-reactive protein in osteoarthritis of the knee. Central Japan Journal of Orthopaedic Surgery and Traumatology, 49(2): 289–90.
10. Wang Y et al (2008) Effect of fatty acids on bone marrow lesions and knee cartilage in healthy, middle-aged subjects without clinical knee osteoarthritis. Osteoarthritis Cartilage, 16(5): 579–83.
11. Fischbach FT. Dunning MB. (2008) A manual of laboratory and diagnostic tests. 8th ed. Philadelphia: Lippincott, Williams & Wilkins.
12. Dingle JT. (1999) The effects of NSAID on the matrix of human articular cartilages. Zeitschrift fur Rheumatologie, 58(3): 125–9.
13. Kimmatkar N et al (2003) Efficacy and tolerability of Boswellia serrata extract in treatment of osteoarthritis of knee: a randomized double blind placebo controlled trial. Phytomedicine, 10(1): 3–7.
14. Kwon YD. Pittler MH. Ernst E. (2006) Acupuncture for peripheral joint osteoarthritis: a systematic review and meta-analysis. Rheumatology, 45(11): 1331–7.
15. Lee HY. Lee KJ. (2008) Effects of Tai Chi exercise in elderly with knee osteoarthritis. Taehan Kanho Hakhoe Chi, 38(1): 11–18.
16. Long L. Ernst E. (2001) Homeopathic remedies for the treatment of osteoarthritis: a systematic review. British Homoeopathic Journal, 90(1): 37–43.
17. Sengupta K et al (2008) A double blind, randomized, placebo controlled study of the efficacy and safety of 5-Loxin(R) for treatment of osteoarthritis of the knee. Arthritis Research and Therapy, 10(4): R85.
18. Song R et al (2007) Effects of a Sun-style tai chi exercise on arthritic symptoms, motivation and the performance of health behaviors in women with osteoarthritis. Taehan Kanho Hakhoe Chi, 37(2): 249–56.
19. Sontakke S et al (2007) Open, randomized, controlled clinical trial of Boswellia serrata extract as compared to valdecoxib in osteoarthritis of knee. Indian Journal of Pharmacology, 39(1): 27–9.
20. Kacar C et al (2004) The association of milk consumption with the occurrence of symptomatic knee osteoarthritis. Clinical and Experimental Rheumatology, 22(4): 473–6.
21. Christensen R. Astrup A. Bliddal H. (2005) Weight loss: the treatment of choice for knee osteoarthritis? A randomized trial. Osteoarthritis and Cartilage, 13(1): 20–7.
22. Miller GD et al (2006) Intensive weight loss program improves physical function in older obese adults with knee osteoarthritis. Obesity, 14(7): 1219–30.
23. Nicklas BJ et al (2004) Diet-induced weight loss, exercise, and chronic inflammation in older, obese adults: a randomized controlled clinical trial. American Journal of Clinical Nutrition, 79(4): 544–51.
24. Baird CL. Sands LP. (2004) A pilot study of the effectiveness of guided imagery with progressive muscle relaxation to reduce chronic pain and mobility difficulties of osteoarthritis. Pain Management Nursing, 5(3): 97–104.
25. Gay MC. Philippot P. Luminet O. (2002) Differential effectiveness of psychological interventions for reducing osteoarthritis pain: a comparison of Erickson hypnosis and Jacobson relaxation. European Journal of Pain, 6(1): 1–16.
26. Baird CL. Sands LP. (2006) Effect of guided imagery with relaxation on health-related quality of life in older women with osteoarthritis. Research in Nursing and Health, 29(5): 442–51.
27. Frye B et al (2007) Tai chi and low impact exercise: effects on the physical functioning and psychological well-being of older people. Journal of Applied Gerontology, 26(5): 433–53.
28. Jin P. (1992) Efficacy of Tai Chi, brisk walking, meditation, and reading in reducing mental and emotional stress. Journal of Psychosomatic Research, 36(4): 361–70.
29. Lee MS. Pittler MH. Ernst E. (2008) Tai chi for osteoarthritis: a systematic review. Clinical Rheumatology, 27(2): 211–18.
30. Brosseau L et al (2004) Efficacy of aerobic exercises for osteoarthritis (part II): a meta-analysis. Physical Therapy Reviews, 9(3): 125–45.
31. Pelland L et al (2004) Efficacy of strengthening exercises for osteoarthritis (part I): a meta-analysis. Physical Therapy Reviews, 9(2): 77–108.
32. Garfinkel MS et al (1994) Evaluation of a yoga based regimen for treatment of osteoarthritis of the hands. Journal of Rheumatology, 21(12): 2341–3.
33. Kolasinski SL et al (2005) Iyengar yoga for treating symptoms of osteoarthritis of the knees: a pilot study. Journal of Alternative and Complementary Medicine, 11(4): 689–93.
34. Monfort J et al (2007) Biochemical basis of the effect of chondroitin sulfate on osteoarthritis articular tissues. Annals of the Rheumatic Diseases, 67: 735–40.
35. Reichenbach S et al (2007) Meta-analysis: chondroitin for osteoarthritis of the knee or hip. Annals of Internal Medicine, 146(8): 580–90.
36. Bassleer C. Rovati L. Franchimont P. (1998). Stimulation of proteoglycan production by glucosamine sulfate in chondrocytes isolated from human osteoarthritic articular cartilage in vitro. Osteoarthritis Cartilage, 6(6): 427–34.

37. Largo R et al (2003) Glucosamine inhibits IL-1beta-induced NFkappaB activation in human osteoarthritic chondrocytes. Osteoarthritis Cartilage, 11(4): 290–8.
38. Uitterlinden EJ et al (2006) Glucosamine decreases expression of anabolic and catabolic genes in human osteoarthritic cartilage explants. Osteoarthritis Cartilage, 14(3): 250–7.
39. Towheed T et al (2005) Glucosamine therapy for treating osteoarthritis. Cochrane Database of Systematic Reviews, (2): CD002946 (updated November 2008).
40. Kim YH et al (2009) The anti-inflammatory effects of methylsulfonylmethane on lipopolysaccharide-induced inflammatory responses in murine macrophages. Biological and Pharmaceutical Bulletin, 32(4): 651–6.
41. Brien S. Prescott P. Lewith G. (2009) Meta-analysis of the related nutritional supplements Dimethyl Sulfoxide and Methylsulfonylmethane in the treatment of osteoarthritis of the knee. Evidence-Based Complementary and Alternative Medicine, early release.
42. Doggrell SA. (2009) Lyprinol – is it a useful anti-inflammatory agent? Evidence-Based Complementary and Alternative Medicine, early release.
43. Murphy KJ et al (2006) Low dose supplementation with two different marine oils does not reduce pro-inflammatory eicosanoids and cytokines in vivo. Asia Pacific Journal of Clinical Nutrition, 15(3): 418–24.
44. Brien S et al (2008) Systematic review of the nutritional supplement Perna Canaliculus (green-lipped mussel) in the treatment of osteoarthritis. QJM, 101(3): 167–79.
45. Blewett HJH. (2008) Exploring the mechanisms behind S-adenosylmethionine (SAMe) in the treatment of osteoarthritis. Critical Reviews in Food Science and Nutrition, 48(5): 458–63.
46. Soeken KL et al (2002) Safety and efficacy of S-adenosylmethionine (SAMe) for osteoarthritis. Journal of Family Practice, 51(5): 425–30.
47. Rutjes AWS et al (2009) S-Adenosylmethionine for osteoarthritis of the knee or hip. Cochrane Database of Systematic Reviews, (4): CD007321.
48. Wannamethee SG et al (2006) Associations of vitamin C status, fruit and vegetable intakes, and markers of inflammation and hemostasis. American Journal of Clinical Nutrition, 83(3): 567–74.
49. Jensen NH. (2003) Reduced pain from osteoarthritis in hip joint or knee joint during treatment with calcium ascorbate. A randomized, placebo-controlled cross-over trial in general practice. Ugeskrift for Laeger, 165(25): 2563–6.
50. Singh U. Devaraj S. Jialal I. (2005) Vitamin E, oxidative stress, and inflammation. Annual Review of Nutrition, 25: 151–74.
51. Blankenhorn G. (1986) Clinical effectiveness of Spondyvit (vitamin E) in activated arthroses: a multicenter placebo-controlled double-blind study. Zeitschrift fur Orthopadie und ihre Grenzgebiete, 124(3): 340–3.
52. Scherak O et al (1990) Therapy with high doses of vitamin E in patients with osteoarthritis. Zeitschrift fur Rheumatologie, 49(6): 369–73.
53. Brand C et al (2001) Vitamin E is ineffective for symptomatic relief of knee osteoarthritis: a six month double blind, randomised, placebo controlled study. Annals of the Rheumatic Diseases, 60(10): 946–9.
54. Wluka AE et al (2002) Supplementary vitamin E does not affect the loss of cartilage volume in knee osteoarthritis: a 2 year double blind randomized placebo controlled study. Journal of Rheumatology, 29(12): 2585–91.
55. Hale JE. Fraser JD. Price PA. (1988) The identification of matrix Gla protein in cartilage. Journal of Biological Chemistry, 263(12): 5820–4.
56. Neogi T et al (2006) Low vitamin K status is associated with osteoarthritis in the hand and knee. Arthritis and Rheumatism, 54(4): 1255–61.
57. Neogi T et al (2008) Vitamin K in hand osteoarthritis: results from a randomised clinical trial. Annals of the Rheumatic Diseases, 67(11): 1570–3.
58. Ammon HP. (2006) Boswellic acids in chronic inflammatory diseases. Planta Medica, 72(12): 1100–16.
59. Cordell GA. Araujo OE. (1993) Capsaicin: identification, nomenclature, and pharmacotherapy. Annals of Pharmacotherapy, 27(3): 330–6.
60. Altman RD et al (1994) Capsaicin cream 0.025% as monotherapy for osteoarthritis: a double-blind study. Seminars in Arthritis and Rheumatism, 23(Suppl 3): 25–33.
61. Deal CL et al (1991) Treatment of arthritis with topical capsaicin: a double-blind trial. Clinical Therapeutics, 13(3): 383–95.
62. McCarthy GM. McCarty DJ. (1992) Effect of topical capsaicin in the therapy of painful osteoarthritis of the hands. Journal of Rheumatology, 19(4): 604–7.
63. McCleane G. (2000) The analgesic efficacy of topical capsaicin is enhanced by glyceryl trinitrate in painful osteoarthritis: a randomized, double blind, placebo controlled study. European Journal of Pain, 4(4): 355–60.
64. Schnitzer T. Morton C. Coker S. (1994) Topical capsaicin therapy for osteoarthritis pain: achieving a maintenance regimen. Seminars in Arthritis and Rheumatism, 23(Suppl 3): 34–40.
65. Bone K. (2003) A clinical guide to blending liquid herbs. St Louis: Churchill Livingstone.
66. Brien S. Lewith GT. McGregor G. (2006) Devil's claw (Harpagophytum procumbens) as a treatment for osteoarthritis: a review of efficacy and safety. Journal of Alternative and Complementary Medicine, 12(10): 981–93.
67. Busserolles J et al (2006) In vivo antioxidant activity of procyanidin-rich extracts from grape seed and pine (Pinus maritima) bark in rats. International Journal for Vitamin and Nutrition Research, 76(1): 22–7.
68. Cho KJ et al (2000) Effect of bioflavonoids extracted from the bark of Pinus maritima on proinflammatory cytokine interleukin-1 production in lipopolysaccharide-stimulated RAW 264.7. Toxicology and Applied Pharmacology, 168(1): 64–71.
69. Belcaro G et al (2008) Pycnogenol may alleviate adverse effects in oncologic treatment. Panminerva Medica, 50(3): 227–34.
70. Cisar P et al (2008) Effect of pine bark extract (Pycnogenol) on symptoms of knee osteoarthritis. Phytotherapy Research, 22(8): 1087–92.
71. Farid R et al (2007) Pycnogenol supplementation reduces pain and stiffness and improves physical function in adults with knee osteoarthritis. Nutrition Research, 27(11): 692–7.
72. Shen CL. Hong KJ. Kim SW. (2005) Comparative effects of ginger root (Zingiber officinale Rosc.) on the production of inflammatory mediators in normal and osteoarthrotic sow chondrocytes. Journal of Medicinal Food, 8(2): 149–53.
73. Blumenthal M. (2003) The ABC clinical guide to herbs. Austin: American Botanical Council.
74. Leach MJ. Kumar S. (2008) The clinical effectiveness of Ginger (Zingiber officinale) in adults with osteoarthritis. International Journal of Evidence-based Healthcare, 6(3): 311–20.
75. O'Brien KA. Xue CC. (2003) Acupuncture. In: Robson T, editor. An introduction to complementary medicine. Sydney: Allen & Unwin.

76. White A et al (2006) The effectiveness of acupuncture for osteoarthritis of the knee: a systematic review. Acupuncture in Medicine, 24(Suppl 1): 40–8.

77. Foster NE et al (2007) Acupuncture as an adjunct to exercise based physiotherapy for osteoarthritis of the knee: randomised controlled trial. British Medical Journal, 335(7617): 436.

78. Jubb RW et al (2008) A blinded randomised trial of acupuncture (manual and electroacupuncture) compared with a non-penetrating sham for the symptoms of osteoarthritis of the knee. Acupuncture in Medicine, 26(2): 69–78.

79. Tsang RC et al (2007) Effects of acupuncture and sham acupuncture in addition to physiotherapy in patients undergoing bilateral total knee arthroplasty: a randomized controlled trial. Clinical Rehabilitation, 21(8): 719–28.

80. Yip YB. Tam AC. (2008) An experimental study on the effectiveness of massage with aromatic ginger and orange essential oil for moderate-to-severe knee pain among the elderly in Hong Kong. Complementary Therapies in Medicine, 16(3): 131–8.

81. Beyerman KL et al (2006) Efficacy of treating low back pain and dysfunction secondary to osteoarthritis: chiropractic care compared with moist heat alone. Journal of Manipulative and Physiological Therapeutics, 29(2): 107–14.

82. Maiko OY. (2002) Homoeopathic therapy of gonarthrosis with Zeel T. Biologische Medizin, 31(2): 68–74.

83. Moyer CA. Rounds J. Hannum JW. (2004) A meta-analysis of massage therapy research. Psychological Bulletin, 130(1): 3–18.

84. Perlman AI et al (2006) Massage therapy for osteoarthritis of the knee: a randomized controlled trial. Archives of Internal Medicine, 166(22): 2533–8.

85. Brosseau L et al (2003) Thermotherapy for treatment of osteoarthritis. Cochrane Database of Systematic Reviews, (4): CD004522.

86. Seto H et al (2008) Effect of heat- and steam-generating sheet on daily activities of living in patients with osteoarthritis of the knee: randomized prospective study. Journal of Orthopaedic Science, 13(3): 187–91.

# Case 10
# Psoriasis

## Description of psoriasis

Definition
Psoriasis is a chronic dermatological condition represented by epidermal thickening, hyperplasia, hyperkeratosis and inflammation. Of the two key types of psoriasis, type 1 is the most severe and the most resistant to treatment. Type 1 usually occurs in early adulthood and family history of the disease is common. Type 2 typically manifests in the fifth to sixth decade of life, is less severe and is not related to family history.[1] Overlapping these two types of psoriasis are a number of subtypes, including the erythrodermic, guttate, plaque and pustular variants.

Epidemiology
Psoriasis affects between one and five per cent of the population,[2] and even though the disease can occur at any age, it has a tendency to peak from late adolescence (i.e. 16 years) to 22 years and again between 57 and 60 years.[1]

Aetiology and pathophysiology
Psoriasis is a disorder with a firm genetic basis.[3] The lifetime prevalence of developing psoriasis in first-degree relatives ranges from four per cent if neither parent has the condition, to twenty-eight per cent if one parent has the condition and up to sixty-five per cent if both parents have psoriasis.[4] Additional to this, almost half of sufferers report a positive family history of the condition.[5]

One factor that may increase the skin's susceptibility to chronic plaque formation is a reduction in cyclic adenosine monophosphate (cAMP) levels. Reduced cAMP elevates proteinase activity, for instance, causing accelerated growth and thickening of the epidermis. Low cAMP levels also increase arachidonic acid production, leukotriene $B_4$ activation, neutrophil migration and epidermal inflammation.[6]

While changes in the levels of these chemical messengers may be genetically predetermined, they could also be influenced by several physiological factors, including incomplete protein digestion, bowel toxaemia and impaired liver function. According to one theory, inadequate protein digestion elevates the quantity of undigested amino acids in the intestinal lumen, which, upon exposure to intestinal flora, leads to the formation of toxic polyamines and a subsequent reduction in cAMP production.[7,8] The presence of gut-derived toxins from intestinal bacteria and fungi is believed to increase levels of cyclic guanidine monophosphate (cGMP), which may, in effect, increase cellular proliferation.[8] Although the accumulation of toxins from abnormal digestive or hepatic function might contribute to and/or aggravate the symptoms of psoriasis, there is insufficient evidence to support these mechanisms of action.

Adding to the complexity of this disease are myriad intrinsic and extrinsic triggers of psoriasis. Some of the extrinsic triggers of this disease include alcohol, beta-hemolytic streptococcal infection, epidermal trauma, gluten, sunburn, viral infection and medications, including angiotensin converting enzyme inhibitors, beta-adrenergic blockers, chloroquine, interferon-alpha, lithium, non-steroidal anti-inflammatory drugs and terbinafine.[1,2] Intrinsic triggers, such as emotional stress, are considered to be a major aggravating factor of the disease.[1,9,10] Exactly how stress affects psoriasis is not clear. Findings from one study suggest it could relate to the adverse effects of cortisol on the immunological and integumentary systems. In this 3-year study of 95 sufferers of progressive psoriasis, stressful life events were found to precede a rise in cortisol levels, which was followed by the development of an infectious illness and the eruption of psoriasis over an average span of 8 weeks.[11] Corroborating evidence from larger studies may help to support this stress–psoriasis hypothesis.

Clinical manifestations

Psoriatic lesions and concomitant symptoms of the disease vary according to the type and subtype of psoriasis. Plaque psoriasis is the most common subtype and usually presents as demarcated, erythematous and thickened plaques covered with fine silvery scales. These lesions are often located on the scalp, trunk and extremities, and are frequently accompanied by pruritus and nail pitting. The pustular variant may manifest as erythematous, pustule-studded lesions to the palmar or plantar surfaces, though in some cases can be associated with pyrexia and malaise. Guttate psoriasis presents as distinct, scaly, erythematous, droplet-like lesions to the scalp, ears, face, trunk and proximal limbs. The other major variant, erythrodermic psoriasis, is a dermatological emergency, manifesting as severe and extensive erythema and exfoliation, malaise and reduced skin function. Sufferers of psoriasis can also develop psoriatic arthritis, although this tends to affect a relatively small proportion of psoriasis cases.[1,12,13]

---

## Clinical case
*24-year-old man with plaque psoriasis*

### Rapport

Adopt the practitioner strategies and behaviours highlighted in Table 2.1 (chapter 2) to improve client trust, communication and rapport, as well as the accuracy and comprehensiveness of the clinical assessment.

### Assessment

Once measures have been put into place to build client–practitioner rapport, the clinician can begin the clinical assessment.

Health history

**History of presenting condition**

A 24-year-old man presents to the clinic after being persuaded by his partner to seek the help of a CAM practitioner for intractable psoriasis. The client developed psoriasis to the elbows 3 years ago, shortly after his grandfather died. Over the past 12 months, new lesions have emerged on the buttocks, knees and scalp. The client's general practitioner diagnosed plaque psoriasis 10 months ago and prescribed calcipotriol/betamethasone ointment. The ointment relieves the pruritus temporarily, as does coal tar and sunlight; however, the psoriatic lesions have not regressed in size over the last 6 months and are still intensely itchy, particularly after showering and on rising, when shedding of scales is most notable. Although the psoriasis did flare 3 months ago, no triggers of the flaring could be identified. The only time the psoriasis went into remission was 18 months ago when the client was on an 8-week working holiday.

**Medical history**

**Family history**

Father has psoriasis, paternal grandmother has rheumatoid arthritis.

**Allergies**

Nil known.

**Medications**

Calcipotriol/betamethasone diproprionate 50/500 ointment twice a day, coal tar three times a week.

**Medical conditions**

Plaque psoriasis, depression (treated with sertraline 3 years ago), asthma (resolved 7 years ago).

**Surgical or investigational procedures**
Removal of four wisdom teeth (2005).

## Lifestyle history

**Tobacco use**
Nil.

**Alcohol consumption**
Drinks 3–4 full strength beers every weekend.

**Illicit drug use**
Smokes marijuana once every 1–2 months.

| Diet and fluid intake | |
|---|---|
| Breakfast | Corn Flakes® with full-cream milk. |
| Morning tea | Coffee. |
| Lunch | Meat pie, white roll with salad, hot chicken roll, iced coffee. |
| Afternoon tea | Coffee. |
| Dinner | Spaghetti bolognaise, meat lover's pizza, beef schnitzel or sausages with mashed potato and peas. |
| Fluid intake | 1 cup of water daily, 2 cups of iced coffee daily, 1–2 cups of soft drink daily, 1 cup of milk daily, 2–3 cups of instant coffee daily. |
| **Food frequency** | |
| Fruit | 0–1 serve daily |
| Vegetables | 1–2 serves daily |
| Dairy | 1–2 serves daily |
| Cereals | 4–5 serves daily |
| Red meat | 8 serves a week |
| Chicken | 2 serves a week |
| Fish | 0 serves a week |
| Takeaway/fast food | 8 times a week |

**Quality and duration of sleep**
Interrupted sleep; average duration is 8 hours.

**Frequency and duration of exercise**
Is not engaged in any sporting activities; engages in exercise (e.g. work-related lifting and walking) less than 2 hours a day and sedentary activities more than 5 hours a day.

## Socioeconomic background
The client is New Zealand-born with New Zealand-born parents, and is a non-practising Christian. Lives with his partner (in a de facto relationship) in rented public housing; they have no children. He has worked full time as a forklift operator at a large super-market warehouse since leaving school at Year 11. The house and work environment are not notably stressful, although the nearby main road and landscaping business generate a substantial amount of noise and air pollution.

Physical examination

## Inspection
Skin lesions are evident on the scalp and both elbows, anterior knees and buttocks, ranging from 5 to 100 mm in diameter. All plaques are demarcated, erythematous,

thickened and covered with fine silvery scales. Excoriation and lichenification are also present around the lesions. There is no exudation, bleeding, papules, pustules or ulceration. Pitting and mild onycholysis is evident to all fingernails.

### Olfaction
There is no abnormal odour to the lesions or patient.

### Palpation
The psoriatic plaques are dry, rough and warm. The surrounding skin is also dry, but demonstrates good turgor and mobility.

### Percussion
Not applicable.

### Auscultation
Crepitus is not detectable.

### Additional signs
Client is afebrile (36.5°C, per oral) and slightly overweight (BMI is 26.2 kg/m$^2$, waist circumference is 89 cm).

### Clinical assessment tools
The simplified psoriasis area and severity index (SPASI) provided a score of 12/72, which included moderate lesion erythema (score = 2), thickness (score = 2) and scaling (score = 2), with fifteen per cent of the skin involved (grade = 2). The SPASI score was calculated by multiplying the area grade with the sum of the three severity scores.

## Diagnostics
CAM practitioners can request, perform and/or interpret findings from a range of diagnostic tests in order to add valuable data to the pool of clinical information. While several investigations are pertinent to this case (as described below), the decision to use these tests should be considered alongside factors such as cost, convenience, comfort, turnaround time, access, practitioner competence and scope of practice, and history of previous investigations.

### Pathology tests
#### Liver function test (LFT)
The LFT can provide useful information about hepatic function but cannot reliably detect impairments in liver detoxification because elevated blood ammonia, a sign of functional liver impairment, is unlikely to rise above the normal range in mild to moderate hepatic disease.[14]

#### Comprehensive digestive stool analysis (CDSA)
CDSA measures gastrointestinal function. While this test may help to determine whether intestinal dysbiosis, incomplete protein digestion, candidiasis and consequent bowel toxaemia are contributing factors in the pathogenesis of psoriasis, the validity of the toxaemia–psoriasis theory is still in question.

#### Endomysial and gliadin antibodies
The accumulation of undigested gliadin and gluten within the intestinal tract can lead to the formation of immunoglobulin A (IgA) endomysial antibodies, and IgA/IgG gliadin antibodies. Elevated serum levels of these antibodies are suggestive of gluten-sensitive enteropathy,[14] a possible trigger of psoriasis.[2]

### Radiology tests
Not applicable.

### Functional tests
The comprehensive detoxification profile (CDP) measures a person's capacity to effectively clear toxic metabolites from the blood, which may help to ascertain whether impaired liver function is a contributing and/or aggravating factor of psoriasis.[15]

**Invasive tests**

A lesion biopsy may be required if a diagnosis of psoriasis is uncertain. Histological findings indicative of psoriatic disease include increased mitosis of endothelial cells, fibroblasts and keratinocytes, evidence of inflammatory cells within the dermis and epidermis, and acanthosis.[16]

**Miscellaneous tests**

Not applicable.

## Diagnosis

Clusters of data extracted from the health history, clinical examination and pertinent diagnostic test results point towards the following differential CAM diagnoses.

- Skin plaques (actual), *secondary to* psoriasis, *related to* elevated inflammatory activity (*the symptoms of psoriasis are alleviated following the administration of calcipotriol/betamethasone ointment and coal tar*), emotional stress (*the death of the client's grandfather preceded the onset of psoriasis and the psoriasis went into remission when the client was on an extended working holiday*), genetic predisposition (*client has a family history of psoriasis*), gluten intolerance (*suspicions of gluten intolerance may be supported by elevated serum levels of IgA endomysial antibodies or IgA/IgG gliadin antibodies*), bowel toxaemia (*suspicions of bowel toxaemia may be corroborated by abnormal CDSA findings*) and/or impaired liver function (*suspicions of impaired liver function may be supported by abnormal CDP findings*).
- Pruritus (actual), *secondary to* psoriasis, *related to* elevated inflammatory activity, emotional stress, genetic predisposition, gluten intolerance, bowel toxaemia, and/or impaired liver function.

## Planning

The goals and expected outcomes that best serve the client's needs, and which are most relevant to the presenting case (as determined by the clinical assessment and CAM diagnoses), are as follows.

Goals

1 Client will demonstrate an improvement in psoriatic plaque number, size and severity (*client is primarily concerned about the intractability of the psoriasis*).
2 Client will demonstrate an improvement in pruritus (*client has indicated that pruritus is the most distressing symptom of psoriasis*).

Expected outcomes

Based on the degree of improvement reported in clinical studies that have used CAM interventions for the management of psoriasis,[17–21] the following are anticipated.

1 Client will report a forty-five per cent reduction in the total number of psoriatic plaques at baseline in 12 weeks or by dd/mm/yyyy (as determined by lesion count).
2 Client will demonstrate a forty-five per cent reduction in baseline total SPASI score in 12 weeks or by dd/mm/yyyy.
3 Client will demonstrate a forty-five per cent reduction in baseline erythema, thickness and/or scaling of psoriatic lesions in 12 weeks or by dd/mm/yyyy (according to SPASI severity subscores).
4 Client will demonstrate a forty-five per cent reduction in baseline psoriasis surface area in 12 weeks or by dd/mm/yyyy (according to the average percentage of skin involved).
5 Client will report a forty-five per cent reduction in baseline lesion pruritus in 12 weeks or by dd/mm/yyyy (as measured by a 0–10 numerical scale).

## Application

The range of interventions reported in the CAM literature that may be used in the treatment of psoriasis are appraised below.

### Diet

**Gluten-free diet (Level III-2, Strength C, Direction + (for AGA-positive persons only))**
There is some suggestion that gluten sensitivity may trigger psoriasis by increasing small intestine permeability and superantigen uptake, and by stimulating the release of cytokines from T-cells.[22] This association between gluten and psoriasis is partly supported by findings from a small unblinded study of 36 adults with chronic psoriasis. In patients with antigliadin antibodies (AGA), the 3-month gluten-free diet significantly reduced psoriasis area and severity index scores ($p = 0.001$, $n = 30$). This was not the case for patients who were AGA negative ($n = 6$).[20] While it is probable that the elimination of gluten-containing foods such as wheat, triticale, barley, oats and rye may benefit some sufferers of psoriasis, the likelihood of selection and placebo bias in this study raises questions about the validity of these findings.

**High-antioxidant diet (Level III-2, Strength C, Direction +)**
Findings from a multicentre, case–control study suggest the consumption of high antioxidant and flavonoid content foods may improve the symptoms of psoriasis, possibly by modulating inflammation and oxidative stress. The study, which involved 316 patients with psoriasis and 366 controls, found that the consumption of fresh fruit, carrots, tomatoes and beta-carotene significantly reduced the odds of developing psoriasis ($p<0.05$), while green vegetable intake demonstrated a marginally significant risk reduction ($p = 0.05$).[23] Whether beta-carotene supplementation or the consumption of a prescribed high antioxidant diet can yield similar findings in clinical practice warrants further investigation.

**High-fibre diet (Level III-3, Strength D, Direction o)**
The adequate consumption of soluble and insoluble fibre from sources such as wholegrain cereals, fruits, vegetables, legumes, nuts, seeds and psyllium may be helpful in reducing colon pH and microbial overgrowth, bowel transit time and bowel toxaemia. Then again, when the dietary intake of 136 Norwegian men and women with stable plaque psoriasis was compared to a reference group of Norwegians without psoriasis, neither fibre nor any other dietary component was found to be correlated with psoriasis area and severity index (PASI) scores.[24] Without prospective data from controlled clinical trials it is difficult to determine whether the administration of therapeutic doses of fibre has any effect on psoriasis area and severity.

### Lifestyle

**Abstinence from alcohol (Level III-2, Strength C, Direction +)**
The consumption of alcohol can cause blood histamine levels to rise,[23] which, in susceptible individuals, could aggravate the symptoms of psoriasis. This association between alcohol intake and psoriasis surface area and severity is supported by a number of studies,[25,26] and is particularly evident among male sufferers. While there is a paucity of evidence from intervention studies, it is probable that the abstinence from or moderate intake of alcohol may help to reduce the severity of psoriasis.

**Meditation (Level II, Strength B, Direction +)**
Emotional stress is a major intrinsic trigger of psoriasis. Thus, it would be reasonable to assume that effective stress management could facilitate remission of the disease. To test this assumption, 37 patients undergoing phototherapy or photochemotherapy for psoriasis were randomly assigned to receive audiotape-guided mindfulness meditation or a non-tape control in conjunction with light therapy. Under RCT conditions, audiotape-guided mindfulness meditation significantly increased the rate

of resolution of psoriatic lesions when compared to the non-tape control.[19] This corroborates findings from an earlier trial (n = 24) that found meditation and a combination of meditation and imagery to be significantly superior to waiting-list and no treatment controls in reducing psoriasis severity scores at 20 weeks.[18] Studies comparing stress management and guided imagery to no treatment[27] or relaxation therapy to no treatment[28] have been inconclusive with regards to changes in psoriasis symptoms. Further research into the effectiveness of other stress-reduction strategies on psoriasis, such as yoga, tai chi and progressive muscle relaxation, is now required.

### Sunlight (Level III-1, Strength D, Direction o)

Sun exposure is often recommended to patients with psoriasis to facilitate recovery. Even though several clinical trials have shown ultraviolet B (UVB) radiation and a combination of ultraviolet A (UVA) radiation and the photosensitising agent psoralen to be effective at reducing the surface area of psoriasis,[29] the evidence for natural sunlight is less convincing. Some studies have found the combination of sunlight and psoralen to be more effective than natural sunlight and placebo at improving psoriasis surface area,[29] although these studies predate 1982 and have major methodological limitations. The paucity of rigorous clinical evidence in this area, together with the amplified risk of skin cancer from increasing sun exposure, suggests practitioners should exercise some caution in recommending this therapy. Encouraging clients to limit sunlight exposure to less than 5 minutes a day in summer and 15–20 minutes a day in winter, for instance, minimises this risk while also addressing the importance of vitamin D in psoriasis and the role of sunlight in enhancing endogenous vitamin D synthesis.

## Nutritional supplementation

### Folic acid (Level III-2, Strength C, Direction o)

Low plasma folate levels have been shown to be inversely related to psoriasis area and severity.[30] Folate antagonists, such as methotrexate, can be prescribed for the management of this disease and may be an associated factor; however, because folate antagonists are effective at improving the symptoms of psoriasis[31] and folic acid may reduce the effectiveness of these drugs,[32] it is advised that folic acid supplementation be withheld while a patient is being treated with a folate antagonist.

### Omega 3 fatty acids (Level II, Strength B, Direction + (intravenous use only))

The anti-inflammatory effects of omega 3 polyunsaturated fatty acids have been well documented in population and clinical studies,[33] although evidence of the effectiveness of orally and topically administered omega 3 fatty acids in psoriasis has been inconsistent. RCTs reporting significant improvements in the surface area and severity of guttate and plaque psoriasis have only been demonstrated with intravenous omega 3 fatty acids.[34,35] This route of administration has limited application in conventional CAM practice.

### Selenium (Level III-1, Strength C, Direction o)

Selenium plays a pivotal role in the regulation of inflammation and immunity, specifically, the inhibition of nuclear factor-kappaB activation[36] and the enhancement of T-cell function and B-cell activation and proliferation.[37] In spite of these actions, evidence from a double-blind controlled trial has shown the administration of 600 µg of selenium for 12 weeks had no statistically significant effect on the severity of psoriasis when compared with placebo.[38] It would be premature to make any firm conclusions about the effectiveness of selenium in psoriasis until further research emerges.

### Vitamin A (Level I, Strength A, Direction +)

Vitamin A is one of several systemic medical treatments used in the treatment of severe psoriasis. This may be because vitamin A plays a key role in normal epithelial cell differentiation and collagen synthesis,[39] but more so because the treatment is supported by six RCTs. A systematic review of these trials found that when compared with placebo, synthetic oral retinoids (75 mg a day) were moderately effective at reducing the surface area and severity of psoriasis.[29] Given that these findings may not be representative of the effects of natural vitamin A or beta-carotene, clinicians should be cautious about using these agents as a substitute for synthetic retinoids.

### Vitamin B₁₂ (Level II, Strength D, Direction o)

Vitamin $B_{12}$ plays an important role in immunomodulation. Experimental data show that this vitamin stimulates helper and suppressor T-cell activity[40] and suppresses T-cell cytokine production.[41] Although these effects may not necessarily manifest in humans, they provide some explanation for the outcomes of a small RCT in 13 patients with plaque psoriasis. The study found the application of a vitamin $B_{12}$ and avocado oil cream for 12 weeks to be as effective as calcipitriol treatment (a vitamin D derivative) at reducing the severity of psoriasis.[42] Given the small sample size, questionable control and the confounding effect of the avocado oil, these results should be interpreted with caution.

### Vitamin D (Level II, Strength A, Direction + (topical use only))

Vitamin D exhibits a range of antipsoriatic effects, including anti-inflammatory, immunomodulatory and keratinocytic activity. Specifically, experimental data have shown that vitamin D downregulates the expression of tissue necrosis factor-alpha, interleukin (IL)-6, IL-1 and IL-8 in monocytes,[43] reduces keratinocyte proliferation and increases cell differentiation.[29] Evidence from a number of RCTs supports these data, with topically administered synthetic vitamin D3 analogues found to be significantly more effective than placebo at reducing the symptoms and severity of plaque psoriasis.[44–46] Despite these encouraging results, these effects are not likely to be representative of orally administered vitamin D and, as such, may not be applicable to conventional CAM practice.

### Zinc (Level III-1, Strength C, Direction o)

Zinc is frequently recommended as a treatment for integumentary disorders, possibly due to the anti-inflammatory, vulnerary and immunomodulatory effects of the mineral, in particular, the capacity to reduce spontaneous cytokine release and improve T-cell response.[47] As a treatment for psoriasis, the evidence is not so convincing. First, it is uncertain whether psoriatic sufferers require zinc supplementation; one study reported low epidermal zinc levels in sufferers[48] and a number of clinical studies demonstrated similar serum zinc levels between sufferers and healthy controls.[49,50] The lack of understanding about the role of zinc in this disorder may explain why oral zinc supplementation has failed to demonstrate a clinical benefit in psoriasis in studies to date.[51,52]

### Ascorbic acid and vitamin E

These nutrients demonstrate anti-inflammatory activity in vitro, yet, due to the paucity of clinical evidence in this area, it is not clear if they offer any clinical benefit to sufferers of psoriasis.

## Herbal medicine

### *Aloe barbadensis* (Level II, Strength C, Direction o)

Aloe vera was traditionally used in Western herbal medicine as a vulnerary, anti-inflammatory and immunostimulant agent. While a number of clinical studies have investigated the effect of this plant in psoriasis, the findings have not been consistent. In a double-blind, placebo-controlled trial of sixty adults with mild to moderate plaque psoriasis, for example, the application of 0.5 per cent aloe vera gel three times a day, 5 days a week for a maximum of 4 weeks, was found to be significantly more effective than placebo at reducing the severity, redness and number of psoriatic lesions.[53] This is in contrast to an RCT of 41 adults with plaque psoriasis that found topically administered aloe vera gel twice daily for 4 weeks to be significantly less effective than placebo gel at reducing the symptoms of psoriasis (p = 0.02).[54] Differences in the frequency of application of aloe may have contributed to these incongruent findings.

### Azadirachta indica (Level III-1, Strength C, Direction +)
The anti-inflammatory, immunomodulatory and antimicrobial effects of neem leaf have been demonstrated in a number of experimental studies.[55–57] These effects have been further supported by evidence from a double-blind placebo-controlled trial. This small study of 44 patients with plaque psoriasis showed the oral administration of an aqueous extract of neem leaves (three times a day for 4 weeks), together with the application of five per cent coal tar ointment (twice a day for 4 weeks), was significantly more effective than placebo and coal tar at reducing psoriasis surface area and severity (p<0.001).[58] As a cautionary note to Australian practitioners, the use of Azadirachta in Australia is restricted to topical use only. These findings therefore may not be relevant to CAM practice in Australia or in other countries with similar restrictions on use.

### Berberis aquifolium (Level II, Strength B, Direction + (topical use only))
Oregon grape was traditionally used as a treatment for psoriasis, possibly due to the depurative, anti-inflammatory, antimicrobial and antipsoriatic effects of the plant. Emerging evidence from clinical trials corroborates this traditional body of knowledge. To exemplify this point, two 12-week, double-blind placebo controlled trials have consistently shown that when compared with placebo, topically administered Oregon grape significantly improves psoriasis symptoms and quality of life.[17,21] Findings from another RCT point out that Oregon grape ointment might benefit psoriasis by improving cellular cutaneous immune mechanisms and keratinocyte hyperproliferation.[59]

### Other herbs
Arctium lappa (burdock), Chamomilla recutita (German chamomile), Centella asiatica (gotu kola), Coleus forskohlii (coleus), Echinacea spp. (echinacea), Glycyrrhiza glabra (licorice), Hydrastis canadensis (goldenseal), Silybum marianum (milk thistle), Smilax ornata (sarsaparilla) and Withania somnifera (ashwaganda) exhibit a number of effects that may be useful in the management of psoriasis, including anti-inflammatory, antipsoriatic, immunomodulatory, hepatic and depurative activity. Even so, there is still uncertainty about the clinical efficacy of these herbs in the treatment of psoriasis due to the lack of current and high-level evidence in this area.

## Other
### Acupuncture (Level II, Strength B, Direction o)
Acupuncture originated in China more than 4000 ago.[60] Since then, a large traditional evidence base for the therapy has been established. Positive findings from case reports have since added to this traditional knowledge, particularly in the area of psoriasis.[61] An RCT of 56 patients with chronic plaque psoriasis challenges this body of evidence; it showed classical acupuncture together with auricular acupuncture twice a week for 10 weeks to be no more effective than sham acupuncture at improving psoriasis area and severity.[62]

### Aromatherapy, chiropractic, homeopathy, massage, osteopathy and reflexology
There is insufficient clinical evidence supporting the use of these therapies in the management of psoriasis.

## CAM prescription
The CAM interventions that are most appropriate for the management of the presenting case – that is, they target the planned goals, expected outcomes and CAM

diagnoses, they are supported by the best available evidence, they are pertinent to the client's needs and they are most relevant to CAM practice – are outlined below.

**Primary treatments**
- Commence audiotape-guided mindfulness meditation, at least 30 minutes three times a week (*meditation induces the relaxation response, and may help to reduce levels of emotional stress, a known trigger of psoriasis; in doing so, meditation may help to reduce the severity of psoriasis*).
- Apply topical *Berberis aquifolium* bark extract ten per cent ointment (standardised to ten per cent berberine) to lesions twice daily (*topically administered Oregon grape ointment is shown to be effective in improving psoriasis symptoms and psoriasis-associated quality of life; this is possibly attributed to the anti-inflammatory and antipsoriatic actions of the plant*).

**Secondary treatments**
- Increase the consumption of high-antioxidant foods such as fruit, carrots, tomatoes and green vegetables (*the regular consumption of these foods may modulate inflammatory activity and help improve the symptoms of psoriasis*).
- Abstain from alcohol, or at least reduce alcohol intake by fifty per cent (*client regularly consumes alcohol, which may increase the severity of psoriasis, particularly in male sufferers; abstinence from or moderate alcohol intake may help to reduce the severity of psoriasis*).
- If the client tests positive for the IgA endomysial antibody test or IgA/IgG gliadin antibody test, commence a gluten-free diet (*a gluten-free diet may improve psoriasis area and severity in people who are anti-gliadin antibody (AGA) positive*).

Referral
- Refer client to a general practitioner, family physician, dermatologist or emergency department if the condition deteriorates, if serious pathology is suspected (e.g. squamous cell carcinoma, secondary syphilis) or if a serious complication or psoriatic variant arises (e.g. erythrodermic psoriasis, generalised pustular psoriasis).
- If the psoriasis does not improve, consider referring the client to a clinician who is authorised to prescribe synthetic oral retinoids at a dose of 75 mg/day.
- If the client tests positive for the IgA endomysial antibody test or IgA/IgG gliadin antibody test, the client should be referred to a physician who can perform an endoscopic-guided small intestine biopsy to confirm a diagnosis of coeliac disease.
- Refer client to another CAM practitioner if psoriasis, or the treatment of psoriasis, is outside the clinician's area of expertise.
- Liaise with the general practitioner about the client's overall management plan.

## Review

To determine whether pertinent client goals and expected outcomes have been achieved at follow-up, and if any aspects of the client's care need to be improved, consider the factors listed in Table 8.2 (chapter 8), as well as the questions listed below.
- Was there a reduction in the total number of psoriatic lesions?
- Was there a decrease in erythema, thickness and/or scaling of psoriatic lesions?
- Was there a reduction in psoriasis surface area or SPASI area score?
- Did the client experience a decrease in lesion pruritus?
- Has the need for beclomethasone decreased?
- Has there been a decline in the volume of shed scales collected on the bed sheets overnight?

# References

1. Weller PA. (2005) Psoriasis. In: Marks R, editor. Dermatology. 2nd ed. Sydney: Australasian Medical Publishing Company.
2. Porter R et al, editors. (2008) The Merck manual. Rahway: Merck Research Laboratories.
3. Gudjonsson JE. (2008) Genetic variation and psoriasis. Giornale Italiano di Dermatologia e Venereologia, 143(5): 299–305.
4. Swanbeck G et al (1997) Genetic counselling in psoriasis: empirical data on psoriasis among first-degree relatives of 3095 psoriatic probands. British Journal of Dermatology, 137(6): 939–42.
5. Altobelli E et al (2007) Family history of psoriasis and age at disease onset in Italian patients with psoriasis. British Journal of Dermatology, 156(6): 1400–1.
6. Rubin R. Strayer DS. (2007) Rubin's pathology: clinicopathologic foundation of medicine. 5th ed. Philadelphia: Lippincott, Williams & Wilkins.
7. Clo C et al (1979) Polyamines and cellular adenosine 3':5'-cyclic monophosphate. Biochemical Journal, 182(3): 641–9.
8. Pizzorno JE. Murray MT. (2006) Textbook of natural medicine. 3rd ed. Philadelphia: Elsevier.
9. O'Leary CJ et al (2004) Perceived stress, stress attributions and psychological distress in psoriasis. Journal of Psychosomatic Research, 57(5): 465–71.
10. Zachariae R et al (2004) Self-reported stress reactivity and psoriasis-related stress of Nordic psoriasis sufferers. Journal of the European Academy of Dermatology and Venereology, 18(1): 27–36.
11. Weigl BA. (2000) The significance of stress hormones (glucocorticoids, catecholamines) for eruptions and spontaneous remission phases in psoriasis. International Journal of Dermatology, 39(9): 678–88.
12. Buchanan P. Courteney M. (2006) Prescribing in dermatology. Cambridge: Cambridge University Press.
13. Levine N. (2007) Dermatology: diseases and therapy. New York: Cambridge University Press.
14. Pagana K. Pagana T. (2005). Mosby's diagnostic and laboratory test reference. 7th ed. St Louis: Elsevier Mosby.
15. Liska D. Lyon M. Jones DS. (2006) Detoxification and biotransformational imbalances. Explore: Journal of Science and Healing, 2(2): 122–40.
16. Tuchman M. Buchholz R. Weinberg JM. (2006) Psoriasis. In: Hall JC, editor. Sauer's manual of skin diseases. 9th ed. Philadelphia: Lippincott, Williams & Wilkins.
17. Bernstein S et al (2006) Treatment of mild to moderate psoriasis with Relieva, a Mahonia aquifolium extract: a double-blind, placebo-controlled study. American Journal of Therapeutics, 13(2): 121–6.
18. Gaston L et al (1991) Psychological stress and psoriasis: experimental and prospective correlational studies. Acta Dermato-Venereologica, 156: 37–43.
19. Kabat-Zinn J et al (1998) Influence of a mindfulness meditation-based stress reduction intervention on rates of skin clearing in patients with moderate to severe psoriasis undergoing phototherapy (UVB) and photochemotherapy (PUVA). Psychosomatic Medicine, 60(5): 625–32.
20. Michaelsson G et al (2000) Psoriasis patients with antibodies to gliadin can be improved by a gluten-free diet. British Journal of Dermatology, 142(1): 44–51.
21. Wiesenauer M. Ldtke R. (1996) Mahonia aquifolium in patients with Psoriasis vulgaris: an intraindividual study. Phytomedicine, 3: 231–5.
22. Wolters M. (2005) Diet and psoriasis: experimental data and clinical evidence. British Journal of Dermatology, 153: 706–14.
23. Naldi L et al (1996) Dietary factors and the risk of psoriasis: results of an Italian case-control study. British Journal of Dermatology, 134(1): 101–6.
24. Solvoll K et al (1997) Dietary intake in relation to clinical status in patients with psoriasis. British Journal of Nutrition, 77: 337–44.
25. Behnam SM. Behnam SE. Koo JY. (2005) Alcohol as a risk factor for plaque-type psoriasis. Cutis, 76(3): 181–5.
26. Kirby B et al (2008) Alcohol consumption and psychological distress in patients with psoriasis. British Journal of Dermatology, 158(1): 138–40.
27. Zachariae R et al (1996) Effects of psychologic intervention on psoriasis: a preliminary report. Journal of the American Academy of Dermatology, 34(6): 1008–15.
28. Keinan G et al (1995) Stress management for psoriasis patients: the effectiveness of biofeedback and relaxation techniques. Stress Medicine, 11(4): 235–41.
29. Griffiths CEM et al (2000) A systematic review of treatments for severe psoriasis. Health Technology Assessment Monograph. Norwich: HMSO.
30. Malerba M et al (2006) Plasma homocysteine and folate levels in patients with chronic plaque psoriasis. British Journal of Dermatology, 155(6): 1165–9.
31. Flytstrom I et al (2008) Methotrexate vs. ciclosporin in psoriasis: effectiveness, quality of life and safety: a randomized controlled trial. British Journal of Dermatology, 158(1): 116–21.
32. Salim A et al (2006) Folic acid supplementation during treatment of psoriasis with methotrexate: a randomized, double-blind, placebo-controlled trial. British Journal of Dermatology, 154(6): 1169–74.
33. Jho DH et al (2004) Role of omega-3 fatty acid supplementation in inflammation and malignancy. Integrative Cancer Therapies, 3(2): 98–111.
34. Grimminger F et al (1993). A double-blind, randomized, placebo-controlled trial of n-3 fatty acid based lipid infusion in acute, extended guttate psoriasis: rapid improvement of clinical manifestations and changes in neutrophil leukotriene profile. Clinical Investigator, 71(8): 634–43.
35. Mayser P et al (1998) Omega-3 fatty acid-based lipid infusion in patients with chronic plaque psoriasis: results of a double-blind, randomized, placebo-controlled, multicenter trial. Journal of the American Academy of Dermatology, 38(4): 539–47.
36. Vunta H et al (2007) The anti-inflammatory effects of selenium are mediated through 15-deoxy-Delta12, 14-prostaglandin J2 in macrophages. Journal of Biological Chemistry, 282(25): 17964–73.
37. Hawkes WC. Kelley DS. Taylor PC. (2001) The effects of dietary selenium on the immune system in healthy men. Biological Trace Element Research, 81(3): 189–213.
38. Fairris GM et al (1989) The effect of supplementation with selenium and vitamin E in psoriasis. Annals of Clinical Biochemistry, 26(1): 83–8.
39. Leach MJ. (2004) A critical review of natural therapies in wound management. Ostomy/Wound Management, 50(2): 36–51.
40. Sakane T et al (1982) Effects of methyl-B12 on the in vitro immune functions of human T lymphocytes. Journal of Clinical Immunology, 2: 101–9.

41. Yamashiki M. Nishimura A. Koska Y. (1992) Effects of methylcobalamin (vitamin B12) on in vitro cytokine production of peripheral blood mononuclear cells. Journal of Clinical Laboratory Immunology, 37: 173–82.

42. Stucker M et al (2001) Vitamin B12 cream containing avocado oil in the therapy of plaque psoriasis. Dermatology, 203: 141–7.

43. Giulietti A et al (2007) Monocytes from type 2 diabetic patients have a pro-inflammatory profile. 1,25-Dihydroxyvitamin D(3) works as anti-inflammatory. Diabetes Research and Clinical Practice, 77(1): 47–57.

44. Helfrich YR et al (2007) Topical becocalcidiol for the treatment of psoriasis vulgaris: a randomized, placebo-controlled, double-blind, multicentre study. British Journal of Dermatology, 157(2): 369–74.

45. Lebwohl M et al (2007) Calcitriol 3 microg/g ointment in the management of mild to moderate plaque type psoriasis: results from 2 placebo-controlled, multicenter, randomized double-blind, clinical studies. Journal of Drugs in Dermatology, 6(4): 428–35.

46. Van de Kerkhof PC et al (1996) Tacalcitol ointment in the treatment of psoriasis vulgaris: a multicentre, placebo-controlled, double-blind study on efficacy and safety. British Journal of Dermatology, 135(5): 758–65.

47. Kahmann L et al (2008) Zinc supplementation in the elderly reduces spontaneous inflammatory cytokine release and restores T-cell functions. Rejuvenation Research, 11(1): 227–37.

48. Michaelsson G. Ljunghall K. (1990) Patients with dermatitis herpetiformis, acne, psoriasis and Darier's disease have low epidermal zinc concentrations. Acta Dermato-Venereologica, 70(4): 304–8.

49. Kreft B et al (2000) Analysis of serum zinc level in patients with atopic dermatitis, psoriasis vulgaris and in probands with healthy skin. Hautarzt, 51(12): 931–4.

50. Ozturk G et al (2001) Natural killer cell activity, serum immunoglobulins, complement proteins, and zinc levels in patients with psoriasis vulgaris. Immunological Investigations, 30(3): 181–90.

51. Burrows NP et al (1994) A trial of oral zinc supplementation in psoriasis. Cutis, 54(2): 117–18.

52. Leibovici V et al (1990) Effect of zinc therapy on neutrophil chemotaxis in psoriasis. Israel Journal of Medical Sciences, 26(6): 306–9.

53. Syed TA et al (1996) Management of psoriasis with Aloe vera extract in a hydrophilic cream: a placebo-controlled, double-blind study. Tropical Medicine and International Health, 1(4): 505–9.

54. Paulsen E. Korsholm L. Brandrup F. (2005) A double-blind, placebo-controlled study of a commercial Aloe vera gel in the treatment of slight to moderate psoriasis vulgaris. Journal of the European Academy of Dermatology and Venereology, 19(3): 326–31.

55. Beuth J. Schneider H. Ko HL. (2006) Enhancement of immune responses to neem leaf extract (Azadirachta indica) correlates with antineoplastic activity in BALB/c-mice. In Vivo, 20(2): 247–51.

56. Bone K. (2003) A clinical guide to blending liquid herbs. St Louis: Churchill Livingstone.

57. Chattopadhyay RR. (1998) Possible biochemical mode of anti-inflammatory action of Azadirachta indica A. Juss. in rats. Indian Journal of Experimental Biology, 36(4): 418–20.

58. Pandey SS. Jha AK. Kaur V. (1994) Aqueous extract of neem leaves in treatment of psoriasis vulgaris. Indian Journal of Dermatology, Venereology and Leprology, 60(2): 63–7.

59. Augustin M et al (1999) Effects of Mahonia aquifolium ointment on the expression of adhesion, proliferation, and activation markers in the skin of patients with psoriasis. Forschende Komplementarmedizin, 6(Suppl 2): 19–21.

60. O'Brien KA. Xue CC. (2003) Acupuncture. In: Robson T, editor. An introduction to complementary medicine. Sydney: Allen & Unwin.

61. Liao SJ. Liao TA. (1992) Acupuncture treatment for psoriasis: a retrospective case report. Acupuncture and Electro-Therapeutics Research, 17(3): 195–208.

62. Jerner B. Skogh M. Vahlquist A. (1997) A controlled trial of acupuncture in psoriasis: no convincing effect. Acta Dermato-Venereologica, 77(2): 154–6.

# Appendix: The DeFCAM template

[Insert business name/logo]

[Insert patient details]

## Decision-making framework for complementary and alternative medicine (DeFCAM)

Date: _____

### Rapport

The following strategies have been/will be put in place to improve client trust, communication and rapport:

a. _____
b. _____
c. _____
d. _____
e. _____

### Assessment

Health history

a. *History of presenting condition*

_____
_____
_____
_____
_____
_____
_____
_____

b. *Medical history*

   i.  Family history

_____
_____

  ii.  Allergies

_____
_____

 iii.  Medications

_____
_____

 iv.  Medical conditions

_____
_____

  v.  Surgical or investigational procedures

_____
_____

c. *Lifestyle history*
  i. Tobacco use

  _____

  _____

  ii. Alcohol consumption

  _____

  _____

  iii Illicit drug use

  _____

  _____

  iv. Diet and fluid intake:
  *Breakfast* _____
  *Morning tea* _____
  *Lunch* _____
  *Afternoon tea* _____
  *Dinner* _____
  *Fluid intake* _____

  Food frequency:

| | | |
|---|---|---|
| *Fruit* | *Red meat* | |
| *Vegetables* | *Chicken* | |
| *Dairy* | *Fish* | |
| *Cereals* | *Takeaway/fast food* | |

  v. Quality and duration of sleep

  _____

  _____

  vi. Frequency and duration of exercise

  _____

  _____

d. *Socioeconomic background*

  _____

  _____

  _____

Physical examination
a. Inspection

  _____

  _____

b. Olfaction

  _____

  _____

c. Palpation

  _____

  _____

d. Percussion

  _____

  _____

e. Auscultation

_____

_____

f. Additional signs

_____

_____

g. Clinical assessment tools

_____

_____

Diagnostics

a. Pathology tests

_____

_____

b. Radiology tests

_____

_____

c. Functional tests

_____

_____

d. Invasive tests

_____

_____

e. Miscellaneous tests

_____

_____

## Diagnosis

1. _____ (_____), _secondary_ to _____, related to _____
2. _____ (_____), _secondary_ to _____, related to _____
3. _____ (_____), _secondary_ to _____, related to _____
4. _____ (_____), _secondary_ to _____, related to _____

## Planning

Goals

1. _____
2. _____
3. _____
4. _____

Expected outcomes

1. _____
2. _____
3. _____
4. _____
5. _____
6. _____

## Application

Diet

_____
_____
_____
_____
_____

Lifestyle

_____
_____
_____
_____
_____

Nutritional supplementation

_____
_____
_____
_____
_____

Herbal medicine

_____
_____
_____
_____
_____

Other

_____
_____
_____
_____

Referral

_____
_____
_____
_____
_____

## Review

_____
_____
_____
_____

Other comments

_____
_____
_____
_____

_Practitioner surname:_ _____     _Signature:_ _____
_Date:_ _____

# Index